ETHICS IN HEALTH CARE
A CANADIAN FOCUS

ETHICS IN HEALTH CARE
A CANADIAN FOCUS

EIKE-HENNER W. KLUGE

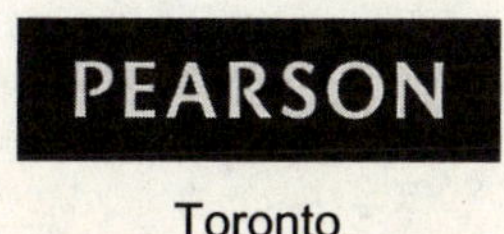

Toronto

Vice-President, Editorial Director: Gary Bennett
Editor-in-Chief: Michelle Sartor
Acquisitions Editor: Deana Sigut
Signing Representative: Carmen Batsford
Marketing Manager: Loula March
Supervising Developmental Editor: Madhu Ranadive
Developmental Editor: Rebecca Ryoji
Project Manager: Jessica Hellen
Production Editor: Sapna Rastogi, Cenveo Publisher Services
Copy Editor: Barbara Kamienski
Proofreader: Deborah Cooper-Bullock
Compositor: Cenveo Publisher Services
Art Director: Julia Hall
Cover Designer: Cenveo Publisher Services
Cover Image: Fotolia

10 9 8 7 6 5 4 3 2 1   [RRD-H]

Library and Archives Canada Cataloguing in Publication

Kluge, Eike-Henner W.
    Ethics in health care : a Canadian focus / Eike-Henner.
W. Kluge.   1st ed.

Includes bibliographical references and index.
ISBN 978-0-13-270847-0

    1. Medical ethics   Canada. 2. Medical care   Canada. I. Title.

R724.K588 2012   174.2   C2012-903758-3

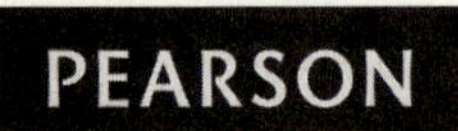

ISBN 978-0-13-270847-0

Brief Contents

Contents

In the past few decades, developments in what might loosely be called the technology of health care have accelerated at an exponential rate and have expanded the scope of health care itself beyond anything that could have been imagined in the past. In many instances, this has left traditional perspectives on the delivery of health care struggling to adjust. For example, traditional perspectives can provide only limited guidance on how to structure telemedicine; similarly, the rules and guidelines that were developed for health care in the mid-20th century are only partly applicable to health care that uses tools such as robo-surgery, gene therapy and pharmacogenetics; and the policies that determined how resources were allocated and health care was structured thirty years ago require fundamental revision in an environment of electronic health records and global epidemiological tracking.

However, *plus ça change, plus ça reste la même chose!* That is to say, while these challenges may be occasioned by technological developments, they are not inherently technological in nature. They are ethical, because they derive their very meaning and significance from the social and professional embedding in which the technology is employed and health care is delivered. That setting, in turn, has inherent ethical dimensions, which remain invariant, no matter how technologically sophisticated the technology itself or the delivery vehicle may be. At its very core, health care centres in the relationship between patients, health care professionals and society. That is why resource allocation is always an ethical problem in health care, because resources are always limited; the professional–patient relationship is always an ethical issue, because without such a relationship, no matter how mediated, there is no health care at all; and similar remarks apply to issues such as research and experimentation, deliberate death, etc.

Moreover, everything that happens in a society is subject to socio-political forces—which is why socio-political considerations must also be taken into account when analyzing the nature and structure of health care. Thus, it is socio-political factors that ultimately determine whether a society treats health care as a commodity or as a right, and this, in turn, conditions how the challenges (and opportunities) presented by technological deployments are solved and what ethical considerations are treated as telling or even as germane. Socio-political parameters, however, ultimately manifest themselves in legal injunctions, and these frequently add a confounding element to the mix. Therefore, when all is said and done, it is the interplay of technological, ethical and legal elements that characterizes the landscape of health care itself. As these elements change, so does what is perceived as an issue, why it is perceived as an issue and how a solution is attempted.

This book attempts to situate the ethics of health care in the context of contemporary technologies and the Canadian social and legal system. It begins with a brief introduction to ethical theory in order to provide the necessary conceptual tools for identifying the issues and dealing with them. The chapters that follow then consider in greater detail issues that are considered important at the present time. An attempt has been made to correlate issues as to type and to deal with them in distinct chapters, even though they may overlap. For example, the ethical issues that are generated by the biotechnologies are treated separately from the ethical issues that are generated by research and experimentation, even though both have an overlapping set of problems, and the ethical issues that arise in the context of informed consent are treated separately from the ethical issues that arise in the professional–patient relationship, even though both are closely interrelated.

It bears emphasizing that health care is not something theoretical. It is hands-on stuff. Therefore when considering the ethics of health care, it is important not simply to look at theory but also to look at how it is actually delivered and what conditions that delivery—in other words, to be clear on what the ethical lay of the land is actually like. Without this, an analysis of health care becomes a study in system building that is removed from reality. That is why, throughout this book, while theoretical analysis and discussion play an important role, the emphasis has not been on pure theory but on theory in relation to reality, and why legal decisions and how they impact on health care have frequently been highlighted. They are important determinants of how care is actually delivered. Canada is very fortunate in that most of its health care law is ethically defensible in terms of the major ethical frameworks that have currency at the present time. However, there are exceptions. These have been identified and possible ethically appropriate alternate ways of structuring the delivery framework have been explored.

Clearly no book can touch on, let alone deal adequately with the myriad of issues and problems that arise in the planning, development and delivery of health care. And that is not the purpose of this book. Its purpose is not, as it were, to "cover all the bases," but to set out in a systematic fashion the major ethical considerations that arise in the Canadian context and to provide an ethical framework for identifying and dealing with them. Its purpose, therefore, is to provide the readers with the conceptual tools for making their own informed judgments.

Throughout most of the book, physicians are at the focus of the discussions involving the actions of health care professionals. This is not an accident or an oversight. Whether we like it or not, physicians are the major players in the arena of health care. All other things being equal, they are the gatekeepers to health care and exercise tremendous control over who has access, the direction that care takes, and how health care decisions are made both at the policy level and at the level of individual persons. It is therefore appropriate that the ethics of medical practice should receive special consideration.

However, this does not mean that the ethics of medical practice is somehow special in itself. With due alteration of detail, what applies to physicians applies to all health care professionals commensurate with their area of expertise and practice, and therefore relevant substitutions should be made as and when appropriate. The *ethics* is the same for all health care professionals; what differs is how it manifests itself in the particulars of the professionals' actions. In other words, there is a host of issues that concern other health care professionals as much as they do physicians. I have already identified some of them. They include informed consent, allocation of resources, competence and so on.

Furthermore, and perhaps much more importantly, most of these issues also concern individual patients and society as a whole. The discussion that follows will attempt to indicate where and why the relevant issues arise, why they are issues, and the considerations that should guide the various players if they are to interact in an ethical fashion. The underlying principle will always be this: All participants, whether they be professionals or patients, are part of society. They are embedded in a social context that defines not only what they can do in a material sense but also what they should (or should not) do, ethically speaking. While the roles that the various individuals play may be different, the ethical principles that should guide how they engage in these roles are the same for all.

As I said, this book covers a host of issues. They range from codes of professional ethics to allocation of resources and reproductive technology. However, just as one cannot hope to deal with these issues from all possible perspectives, neither can one deal with all of them in any great depth. I have therefore been selective in what I have included; and even topics that I have selected I have considered only as far as is necessary to allow some insight into the ethical principles that are generally considered relevant when dealing with the issues. My primary concern has been to provide some feel for how these principles function when one is trying to develop an ethically defensible solution to a particular issue. Readers who wish to pursue particular topics in greater depth should consult the list of Further Readings at the end of each chapter. I have also illustrated many of the more important issues by adducing cases taken from actual life, and have appended several more cases to most of the chapters. Finally, I have prefaced each chapter with a set of questions that should be useful in identifying major themes and that may serve as guidelines when reading the chapters themselves.

I owe thanks to the many persons who, over the years, have assisted me in developing and refining my views on health care ethics. Paramount thanks are of course due to the patients who had faith in the process of ethical consultation. Special thanks are due to the physicians and hospitals who, over the years, entrusted me with the responsibility of giving ethics advice—and for making sure that I experienced at first-hand what the implications of that advice would look like; and to my legal colleagues, whose unfailing counsel has always been a source of joy. While court work has often been challenging, it has also served to sharpen my appreciation of the socio-legal implications of ethical analysis. Thanks are also due to my students who, over the years, forced me to clarify a lot of my analyses. Thank you to the editors at Pearson Canada without whose supportive work this book would never have come to completion. Finally, I would like to thank the reviewers who read the published edition and penultimate draft of this book and offered helpful criticism and suggestions: Jason P. Blahuta, Lakehead University;

Kenneth Kirkwood, University of Western Ontario; Bernie Koenig, Fanshawe College; Brian Lightbody, Brock University; Marc Ramsay, Acadia University; and Andrew Sneddon, University of Ottawa.

Eike-Henner W. Kluge

Victoria, 2012

SUPPLEMENTS FOR *ETHICS IN HEALTH CARE: A CANADIAN FOCUS*

Readings in Health Care Ethics, Fourth Edition (ISBN 978-0-13-276670-8)

An up-to-date, balanced collection of readings that examine the diversity of opinion surrounding current issues in health care ethics. This anthology focuses largely on the Canadian perspective, covering the political and social aspects of Canadian access to health care and the distinct nature of Canadian legislation.

CourseSmart for Instructors (ISBN 978-0-13-270797-8)

CourseSmart goes beyond traditional expectations—providing instant, online access to the textbooks and course materials you need at a lower cost for students. And even as students save money, you can save time and hassle with a digital eTextbook that allows you to search for the most relevant content at the very moment you need it. Whether you are evaluating textbooks or creating lecture notes to help students with difficult concepts, CourseSmart can make life a little easier. See how when you visit www.coursesmart.com/instructors.

CourseSmart for Students (ISBN 978-0-13-270797-8)

CourseSmart goes beyond traditional expectations—providing instant, online access to the textbooks and course materials you need at an average savings of 60 percent. With instant access from any computer and the ability to search your text, you'll find the content you need quickly, no matter where you are. And with online tools like highlighting and note-taking, you can save time and study efficiently. See all the benefits at www.coursesmart.com/students.

Generic MySearchLab

MySearchLab contains writing, grammar, and research tools, and access to a variety of academic journals, Associated Press news feeds, and discipline-specific readings to help you hone your writing and research skills. For more information and to redeem or purchase an access code, please visit www.mysearchlab.com.

Pearson Custom Library

For enrollments of at least 25 students, you can create your own textbook by choosing the chapters that best suit your own course needs. To begin building your custom text, visit www.pearsoncustomlibrary.com. You may also work with a dedicated Pearson custom editor to create your ideal text—publishing your own original content or mixing and matching Pearson content. Contact your local Pearson representative to get started.

Technology Specialists

Pearson's technology specialists work with faculty and campus course designers to ensure that Pearson technology products, assessment tools, and online course materials are tailored to meet your specific needs. This highly qualified team is dedicated to helping schools take full advantage of a wide range of educational resources, by assisting in the integration of a variety of instructional materials and media formats. Your local Pearson Canada sales representative can provide you with more details on this service program.

Chapter 1
Ethics as a Discipline

Human beings are unusual in the animal kingdom. They are self-aware, and they use their reason to understand their surroundings and to plan their lives. They are also social animals, which means that they interact with other human beings and realize their full potential only in a social setting. Because they are self-aware and rational social animals, their interactions have a qualitative dimension that is not shared by other social animals such as ants or hyenas. Ethics is the discipline that studies this qualitative dimension; and since this book deals with ethics in health care, it is only appropriate that it begins with a closer look at what ethics is all about.

This chapter, then, introduces ethics as a discipline. It begins with a discussion of several approaches to the very concept of ethics itself and then goes on to briefly sketch the major (and competing) ethical theories that dominate health care decision-making. At the end of this chapter the reader should have some understanding of what ethics is all about, how ethical decision-making differs from other decision-making and what all of this means for the health care setting.

Questions to Keep in Mind While Reading this Chapter:

1. What is meta-ethics, and how does it differ from ethics?

2. What meta-ethical theories are most commonly encountered in social practice in our society—and why?

3. What are some of the major contemporary ethical theories, and how do they differ?

4. What is attractive about utilitarian theories? What are some of their disadvantages?

5. What is attractive about deontological theories? What are some of their disadvantages?

6. What is meant by ethical justification, and how does it differ from the psychological account of ethical decision-making?

INTRODUCTION

The *Universal Declaration of Human Rights*[1] begins with the assertion that the "recognition of the inherent dignity and of the equal and inalienable rights of all members of the human family is the foundation of freedom, justice and peace in the world." The Declaration further states that these rights hold for all people, irrespective of their national, ethnic or religious affiliations or origins, and that they apply irrespective of gender, age or condition. The Declaration therefore assumes that the world has an objective moral structure, since otherwise one cannot meaningfully talk about inherent dignity and inalienable rights. Further, the International Criminal Court in The Hague tries people for crimes against humanity. It tries them irrespective of whether their own culture legitimated such actions.[2] It is generally assumed—although this assumption is by no means universally shared[3]—that this presupposes that the world has an objective moral structure and that there are fundamental ethical principles that no one may contravene without becoming morally guilty. The *International Code of Medical Ethics* of the World Medical Association[4] appears to be based on the same assumption; and the *Code of Ethics* of the Canadian Medical Association states that it is grounded on the "fundamental ethical principles and values of medical ethics."[5] Nor is this stance confined to medicine: Nursing, law and indeed most other professions hold to a similar perspective.

Clearly, then, the assumption that the world has an objective moral structure is fairly widespread. The question, of course, is whether this assumption is correct. Are there really actions that are ethically acceptable or unacceptable in some objective sense, no matter what, or is this merely the position of cultural imperialists who want to impose their views on others?

META-ETHICS AND CULTURAL PLURALITY

While it may not be obvious at first glance, the question itself assumes something very important. It assumes that ethical statements are more than merely sophisticated expressions of emotions or feelings but are cognitively meaningful, and that they say something true or false about the world. If this assumption is false, then a code of medical ethics stating that it is unethical for physicians to kill their incurably ill patients would not be saying anything true or false. It would merely be expressing how the drafters of the code (or the people who accepted it) feel about such an act. Similarly, if the code said that abandoning a patient was unethical, it would not be stating an objective truth. It would only be expressing the profession's aversion to such behaviour. On the other hand, if the assumption is correct, then these statements not only are cognitively meaningful but also say something true or false about the world.

Not only that: If the assumption is false, then saying that someone is unethical or is doing something immoral would not be to say anything about that person or about what he or she does. It would be to say something about us—about how we feel. By contrast, if the assumption is correct, then saying that someone is unethical would be to say something about the other person. Specifically, it would be to say that the other person possesses a negative ethical property or quality. However, it would say nothing about how we feel about the matter.

The Meaning of Ethical Statements

These two positions are not ethical theories but theories about ethics. In other words, they are meta-ethical theories. The first is called *ethical non-cognitivism*, the second is called *ethical cognitivism*—and they have fundamentally distinct implications. If ethical non-cognitivism is correct, then ethical disagreements essentially reduce to more or less sophisticated shouting matches, and the way to resolve such disagreements is not through reasoning but by somehow getting people to change how they feel. On the other hand, if ethical cognitivism is correct, then people who make opposing ethical statements are making meaningful claims, and the way to resolve their disagreement is not to change how they feel but to reason with them and try to get them to come to the same understanding.

The question, of course, is which of these positions (if any) is correct. The long and the short of it is that there is no way—no objective way—to tell. In the end, one simply has to decide. Of course, this does not mean that people actually choose their meta-ethical stance—how they treat ethical claims and considerations—on the basis of careful reflection and deliberation. It is merely to say that the question of which meta-ethical stance is correct is objectively undecidable. In real life, the meta-ethical framework that grounds peoples' ethical decision-making and how they view ethics is at least as much a result of conditioning and socio-cultural factors as of deliberation.

What ethical non-cognitivism has going for it is that ethical disagreement can be a highly emotional affair. All of us have found on occasion that disagreement over what we consider unethical can easily turn into a highly charged confrontation of attitudes in which no amount of reasoning is likely to convince the other party. Even when their logic is shown to be faulty or to lead to unacceptable consequences, people still tend to insist on their ethical position because it just feels right. "I just know I'm right" or "I can't argue with you—you just don't see!" are expressions that reflect this attitude. This fact of intense emotional commitment has led ethical non-cognitivists to conclude that the core of ethical assertions is really emotional commitment: Ethical judgments are nothing more than sophisticated verbal expressions of emotional convictions. According to them, "Murder is wrong!" really amounts to "Murder: Boo!"; "Kindness is ethically praiseworthy" is really a stance that could just as validly have been expressed by saying "Kindness: Yeah!"[6]

Of course, not all non-cognitivists have gone this far. Some have admitted that ethical statements do have cognitive components. They have said that while ethical judgments are essentially nothing more than sophisticated emotional exclamations, they also involve an attempt to evoke similar attitudes in others.[7] Some have gone even further and said that ethical statements are also convoluted attempts to recommend a certain kind of behaviour to others—that they are linguistic expressions of a willingness to generalize or universalize the attitudes that are expressed in them.[8]

However, there are some very good reasons why society generally tends to reject ethical non-cognitivism. *First*, feelings aside, when people make competing ethical claims, they generally do take themselves to be genuinely disagreeing, and they also think that this disagreement is more than merely a matter of feelings. For instance, when someone says "Euthanasia is wrong!" or "Physicians have a duty to treat people with AIDS!" and someone responds by saying "So that is how you feel about the matter," people think it is perfectly appropriate to reply "No, it's not merely how I feel about it—although, of course, it is—it's also true!"

In other words, the fact that people distinguish between the emotive aspect of ethical assertions and the claim that they are true does not strike anyone as confused, and to insist on the difference—as in the examples above—would be seen as simply setting the record straight. While people would agree that ethical claims may involve or evoke emotional reactions, people do not generally feel that it is these emotive parameters that are at issue. Rather, the real issue is which one of the competing claims is correct. This would be nonsense if there were no difference between the emotive and the cognitive parameters of ethical assertions.

Second, if ethical non-cognitivism were correct, people who felt negatively about some ethical matter could not reasonably and at the same time say that others had a right to do what they themselves felt negatively about. For instance, physicians who rejected abortions on ethical grounds could then not say to their patients—as some physicians do—"I feel abortions are wrong, but you have the right to an abortion, and I shall refer you to someone who performs them." If ethics were really about feelings and emotions, the two parts of the statement would contradict each other. It would amount to what has been called a pragmatic contradiction.[9]

Third, if ethical non-cognitivism were correct, then all that would be necessary for something to be morally acceptable would be to make people feel positive about it. That would legitimate such things as racial cleansing, slavery and child labour. All one would have to do to turn these from something unethical into something ethical would be to make people feel good about them. Dialogue and discourse would go by the board. What was right or wrong would become purely a function of emotional manipulation.

Ethical Relativism and Cultural Plurality

However, even if one rejected ethical non-cognitivism and said that ethical statements are cognitively meaningful, that would still leave two options.

On the one hand, one could argue that different people and different cultures have different points of view, and that while what they say is meaningful and indeed true or false, it is true or false only *relative to the conceptual framework of the speaker*. In other words, from a relativistic perspective, the ethical nature of the world—i.e., what would be ethically right or wrong—would not be an objective fact but a function of how the conceptual frameworks of the respective interlocutors interpreted the world. Moral claims would then always carry the hidden rider, "from my (our) point of view," and moral facts would always be moral facts "from my (our) point of view." Therefore, even though the people (or cultures) who disagreed in their ethical claims might use the same vocabulary and might even be talking about the same *material* state of affairs, they would be talking about a different *ethical* state of affairs because the ethical state of affairs would always be the state-of-affairs-as-perceived. It follows that what at first glance looked like a meaningful ethical disagreement would actually be a case of crossed monologues.[10]

On the other hand, one could argue that ethical statements are not true relative to a conceptual framework but true in an objective sense. That is to say, one could argue that ethical statements are objectively true or false because, as a matter of fact, the world objectively includes more than merely material properties. It also includes ethical or moral properties, and while these properties are different from such things as colours, hardness or size, they are perfectly objective and real. Moreover, one could argue that because these properties are objective, they are independent of how—or even of whether—people perceive or understand them. The fact that not everybody sees them, or that not everybody understands them the same way, says nothing about the moral structure of the world. It says something about the people who do the perceiving.

These two opposing views are called *ethical relativism* and *ethical realism* or *objectivism* respectively. To illustrate the difference, consider female circumcision. The World Health Organization (WHO) has condemned female circumcision as "a violation of the human rights of girls and women."[11] Ethical relativists would say that this was cultural imperialism on a global scale; that what was right for people who accept such a practice—for instance, aboriginal peoples in Somalia or in Australia—was perfectly legitimate because there are no objective moral facts. It all comes down to a matter of viewpoint, culture or religion.[12] In fact, ethical relativists would argue that the WHO's condemnation of the practice had validity only within the WHO's frame of reference, and that to impose it on people who did not share that frame of reference would be a clear case of cultural hegemony.

By contrast, ethical objectivists would agree with the WHO. They would say that female circumcision (and male circumcision for non-medical reasons) was objectively wrong and was a violation of human rights. They would probably also say that while it was understandable that someone from a particular culture or religion might accept such a practice, that would not make it right in any objective sense—any more than the fact that the people who were raised to believe in leprechauns or in sympathetic magic were right simply because they were raised that way. Being raised with a certain world view or within a certain religious framework and making claims that are consistent with that world view or framework is not the same as being right.

Critique of Ethical Relativism

As an ethical theory, ethical relativism has a fairly ancient lineage. Already in ancient Greece, well-travelled individuals called Sophists noted that the customs and laws of the various countries and city states frequently differed, sometimes even fundamentally. What was considered right or wrong in one society was not necessarily considered so in another society and *vice versa*; neither moral nor legal standards and injunctions could be generalized for all societies. In fact, they found that the only safe generalization they could make was that conceptions of right and wrong were society relative. On this basis they concluded that there were no objective universal ethical standards, and that ethical judgments were relative to their particular social dimensions.

In more recent times, social scientists have adopted a similar line of reasoning. They have argued that because some cultures practise infanticide, infanticide cannot be wrong absolutely speaking, but only from our perspective; that because public execution by stoning for marital infidelity is practised in some cultures, it cannot be ethically objectionable in an absolute sense but only from our particular point of view, and so on. Their bottom line is the same as that of the Sophists: There are no universally applicable moral laws and no universally applicable ethical standards because, as a matter of fact, none are universally shared.

There is something very comforting and convenient about ethical relativism. If ethical judgments are framework relative, and if the fact that different cultures operate with different ethical standards has no objective implications, then no matter how heinous the practices of a given culture may seem to others, so long as they are justifiable in terms of the ethical concepts of that culture, they are above reproach. The fact that another society condemns the practice might be anthropologically interesting, but matters can go no further, at least not in any ethically relevant sense. Therefore, all other things being equal, ethical relativism leaves the actions of individuals and of groups of people immune from outside attack. Politically, that is very convenient.

Again, the question becomes who is right—the relativist or the objectivist? And once more, the answer is that there is no objective way of proving either position. However, there are some weighty reasons for questioning ethical relativism. For instance, if ethical relativism were correct, then ethical disagreement between people who do not share the same conceptual framework would quite literally be impossible. From this perspective, right and wrong would be framework relative, and different individuals or different cultures would have different conceptual frameworks—which means that, logically and conceptually, they would really be making entirely different claims.

Moreover, as was already pointed out over two thousand years ago by Socrates, ethical relativism confuses the question of what is believed, legislated or otherwise promulgated by a group of individuals with the question of whether what they believe, legislate or otherwise promulgate is ethically correct. Believing that one is right does not necessarily make one right—in ethics any more than in mathematics or embryology.

In addition to this, by arguing that there is no objective right or wrong because cultures differ in their ethical standards, ethical relativism assumes something very much like a consensus theory of truth. This is the theory that something is true if, and only if, there is consensus on the matter. However, consensus on something does not make it true. One need merely recall the history of witchcraft, chemistry and physics—and even the history of medicine itself, with its theory of the four humours. Once upon a time, there was consensus that witches could change into cats, that combustion was due to phlogiston, that nature abhorred a vacuum and that melancholy was due to an imbalance of the four humours. That consensus did not make these propositions true. With due alteration of detail, the same thing could be said about ethical relativism.

Furthermore, the fact that there is no consensus on matters of ethics does not logically entail that therefore there are no universally valid ethical propositions. There could be all sorts of reasons for a lack of consensus. These could include the dominance of traditions, the conditioning power of education or of religious influences, etc. It might even be possible that there is no consensus because people are just not sufficiently sophisticated to appreciate and understand the ethical nature of reality. Whatever one might think of the work of Kohlberg and others in this regard,[13] few would reject his claim that moral sophistication and understanding undergo development;[14] and as some have argued in defence of evolutionary ethics, something similar applies to groups of people.[15]

Finally, one could point to the fact that, as was already mentioned, the International Criminal Court in The Hague tries people for crimes against humanity irrespective of whether their culture or their laws legitimated such actions.[16] The judges of the International Criminal Court do not justify their decisions by pointing to the superior power of the world community that has underwritten the Court; nor did the judges who prosecuted Nazi physicians as war criminals in the Nuremberg Tribunal base themselves on a might-is-right approach to ethics, as Thrasymachus did in Plato's *Republic*.[17] In other words, they did not justify the validity of their judgments by saying, "We are the victors, therefore we will judge you according to our own standards. Your actions are ethically above reproach when considered from the viewpoint of your own system; but since we have prevailed over you by force of arms and can enforce our standards, we will judge you according to our's." Rather, their judgment was based on the position that no matter what was accepted or legitimate according to the standards of the accused, what the accused did was ethically wrong in an absolute sense that transcended individual ethical (and legal) frameworks. In other words, they maintained that the Nazi physicians who were convicted knew (or should have known) that what they were doing was wrong. The fact that Nazi society at the time condoned their behaviour was not considered an acceptable excuse.

Therefore, when it comes to actual practice, ethical relativism ceases to be fashionable and goes by the board. There is a reason for this. It lies in the fact that at some level, most people believe that ethical judgments are not moves in a game in which different players operate according to different rules. People generally believe that, in some way or another, ethical judgments are statements about the world. They tend to believe that opposing ethical judgments about people are genuinely in conflict with each other. They also tend to accept that opposing statements cannot both be true, and that at least one of them must be unacceptable. And here it is no good replying that ethical judgments always carry the rider "according to my point of view," "according to system x" or some such. We still want to ask, "But does your point of view (system x, etc.) correctly characterize the ethical state of affairs?" This question lies at the heart of ethical disagreement. It is not answered by pointing to the fact of disagreement itself.

In other words, when people disagree in their ethical assessments of a given situation—say, of the acceptability of abortion—it is pointless to show them that their competing claims follow from their respective moral premises. It is the acceptability of these very premises that is at issue. That is why ethical disagreements cannot be solved by showing the internal consistency of the relevant ethical frameworks, or by showing that certain ethical injunctions or claims follow logically within these frameworks. That would be to confuse validity with soundness. It would be to confuse the question of whether certain judgments follow from the basic concepts of a particular ethical framework with the question of whether the framework, with its principles and concepts, correctly captures the ethical aspects of the world.

Putting the matter this way may give the impression that ethical non-cognitivism and ethical relativism are silly. That, however, would be short-sighted and unfair. Both make some important points. For example, ethical non-cognitivism picks up on the fact that ethical claims tend to be emotionally charged: People tend to feel strongly about what they think is right or wrong. That is why ethical disagreements over such things as abortion or euthanasia frequently devolve into sophisticated shouting matches. Any theory of ethics that does not take this emotional factor into account will be incomplete. For this reason, some contemporary ethical theorists have distinguished between the rights and duties that people have (which identify the direction that their actions should take) and their values (which are the—frequently emotion-laden—action-potentials that motivate people to act in the first place).[18]

It is also fairly obvious that ethical relativism is quite right when it says that no one set of ethical standards or imperatives is accepted by all people. Different cultures often have quite different standards of what is considered right or wrong, and what is approved in one setting may be strongly disapproved of in another. For instance, judicial amputation and flogging are considered unethical in Canada and most of the Western world, whereas they are considered ethically appropriate judicial remedies in countries such as Saudi Arabia[19] and Yemen.[20] For that matter, something may not even be considered right (or wrong) in the same culture at different times in its own history. Capital punishment, slavery and discrimination on the basis of sexual orientation are three of many issues on which not only Canada but the rest of world has changed its ethical stance.

Ethical Realism (Objectivism)

By contrast, ethical realism assumes that there are ethical facts, that actions have moral properties and that these constitute—or at least *should* constitute—the basis of our moral judgments. However, in order to make sense of this position, one has to have some explanation of what these moral properties and ethical facts are like.

One answer was given by G.E. Moore and the so-called *non-naturalists*.[21] Moore maintained that ethical properties are irreducible to material properties and therefore cannot be apprehended through the senses. They are non-sensible, metaphysically unique and can be apprehended only through our understanding.[22] Another answer is given by the *naturalists* or, as they are also frequently called, *reductionists*. They deny that moral properties are somehow metaphysically unique. Instead, reductionists argue that on closer analysis, ethical properties reduce to or can be analyzed in terms of ordinary properties.[23]

A theory that lies somewhere between these two holds that ethical properties are emergent in nature.[24] The notion of emergence can be illustrated by considering ordinary material objects such as kumquats and aardvarks. Kumquats and aardvarks are composed of molecules and atoms, which in turn are composed of subatomic entities such as leptons and quarks, etc. The behaviour of material objects is subject to causal laws and is quite predictable. By contrast, the behaviour of subatomic particles is not subject to causal laws and is not predictable in any ordinary sense. However, even though the ordinary properties and causally predictable behaviour of material objects are not reducible to the properties of the subatomic particles and their non-causal relationships, the latter give rise to the former. The former, so to speak, emerge at the higher level of complex interrelationship between these basic entities.

Another (somewhat more controversial) example is the human brain. The individual neurons that make up the brain are not themselves in any sense conscious or aware. They are merely electrochemically active. However, the integrated firing of these neurons gives rise to the wholly new phenomenon of conscious awareness. The conscious and aware mind emerges as a totally different, totally new entity at the level of the brain functioning as a whole. However, even though it emerges from the activities, natures and qualities of its constitutive neurons and structures, it cannot be causally reduced to them.

Still another illustration comes from the behaviour of groups and populations. The behaviour of these groups is real and, to a degree, predictable. Social psychology and sociology are based on this fact. However, the behaviour of a population or group is not merely a summation of the behaviour of its individual members. The mutually affective interrelations among individual members give rise to social profiles whose qualitative nature is quite distinct from that of the individual persons.

If this understanding of ethics and of the moral nature of the world as emergent is correct, then it has several important implications for ethics in general and for biomedical ethics in particular. *First*, emergent properties can arise only between entities that have a certain qualitative nature. For instance, no matter how cookies and marbles are combined, they will not give rise to something that is consciously aware. By the same token, ethical properties could then arise only in the context of persons: of beings that have a will and the capacity for awareness and reasoning. That is why the relationships between ants or hyenas may be complex, but they are not ethical relations, and why it would be absurd to say that an ant that killed another ant was guilty of murder or that a hyena that bit another hyena was guilty of assault and battery. And closer to the subject of this text, the fact that ethical relations can hold only between certain kinds of entities gives an explanation of why, ethically, one would be justified in saying that a three-month old fetus, while certainly human, is not yet a person—which is why aborting it at that point would not be murder; and it would allow us to say that brain-dead patients, while human beings, are no longer persons—and therefore may be used as cadaveric organ donors. (See Chapter 8.)

Second, since emergence is a function of relations among more basic entities, an awareness of emergent properties would require a perspective that was logically of a higher order than the logic of the more basic entities that give rise to what emerges. Applied to moral properties, this would explain why not all people are aware of moral properties—or aware of them in the same way. The most flagrant example here is that of children. Moral relations do not hold between merely biological or material objects but between sentient cognitive beings, which is to say between persons. That is why children have to develop conceptually to the stage at which they see other human beings *as persons* before they can see them as persons-in-relation and can distinguish right from wrong actions. That is also the ultimate point of Kohlberg's analysis of the moral development of the child. Therefore, as long as someone remains conceptually at a level where they see social interactions merely as interactions between material organisms, they will be unaware of the ethical properties that hold between human beings *as persons.* Such individuals are ethically blind.

Third, it would follow that ethical rights and obligations, etc., could not be discussed in the same way and on the same level as other things such as hot dogs, cats or paper airplanes, nor could they be treated as contractual arrangements. Their logic would be different. That is why, as Hume put it, one cannot get an "ought" from an "is," and why the logic of ethics is a deontic logic, not a straightforward truth-functional logic.[25]

Fourth, since ethical properties and relations would depend on the natures of the individuals who give rise to them through their interrelationships, and on the natures of these relationships themselves, one would expect that variations in any one of these would yield different ethical facts. This would explain the fact that the way in which ethical principles apply depends on the context, and it would explain why a different set of circumstances will give rise to different rights or obligations or both. It would also explain why making ethical judgments always demands attention to the particulars of the specific cases.

The Nature of Ethics

What, then, is ethics? That is to say, what is ethics in this realist or objectivist sense? As a discipline, it is a branch of philosophy. It deals with questions of right and wrong conduct, with what one ought to do or refrain from doing, and with what one may do if one pleases. It considers issues of rights and obligations, and tries to determine what this means for individual people and how such rights and obligations are related to the social context in which the people are embedded.

Of course, ethics is not the only discipline that deals with such issues. Law and theology, psychology and sociology, as well as other disciplines also deal with them. However, what distinguishes ethics from these disciplines is its methodology, its basic operating assumption and the nature of its claims.

Ethics differs from psychology and sociology in that it is prescriptive, not descriptive, in nature.[26] What this means is that ethics is not centrally concerned with how individuals or groups of people feel—or even the reasons why they feel in a certain way. Nor, unlike anthropology, does it focus on the customs that groups of people follow or that they have adopted as a matter of historical fact. Such data are of interest to ethics only insofar as they are the basis of a quite different question: whether people *ought* to follow these customs or *ought* to behave in these ways.

Moreover, ethics does not try to answer these questions by looking at what people have decided to do as a matter of social rules or conventions, or by considering the nature and origin of the psychological makeup that characterizes a certain point of view. Instead, ethics—at least ethics in this realist sense—tries to show how ethical claims follow from basic ethical principles that constitute the moral framework of the world of rational agents.

In this sense, ethics does have something in common with law and religion. Law and religion are also normative or prescriptive. They also lay out what people ought to do and how they ought to behave. However, both law and religion differ from ethics in the source and nature of their pronouncements. Law is largely concerned with the rules that a particular society has chosen in order to govern the behaviour of its members. These rules may be rooted in tradition, as in the common-law tradition of the English-speaking world; or they may be the outcome of conscious decisions by a legislative body, as in statute or civil law countries like France and Germany; or they may be the result of a combination of both, as in Canada, with its civil tradition in Quebec and its common-law tradition in the other provinces. However, except for what is called the natural law tradition (which argues that all genuine laws are based on the moral structure of the universe and that this structure can be understood rationally simply by use of reason),[27] laws are not generally thought to be the result of an objective analysis of ethical principles or values. Moreover, they are generally understood to have binding power only within the political boundaries that define a nation. If they have applicability beyond that—as, for example, with some so-called international laws like those that prohibit slavery—this is rooted in an agreement among the nations themselves.[28]

As to religion, it also tells people what they ought to do or what they ought to refrain from doing. However, religious injunctions find their basis in some belief or series of beliefs whose acceptability is not open to debate. The believer must either accept them or cease to be a member of that religion. An example would be the belief of Christian

Science that disease is the result of insufficient faith and therefore can be cured by restoring faith to an appropriate level and in an appropriate fashion; or the belief of Jehovah's Witnesses that the use of blood contravenes a fundamental law of God; or, finally, the belief of some traditional Christian sects that contraception is against God's dictates. While religion allows reasoning about rules and prescriptions of behaviour, it allows this only within the framework of beliefs that are fundamental to the religion itself. This does not mean that religions may not contain ethical rules and principles. Most religions do. It just means that the way these principles function, and their ultimate justification, is fundamentally different.

Ethics realism does not, of course, maintain that just because the world has an objective moral structure, everyone will behave ethically or everyone will accept the same ethical standards. That requires the appropriate will and the appropriate insight—and not everyone has that.

ETHICAL THEORIES AND THEIR RELEVANCE TO HEALTH CARE

Some Preliminary Remarks

Scientific and academic disciplines often see bitter controversies between rival theories. Physics is a good example. The debate between quantum mechanics and relativistic physics is as long-standing as it is well-known. Quantum mechanics provides a satisfactory description of the world at the subatomic level. However, it is essentially useless at the macro-level of stars and galaxies. Here, relativistic physics comes into its own. Unfortunately, relativistic physics fails at the level of atoms. A great deal of current theorizing in physics is devoted to developing a theory that combines both quantum physics and relativistic physics into one overall and consistent scheme. As yet, there is no generally accepted candidate, although Brane theory[29] seems a good contender in this regard, and others may be developed.[30] However, the point is that an overall theory that links the micro-level of the world (which is described by quantum theory) to the macro-level (which is described by relativistic physics) must be possible, because there is only one world.

The relevance of all this to ethics is that ethics finds itself in a similar position. There are several competing ethical theories, each of which seems to fit some aspect of health care very well but to work not quite so well in others. Thus, so far as health care planning at the policy level and health care delivery at the hands-on level are concerned, deontological and utilitarian[31] ethics are the major contenders. Deontological ethics is generally thought to provide a good account of why the rights of individual persons should figure prominently when it comes to such matters as informed consent, and of how competing rights claims should be balanced on a given occasion; but it seems to fail when it comes to resource allocation at the level of health policy. By contrast, utilitarian ethics is generally considered more appropriate—and more workable—for dealing with resource allocation at the level of health policy and overall planning, but it seems to falter when dealing with such individual rights as informed consent. In other words, just like quantum mechanics and relativistic physics, these competing theoretical approaches seem to do quite well in their respective domains but are fundamentally incompatible in their overall logics. This is not to say that there are no deontological theories that try to answer the question of how health care budgets should be developed.

If these are the major ethical theories that structure health care—and as the subsequent chapters will show, there are some reasons for thinking that, in practical terms, this is in fact the case—then ideally, one would want a theoretical framework that would bring the two together into a single, consistent system. At present, there is no generally accepted theoretical framework that accomplishes this. It is just as possible that the theory about the emergent nature of moral properties that was sketched above might provide a way of reconciling the two. One could then argue that deontological ethics is appropriate at the level of individuals, and that utilitarian ethics is appropriate at the level of aggregates or groups of persons—and one could then explain the apparent incompatibility between the two simply by pointing out that the two theories have different domains of application. It would then not be surprising that statements from a deontological analysis cannot simply be transposed into a utilitarian analysis, and *vice versa*. Because the two have different domains, the deontic properties and relations that they describe not only are different but also have different logics—just as in quantum mechanics and relativistic physics. However, there is no fully worked-out theory to that effect, and the conflict between utilitarian and deontological considerations manifests itself in terms of a *vertical ethical conflict* between considerations that dominate policy-making and considerations that rule hands-on health care delivery. (For more on this, see Chapter 10.)

Of course, deontological and utilitarian theories are not the only ones involved in health care decision-making in Canada. At the institutional level, religiously based ethics is foundational to the care that is delivered in denominational hospitals; and at the level of individual decision-making, both religious health care professionals and patients make ethical decisions based on their religiously grounded beliefs. One also encounters ethical decision-making that finds its theoretical basis in virtue ethics; and feminist ethical theory not only seems to underlie at least part of the reasoning involved in many discussions in reproductive ethics but also is encountered in debates surrounding such issues as research and experimentation, informed consent and the physician–patient relationship.

However—and this is not to equate what is ethical with what is legal—there is a very simple reason for not considering religiously based ethics in this sketch of the major ethical theories. Section 15 of the *Canadian Charter of Rights and Freedoms* rules out any law or public policy that is based on a particular religious perspective. This does not mean that individual persons cannot make health care decisions based on their own religious beliefs. As will be explained more fully in Chapter 4, all people have the right to use their own values and beliefs when making health care decisions for themselves. Nor does it mean that health care professionals may not structure their professional lives in a similar way, or that wholly funded private health care institutions may not have religiously based policies. However, it does mean that health care professionals may not use their own religious beliefs when structuring the care they deliver to patients if the patients are unaware of the professional's beliefs and have not agreed to this. (See Chapter 3 for details on the physician–patient relationship and Chapter 4 for more on informed consent.) It also means that while denominational health care institutions need not deliver health care services that are rejected by their particular religion—for instance, a Catholic hospital need not provide abortion services—they may not structure the services they do deliver along particular religious lines if they receive public funds. Therefore, religiously based ethics plays only a very limited role in the public health care sector in Canada and is essentially confined to the level of individual decision-making.

Virtue-based ethics, in turn, may be subject to similar considerations insofar as (with the exception of a few theorists, who will be identified below) it is generally held that there is no universally accepted set of virtues—because virtues are characteristically tied to a particular view of what it is to be human, and this may in turn be culture relative. If this is true, then virtue ethics–based policies would also fall under section 15. In that case, also, virtue ethics may be fine at the level of individual decision-making —and as such will be dealt with in Chapters 4 and 5, which deal with consent—but could not legitimately play a role in the development of health care policy.

Insofar as feminist ethics is concerned—and there is a wide variety of feminist ethical approaches—it has traditionally tended to focus on issues of paternalism at the hands-on level and on issues revolving around reproductive matters at the policy level. This is no longer the case. Feminist ethics has expanded beyond the "philosophy of care" and issues of reproductive ethics or women's health to include issues of social justice and even the very nature of appropriate ethical analysis itself. The brief sketch of feminist ethics that follows below will show how that is the case.

Finally, in the last few years, two theoretical approaches known as communitarianism and liberalism have emerged as additional contenders. Communitarianism essentially combines the insights of feminist reasoning about social embedding with utilitarianism and virtue theory. It suggests that ethical decision-making in health care, whether at the micro-level of individuals or the macro-level of policy, should be goal oriented. It also suggests that the good to be aimed at cannot be divorced from the overall good in which the individual lives, and therefore cannot be defined simply in terms of individual values.[32] By contrast, liberalism maintains that there is no single conception of the good that all persons share, and that the rights and interests of the individual should not be sacrificed on the altar of the common good.[33] Essentially, therefore, it is a version of deontological ethics.

However, when all is said and done, and whatever the attractions and advantages of the various other ethical theories may be, in terms of policy-making and hands-on health care delivery and health care law, deontology and utilitarianism are the dominant ethical theories in the Canadian health care setting. The discussion of ethical theory that follows, therefore, will begin with a sketch of deontological and utilitarian ethical theories before moving on to give a brief outline of virtue and feminist ethics.

Utilitarianism

Utilitarianism is a *teleological*, outcome-oriented or consequentialist ethical theory. Its main focus is the outcome that a particular action or policy would have for the majority of people. For this reason, it structures a lot of health care decision-making at the administrative or policy level. For instance, it underlies the cost/benefit considerations that go into deciding whether to expand an emergency department or to add a psychiatric wing to a hospital. Theoretically, it could also be used at the level of hands-on decision-making: For instance, in theory it could be used to decide whether a kidney should go to a homeless heroin addict as opposed to a hardworking welder who is the backbone of his or her family, pays taxes and is an involved member of the community. However, as we shall see later, using utilitarianism in this way would encounter serious legal problems.

By its very nature—precisely because it looks at outcomes—utilitarianism is a calculative approach to ethical decision-making. It identifies what is right or wrong by looking at what is likely to produce the best outcome for the greatest number of people, and of course this can be done only by comparing competing options and estimating what their likely effects are going to be. It is based on one principle, the *principle of utility*, which says that something is ethically right if it produces, or is likely to produce, the best outcome—also called the greatest good—for the greatest number.

Principle of Utility

> *Always act in such a way as to maximize the chances of achieving the greatest good for the greatest number of people.*

In itself, the principle leaves open the question of what counts as "the good." Here, there are several candidates. One approach considers what is best in terms of pleasure or happiness; this is called *hedonism* (from the Greek word for pleasure). Hedonistic utilitarianism identifies as good that which is likely to produce the greatest amount of pleasure for the greatest number.

By contrast, *eudaemonistic* utilitarianism—the word comes from the Greek for happiness—identifies the good in terms of happiness. It argues that the principle of utility is satisfied only by something that is likely to maximize the chance of happiness for the greatest number. That is why Jeremy Bentham, one of the original advocates of utilitarianism in the English-speaking world, called the principle of utility the "the greatest happiness or greatest felicity principle."[34]

Finally, some utilitarians distinguish between purely physical pleasures on the one hand and intellectual (or ideal) goods such as justice, equality or liberty on the other. They then maintain that the real good is not something material, as hedonism would say, or happiness, however it may be defined, but the ideal goods just mentioned. Not surprisingly, those who advocate this position are called *ideal utilitarians*. They calculate utility in terms of what is likely to produce the greatest amount of justice, equality or liberty, etc., for the greatest number.

All utilitarians agree that whatever "the good" may be, it may vary in intensity, duration, the certainty or uncertainty of its actually coming about, the temporal remoteness of when the outcome is likely to occur, the chance it has of being followed by similar sensations or states of affairs, the chance of it being followed by its opposite, and of course the number of people who are likely to be affected by it.

Utilitarians, however, may differ in their views on the nature of utility scales themselves. Cardinal utilitarians consider utility to be something that can be assigned on the basis of an objective ranking scale, such as preference or even intrinsic values, and therefore can be used in decision-making by engaging in an objective and absolute comparative ranking. By contrast, ordinal utilitarians claim that ranking based on cardinal values is not really possible, because there is no absolute scale of values. It therefore claims that it is possible to compare and rank what are otherwise considered goods relative to each other, thus allowing one to be considered worse than, equal to or better than the other.[35]

Utilitarianism can also differ on how to actually calculate what is likely to achieve the good in question. *Act-utilitarianism* proceeds on a case-by-case basis by looking at the facts of each case and deciding on that basis, for that case, what is likely to produce the greatest good for the greatest number.[36] This means that health care professionals who are act-utilitarians would not follow general rules or guidelines. Instead, they would calculate the likely proportion of good that would be achieved—the utility—of each situation separately and on the basis of the best data available for that particular case.

This, of course, assumes that one always has the relevant data and that the data are qualitatively adequate for calculative decision-making—which frequently is not the case in health care, an area characterized by considerable uncertainty. It can also be time-consuming. Another disadvantage is that case-by-case decision-making makes it impossible to plan ahead for any length of time at the administrative level—in other words, it makes it impossible to develop long-range health budgets and health policies. However, one cannot develop and maintain a health care system without such budgets and policies. This is where *rule utilitarianism* comes into its own. It says that utility should not be calculated on a case-by-case basis but for general rules of conduct. Therefore, it would express the principle of utility like this: "Those rules of conduct are morally correct which, if implemented, would produce or be likely to produce the greatest amount of good for the greatest number of people."[37] Therefore, when it came to actual decision-making, the rule-utilitarian professional would identify the relevant rule that would apply to the situation and decide on that basis.

Moreover, utilitarianism may also differ on how the nature of these goals is to be determined. Some say that a special sort of insight or intuition is involved. This intuition is supposed to show that whatever is identified as the good has intrinsic value—i.e., that it has value in and of itself, whether or not anyone actually values it or finds it valuable. Others focus on the nature of human beings and maintain that the good can be identified only by looking at human nature and at the capabilities and potentials that are grounded in it. Still others look to the current preferences of society, and say that the nature of the good is a matter of socially accepted preference. While the first two viewpoints allow for *a priori* reasoning, independent of considerations of social practice, social preference utilitarianism is empirical in outlook and finds the basis for its claims in social attitudes. Furthermore, while the first two types of approaches would yield an absolutistic sort of answer about the nature of the good, the preference-based approach has to admit that the good aimed at may change over time.

One of the problems with preference utilitarianism is that it has to come up with some way to aggregate preferences and to determine which of a conflicting set of preferences takes priority. When the desires are of the same sort, this can be done rather easily in purely numerical terms that involve counting the number of people involved and the strength of their relevant desires, or by taking into account the effect of fulfilling the relevant desires and seeing how that would balance out in terms of satisfying the basic preferences. However, when they are not of the same sort it becomes extremely difficult to assign any rational kind of priority ranking.

Another problem with preference utilitarianism is that all preferences and desires are creatures of perspective and upbringing, and that one can move to absolute rights only if one has a value theory that makes the ranking of certain rights possible in objective and absolute terms that are independent of such relativistic conditions. Otherwise, one could not reasonably claim that it is ethically wrong to kill minorities for their organs to save the majority (each human body can save a great number of persons because the organs can be distributed, the blood can be used by many persons, etc.) even if the preferences of the majority (which has the same strong preference to stay alive) outweigh the preferences of the minority. Therefore, it seems that the moral rights of the individual person cannot be protected by classical or preference utilitarianism.[38]

In Canadian health care, utilitarian considerations are essentially confined to matters of policy and resource allocation at the level of groups of persons. For instance, they play a role in decisions on how much of the available resources to allocate to acute care as opposed to chronic care, how much money to put into a pediatric coronary care unit as opposed to an infectious disease ward, etc. The reason they do not really play any role at the level of hands-on health care is that there are legal considerations that enter into play: considerations that fall under the rubric of duty-of-care and negligence, and ethical considerations that derive from the nature of the fiduciary physician–patient relationship. These issues will be explored further in Chapters 3, 9 and 10, which deal with the health care professional–patient relationship, the right to health care and resource allocation respectively.

Deontological Theories

As was mentioned before, health care administrators frequently use a rule-utilitarian approach when deciding what to do. This is scarcely surprising. The job of health care administrators is to develop and implement policies that are likely to ensure the greatest amount of quality health care for the greatest number of people.

However, the picture changes at the hands-on level of actual care. Here, the individual patient is the focus of primary concern. That is why at the hands-on level, deontological ethics is the theory of choice, because the deontological perspective is oriented towards the individual as a person and around the rights and duties that belong to each individual as a person.

Like utilitarianism, deontological theories come in various versions. Three in particular have attracted much attention. One dispenses entirely with particular ethical principles. Instead, it says that the way to determine whether an action is ethically acceptable is to generalize the maxim of the act—i.e., to generalize the logic of the particular action—and to see whether it can function as a universal law without either doing away with itself or contradicting itself. This is called the *universalizability criterion*. It was most famously expressed by Immanuel Kant in what he called the *categorical imperative*: "Act only according to that maxim by which you can at the same time will that it should become a universal law."[39] Another version, which Kant called the *practical imperative*, was "Act so that you treat humanity, whether in your own person or in that of another, always as an end and never as a means only."[40] Kant gave several other formulations of his categorical imperative—three more, to be exact[41]—and he claimed that they were all equivalent. For health care ethics, however, the first two formulations are the most important because, as will become apparent in the next few chapters, they provide the foundation of almost all hands-on ethical decision-making.

The important thing about them is not their particular content but the fact that they state the logical form that the maxim of an act must have to be an ethical imperative.[42] Perhaps one can clarify the meaning of this by means of an example. Consider the case of a patient with metastasized and inoperable cancer of the lungs who is too weak to undergo chemotherapy and radiation treatment. Let us suppose that both the physician who is responsible for the case and the patient's family know that the patient is psychologically labile. Let us suppose further that the physician and the family want to spare the patient the psychological trauma they are convinced she would suffer if she were to be told the true state of affairs before the disease had progressed to the point of seriously incapacitating her. The physician and the family therefore lie to the patient about the diagnosis and prognosis.

While this sort of action might be defensible from a humanitarian perspective, Kant would argue that it is unethical because it fails the first test. The maxim of the act—the general rule according to which the physician would here be acting—would be something like "Lie when motivated by humanitarian considerations." However—so Kant would argue—if this maxim were to be elevated to the level of a universal law, it would become the precept that anyone, on any occasion involving humanitarian motives, should lie. However, what counts as a humanitarian motive is an idiosyncratic matter that depends on the perception and on the private values of the relevant individual. Therefore, if the maxim became a law, no one could ever be sure that in fact he or she was not being lied to by other people on all sorts of occasions. Not only would that completely erode our confidence in what we are told by others[43]—something a utilitarian might also say—it would also mean that, for all practical purposes, the distinction between lying and telling the truth would disappear. The maxim would thus fail the universalizability test and defeat itself.

Kant would further argue—and this would reflect the second formulation of the categorical imperative—that to lie to patients, even under circumstances such as these, is to withhold from them the information that they should have if they are to be able to make reasonable, rational and appropriate decisions about how to conduct the rest of their lives. In other words, it would be to treat them not as what they really are—namely, autonomous, rational beings who are ends in themselves—but as objects, something to be manipulated. (See Chapter 3.)

Kantian deontology presents several problems, perhaps most notoriously the question of what to do when to act in accordance with the imperative would lead to serious negative consequences. For instance, if one does not lie to a Nazi who is searching for Jews hiding in one's house but tells the truth—as the categorical imperative would demand—then the Jews will be killed. There is something very counterintuitive about an ethical theory that would lead to such an outcome.

Of course, there are ways of dealing with this problem. One of them is to point out that the requirement to always speak truly (i.e., not to lie) is not the same as the requirement to talk in the first place. If one keeps quiet or does not answer the Nazi's question, one will not be lying. But even if that solved the problem, people usually have neither the time nor the training to engage in the necessary reasoning, which is why *deontological pluralism*—a version of deontology that identifies several ethical principles—is the version that tends to structure most hands-on health care decision-making.

The best-known historical example of a pluralistic deontological theory is that of Plato, who identified several principles such as equality and justice. A more modern version was proposed by W.D. Ross.[44] Ross suggested that not only are there several fundamental ethical principles, but they do not hold absolutely speaking and without exception. Instead, they hold *prima facie*—which is to say, they are abstract and general approximations that serve as guides, and their actual force or effectiveness depends on the facts of the case and on the relative strengths of the conflicting duties that one has on a given occasion. In other words, the actual force of an ethical principle is functionally determined by the context. This would include not only the nature of the acts themselves but the personal, social and material factors of the situation. Only when all of this is taken into account can one say whether a right or duty actually holds.

A still more recent deontological theory is that of John Rawls.[45] Rawls's main focus in analyzing ethical relationships is justice as fairness, and he suggests that there are two fundamental parts to this principle of justice: *First*, everyone has the same indefeasible claim to equal basic liberties and freedoms that are mutually compatible; and *second*, that everyone has the same right to equality of opportunity, whereby any inequalities must be resolved to the benefit of the least advantaged. Rawls further suggests that ethically acceptable decisions should be made from behind what he calls a *veil of ignorance*— which means that all particular information about decision-makers, their society and their special interests should be ignored; only generalizable aspects of the situation should enter into their decision-making. The purpose of this device is to situate people fairly with respect to one another. At the same time, Rawls maintains that his version of deontology is only a partial theory, because it deals only with justice and does not attempt to explain all ethical concerns such as those that arise in hands-on health care. However, it has attracted considerable attention in health care decision-making at the policy level, because it seems to provide a way of integrating outcome concerns into rights-based reasoning.[46]

ETHICAL PRINCIPLES IN HEALTH CARE

The important question to ask at this juncture is what all of this means for health care ethics. The answer was already hinted at above. Because health care involves both individual patients and groups of patients, and because ethical issues arise at each level, both deontological and utilitarian ethics have their place. Of course, as was also mentioned, the problem is how to integrate them—and here there is no agreement. One thing, however, is certain: Unless one can somehow come up with a way of reconciling the two—perhaps by developing a "grand theory of everything" for ethics in the way that physics is trying to develop a "grand theory of everything" for physics—the stage is set for what might be called vertical ethical conflict. What is an ethically appropriate decision or consideration at the macro-level of groups (or indeed of society as a whole) will conflict with what is an ethically appropriate decision or consideration at the micro-level of individual health care delivery, and *vice versa*.

This does not mean that health care ethics—and indeed biomedical ethics as a whole, of which health care ethics is only a part—is an ad hoc and disconnected affair. There is general agreement that even though utilitarian considerations are valid at the macro-level, they must always be tempered by considerations that derive from the deontological principles that apply at the micro-level. Moreover, there is fairly general agreement on what these deontological principles are. They are the substantive principles of autonomy and respect for persons, equality and justice, beneficence, non-malfeasance and fidelity; and these are conditioned by the more formal principles of impossibility and priority. In a sense, they are the application of Kant's idea of the categorical imperative to the particular sphere of biomedicine and health care; and just as Ross had suggested, they hold *prima facie*, depending on the facts of the situation and the nature of the case. The rest of this chapter is devoted to presenting these principles in detail.

Autonomy and Respect for Persons

All persons are autonomous beings worthy of respect, and as such have a fundamental right to self-determination that is limited only by unjust infringement on the rights of others.

In the health care context, the Principle may also be phrased as follows:

Always treat persons as autonomous decision-makers who have the right to accept or reject any health care intervention.

Logically, this principle is tightly connected to the notion of a right. A right is an entitlement or "justified claim."[47] The important thing about this is that a right-holder need not exercise an entitlement or claim. That is something that the right-holder *may* do, but does not have to. For example, the fact that someone has a right to move about freely doesn't mean that they have to. They may decide simply to stay put wherever they are. Or, the fact that someone with an acute appendicitis has a right to an appendectomy does not mean that he or she has to have an appendectomy. He or she may choose to deal with the acute appendicitis some other way, trying traditional native medicine, applying homeopathic interventions or faith-based interventions such as those used by Christian Scientists—or by deciding to refuse all health care and instead let nature take its course.

It is this freedom to choose that is logically inherent in the nature of a right. One cannot have a right if, by one's nature, one is not free and cannot choose, because if by one's nature one is not free and cannot choose, then whether or not one exercises the entitlement or claim is not a matter of will but of strict causality. The individual will automatically exercise the claim or entitlement when the enabling conditions are present. That is why robots cannot have rights. This of course does not mean that, if one cannot choose at that point in time because of some incapacity or other, or because one has not yet developed sufficiently to exercise the ability that is inherent in one's nature (as in the case of a young child), one does not have rights.

The point is sufficiently important to deserve restating. The notion of moral responsibility is different from the notion of causal responsibility. Moral or ethical responsibility involves choice. In causal responsibility—for example, when we say that the earthquake is responsible for the collapse of the buildings—the outcome is the inescapable consequence of the initial conditions and the laws of nature. There is no choice. Earthquakes do not choose to collapse buildings, and tectonic stresses do not choose to cause earthquakes. They are simply the outcome of a confluence of factors that are governed by the laws of nature. This does not mean that when one is morally responsible for a particular outcome or event one has acted outside of the laws of nature. Rather, it means that one has the ability to interfere in the causal sequence or causal chain of events and thereby to determine the outcome by *using* the causal chain either positively (by interfering) or negatively (by refraining from interfering when one could) *and that one can choose to do so*. (This becomes important when we consider active versus passive euthanasia in Chapter 7, The Ethics of Deliberate Death.) Therefore, the notion of moral responsibility is ineluctably tied to the notion of freedom or autonomy. Things that are not free in this sense cannot be morally responsible for what they do, for what they produce or what they bring about. That is why deciduous trees aren't morally responsible for dropping their leaves or why moths aren't morally responsible for following pheromone cues.

However, autonomy is not the same as licence. As we shall see later, every right is subject to the equal and competing rights of others. There is an old legal saying that captures this very well: "Your right to swing your fist stops where my face begins!" So, for instance, people who are carriers of serious infectious diseases do not have the right to ignore that fact and to go about their normal routines, interacting with other people and not taking "proper precautions." To quote a noted jurist[48]

> The most stringent protection of free speech would not protect a man falsely shouting
> fire in a theater and causing a panic.

It also does not mean that the health care decision of incompetent persons (or, in legal parlance, of persons who "lack capacity") should be respected if they were made while the persons were incompetent. For example, the decisions of young children and of the mentally disabled should not be respected, even though young children and the mentally disabled are persons and, as persons, are equal to any other person. The reason is that such individuals cannot be autonomous decision-makers in any genuine sense. They lack the necessary qualities for making genuine choices. More colloquially, while they can "pick," they cannot choose. The reason they cannot choose (in the genuine sense of that term) is that to choose is not only to have freedom but also to be aware of the available options and understand their implications, and on that basis select one of these options by using one's values. The problem with individuals who are incompetent (lack capacity) is that they lack either understanding or (competent) values—or both. Therefore, even though they are persons, and even though as persons they have the right to autonomous decision-making, their inability to exercise that right means that someone else must make relevant decisions for them. (For more on this, see Chapter 5.)

Equality and Justice

All persons, insofar as they are persons, are equal and should be treated the same. Exceptions to this must always be based on ethically relevant differences in the nature or status of the person in question.

When one stops to think about it, this principle is really a matter of logic. If two things are the same—if x is the same as y—then what one does to x will have the same effect on y if one does the same thing to y and *vice versa*. Since persons, insofar as they are persons, are the same, what applies to the one also applies to the other and *vice versa*. Of course, persons are also individuals with certain physical and mental characteristics, and they don't all do the same things, so in that sense there are differences between them. As *persons*, murderers are persons like any other persons; but murderers have done something that non-murderers have not done—namely, murdered—and that is why murderers have a different ethical status. Or, to put it in terms of the Principle of Autonomy, murderers have exercised their autonomy differently than non-murderers have. This is an ethically relevant difference. Likewise, persons confined to wheelchairs *cannot* exercise their autonomy the way non-disabled persons can. This is another relevant ethical difference. Or, still differently, mentally disabled persons cannot exercise their autonomy because they lack certain requirements for fully autonomous decision-making. This is still another ethically relevant difference.

Ethically relevant differences between persons legitimate—indeed, they *require*—that we treat the persons who have these ethically relevant differences differently. As we shall see later in Chapter 5, this is central to the whole notion of proxy or substitute decision-making. If one were to treat persons who lacked competence as though they were in fact competent, one would not be taking this crucial relevant difference into account. One would indeed be treating them the same as other persons, but that very sameness of treatment would be unethical and would amount to discrimination on the basis of disability. Likewise, if one were to treat an irresponsible person whose irresponsible lifestyle has led to a particular health care need (for example, someone who has had unprotected promiscuous sex with multiple partners and because of this has contracted AIDS) the same as a responsible person who has developed the same health care need by an uncontrollable accident (say, a surgeon who has contracted AIDS because a bone splinter has punctured his or her glove during an emergency and life-saving thoracic operation), then one would be acting unethically. Being responsible is different from being irresponsible. The choices we make affect our ethical standing. This becomes important when the right to health care and the issue of health care resource allocation are considered (see Chapters 9 and 10).

One could go on to multiple examples; however, the point is simply this: Equality does not mean sameness. It means treating people the same *taking their ethically relevant differences into account.* In other words, one should not treat them the same but *equitably*. This is not simply an ethical issue. It finds reflection in human rights legislation and in anti-discrimination cases.

Fidelity (or Integrity or Best Action)

Whoever has an obligation also has the ethical duty to discharge that obligation to the best of their ability.

This principle is closely connected with the notion of a right and the concept of a duty, and is really quite commonsensical. If one has a right, then one has a justified claim towards others. However, such a claim is not met if the relevant action is performed only haphazardly or in a way that is qualitatively different from what is contained in the claim itself. This is not simply a matter of ethics. It also finds reflection in law—for example, in the law of contracts and in the law of negligence. In health care it underlies the notion of *due care*. An interesting example in which this principle is front and centre is the case of the crash team (a team especially trained to respond to emergency codes in a hospital) that "walks to the code" instead of running or going as quickly as possible. Since time is of the essence in such situations, walking to the code violates integrity and constitutes professional negligence.

There are two other principles that are frequently appealed to in biomedical ethics: They are the Principle of Beneficence and the Principle of non-Malfeasance (or Nonmaleficence). Instead of dealing with what might be called the quality of actions, they deal with their direction.

Beneficence

> *Everyone has a duty to advance the good of others if it is possible to do so without undue risk to oneself, where the nature of the good is in keeping with the competently held values of the recipients of the action in question.*

There are several things about this principle that are important. The *first* is that it effectively acknowledges that, as Aristotle said, human beings are social animals and can realize their potentials only within a social context. However—and this is one of the underlying premises of the Principle—that social context cannot exist if people do not interact in a way that allows the members of society to function as persons; and that, in turn, means that they must be able to realize *their own* potentials as persons well. Therefore, what this principle amounts to is an acknowledgement that personhood involves mutuality.

The *second* thing that is important about this principle is that it ties the realization of human potential not to some objective and absolute standard that is the same for all people but to individuals themselves. In other words, it acknowledges that although people as biological organisms have many things in common, as individuals they are situated in a world that is determined by their conceptual framework, which in turn is structured by their values. Therefore, how their potentials should be realized—and indeed, what potentials should be realized—is partly determined by these values. That is why what counts as advancing the good of an individual is always relative to that individual's values.

Third, the principle talks about competently held values. The notion of competently held values will become important later in Chapter 4, when we deal with the issue of informed consent. For now, suffice it to say that not all values are ethically on a par. For instance, values that treat persons solely as workers or production units (and who therefore no longer have a right to health care when they can no longer contribute to the welfare of a family or social grouping) or values that treat others solely as walking organ banks (and therefore allow the exploitation of people who are in desperate financial straits and therefore are willing to sell their organs) are not ethically acceptable or competently held values. Also, values that people hold only because they have been conditioned to hold them are not competently held values. In the language of philosophy, they are not *authentic* values. This, too, will become important in the context of informed consent.

Finally—and this ties in with the first point—the principle acknowledges that if all people were to advance the good of others at undue risk to themselves, this would also jeopardize the social fabric, because this would mean that the very actions intended to safeguard the existence of the social fabric would threaten the existence of the fabric. Moreover, each member of society, as a person, has the same rights as any other, and that includes the right to advance their own (legitimate) interests. Therefore, if we were required to advance the good of others at the cost of undue risk to ourselves, then we as persons would count less than other persons.

Non-Malfeasance or Nonmaleficence

The Principle of Beneficence finds reflection in the first clause of the Canadian Medical Association's Code of Ethics:[49] "Consider first the well-being of the patient," and forms part of the Code of Ethics of most national medical associations. Its flip side—the Principle of non-Malfeasance or Nonmaleficence—may be expressed as follows:

> *Everyone has a duty to prevent harm to others insofar as this is possible without undue risk to oneself, where the nature of the harm is in keeping with the competent values of the recipient of the action in question.*

This is one of the oldest clearly stated principles in the history of medicine. It was already encountered in the Hippocratic tradition, which admonished physicians to "keep [patients] from harm,"[50] and it is reflected in most later codes of ethics for physicians and other health care providers.

This principle also contains several tacit limiting riders. Specifically, what counts as harm is not something objective and absolute that holds for all, but is relative to the values of the recipient of the action. In the biomedical context, this means that what counts as harm is defined not by the health care professionals but by the competently held values of the patient. As we shall see later in Chapter 3, when this rider is ignored the result is paternalism. An example of this would be the case of a patient who is undergoing chemotherapy and radiotherapy for a sarcoma and for whom a blood transfusion is medically indicated because the resultant anemia and hypoxia would otherwise interfere with the response of tumours to the chemotherapy and the radiotherapy.[51] If the patient has competently refused the use of blood and blood products because of (competently held) religious values and the health care professionals transfused blood despite this, they would be acting paternalistically. They would be producing harm as defined by the patient. Not only would that be unethical, it would also be illegal. (For more on this, see Chapter 3, as well as the landmark case of *Malette v. Shulman et al.* [1990] 72 O.R. [2d] 417 [Ont. C.A.])

For reasons that have already been discussed in reference to beneficence, the Principle also limits the extent of duties that fall under it to actions that do not involve undue danger to the agent.

CONFLICT AMONG DEONTOLOGICAL PRINCIPLES AND THEIR DERIVATIVE RIGHTS AND DUTIES

Of course, the fact that there are several ethical principles raises the question of what happens when they conflict with each other.[52] To consider an actual case, suppose someone is a typhoid carrier without being ill—this was the case with Mary Mallon, who entered history as "Typhoid Mary"[53]—and refuses to enter quarantine or otherwise limit interaction with other persons because he or she considers that to be an interference with his or her autonomy. The Principle of Autonomy suggests that such persons have the right not to be quarantined and that they may do as they please, but the Principles of non-Malfeasance (and possibly Fidelity) entail the duty of health care professionals to prevent them from spreading disease. Which principle wins—and why?

The Return of *Prima Facie*

It is here that the notion of *prima facie* developed by Ross comes into its own. According to this notion, all principles are general approximations that can serve as guides, but the rights they entail hold only subject to existing conditions. Therefore, when trying to decide which principle takes priority in a given case—and therefore which right or duty is *in fact* a right or a duty—one should take into account not only the nature of the relevant act in question but also the personal, social and material parameters in which the relevant individuals are embedded.

And this, surely, is correct. Ethical principles apply to human situations and actions. However, human situations and actions are not isolated. They always involve particular circumstances or facts. Therefore, how the principles apply always depends on the facts. An analogy from physics may here be of use. The law of gravity says, roughly, that the strength of gravitational attraction between two bodies is directly proportional to the product of the masses of the two bodies and inversely proportional to the distance between them. This holds true whether the bodies are Jupiter and the Sun or asteroids. The *strength* of their respective gravitational attraction—in other words, what the law means in actual practice—will therefore not be the same, but the *law of gravity* is the same. It merely expresses itself differently depending on the material circumstances. The same thing is true of ethical principles. How they express themselves depends on the circumstances. That is why the very same principles will have different consequences when different circumstances are taken into account.

The Ranking of Rights

This notion of *prima facie* can be spelled out further by considering that sometimes rights can be ranked logically. Thus, purely logically speaking, if a right can be exercised only if a particular condition is satisfied, then the existence of that right entails a right to bring about that necessary condition, and the latter is logically prior to and more fundamental than the former. For example, the right to a certain quality of life presupposes that the person who has that right is alive. Therefore, the right to life is logically prior to and trumps the right to a certain quality of life. This becomes important when dealing with resource allocation and triage under conditions of resource limitation.

At the same time, every competent person may voluntarily give up a right to someone else, or may subordinate a logically prior right to a lower one. This follows from the very nature of rights as justified claims. One does not have to exercise a claim. A particularly graphic example of this ranking device was the case of the pregnant young woman who suffered a ruptured uterus. The woman was informed that it would be possible to save either her or her baby, but not both. She asked that her baby be saved and that she receive only comfort measures. In other words, she voluntarily gave up her right to life-saving treatment in favour of delivering a live baby.[54]

Impossibility and Futility

Another consideration that is relevant when dealing with ranking or ordering rights and duties centres in a logical condition that applies to all right and duties. It simply says that one cannot have a duty to do the impossible. In the legal context it is called the Principle of Common Law Impossibility.[55] In ethics it can be expressed like this:

> *A right that cannot be fulfilled under the circumstances is ineffective as a right, and an obligation that cannot be met under the circumstances ceases to be effective as an obligation.*

This principle is sometimes confused in the bioethical literature with the *doctrine of futility*,[56] but it is actually quite different. The Principle of Impossibility applies only to situations in which fulfilling what would otherwise be a duty is actually impossible. For instance, if no surgical team and no operating facility are available, then not operating on a patient who needs surgery here and now is not failing in one's duty. It simply cannot be done. Likewise, not providing an intervention when that intervention is available but has no chance whatever of being successful—for instance, not attempting to resuscitate a patient who has been found more than ten minutes after the patient has arrested and whose body is at room temperature—is not failing in one's duty of fidelity. It is impossible to resuscitate a person in that condition.

By contrast, futility looks at whether the relevant intervention will be successful in producing the intended or expected result. It has a long history in medical ethics, going back all the way to Hippocrates.[57] An example would be whether one should resuscitate someone whose circulation has already been stopped for five minutes in the absence of hypothermia and central nervous system depressants. One could do it, but to do so would essentially be futile, because the likelihood that the individual would ever be in more than a permanent vegetative state is very low. (For more on this, see the discussion of personhood in Chapter 7.) A slightly different example would be the case of someone dying of inoperable metastasized cancer of the colon that has spread through the whole body, where surgery, chemotherapy and radiation have proven ineffective. Even though one could engage in further aggressive therapy, it would be futile to do so because it would not change the fact of impending death. (However, this does not mean that the patient does not have the right to other health care.)

OTHER ETHICAL THEORIES

As was mentioned above, there are two other ethical theories that play a role in either health care decision-making at the policy level in Canada or in hands-on decision-making by individual patients. They are feminism and virtue ethics respectively.

Feminist Ethics

Feminist ethics has sometimes been described as the "ethics of caring and response."[58] It rose to prominence in the 1960s and '70s with a particular focus on reproductive ethics, power relationships and the unique place of women in society. Originally, its driving idea was the moral experience of women in what was described as a male-dominated and male-oriented world. It argued that the moral and social experiences of women differ from those of men, and that one must take these differences into account when ethically evaluating a particular situation. The seminal writings of Nel Noddings,[59] Carol Gilligan[60] and Annette Baier[61] are particularly noteworthy in this regard. They also argued that the female experience in most societies traditionally involved a greater or lesser degree of discrimination, leaving women disproportionately powerless, and that this could be corrected only by developing a new ethics.[62]

In the health care sector, feminism has been influential in the shaping of policy directions and in the context of health law, most notably regarding abortion. Thus, feminists pointed out—and this found resonance in the Supreme Court case of *Morgentaler*, which will be discussed further in Chapter 8—that the laws on abortion (as well as the traditional medical-social perspective) were unfair to women because they treated pregnant women not as persons but as fetal containers, and their rights were subordinated to those of the developing fetus.[63]

Another example comes from the field of medical research and experimentation. Medical researchers, so feminists argued, did not pay appropriate attention to women's health care needs and excluded them as experimental subjects because, so it was felt, participating in experiments might pose a special risk to their ability to bear (healthy) children.[64] By contrast, no such considerations were raised against the inclusion of fertile men in medical experimentation even though their ability to father (healthy) children might also be impaired. Not only did this reflect an inherent sexist bias at the very heart of traditional experimental protocols, it was also discriminatory in a much more profound fashion, because it resulted in important female health care needs remaining essentially underserviced or even unmet.

Feminist ethics has not remained focused solely on women's actual experiences. One of its more important developments was an examination of the appropriate nature of ethical analysis itself, and of how one should go about dealing with ethical dilemmas. Its cardinal insight in this context was that ethical issues and dilemmas cannot legitimately be resolved by blindly balancing competing rights and duties, or by automatically turning to virtues or applying principles such as autonomy, equality and impartiality. Instead, the particulars of each situation as well as the relationships in which the various stakeholders are embedded importantly determine the ethical nature of each case and therefore have to be taken into account.[65] Moreover, disagreements and problems should not be approached in the spirit of exclusionary decision-making but in the spirit of cooperative resolution. It is in this sense that feminism advocates a departure from traditional principled ethical decision-making.[66] Feminist ethics therefore considers individual narratives an integral part of any ethically defensible deliberative process, because only these can provide depth or substance to what otherwise would be abstract, theoretically grounded considerations.[67] Not surprisingly, feminism also rejects the categorization of people into rigid groups (race, sex, gender, age, disability, susceptibility to disease, etc.) because these tend to obscure important parameters that derive from the felt experience of social embedding.

Feminist ethics is not a monolithic movement but has come to include a variety of ethical perspectives. Some feminist theorists have expanded on the foundational work of Carol Gilligan.[68] Gilligan had claimed that there is a uniquely female ethical perspective that emerges at an early stage and results in differential ethical development in female and male children,[69] where the female perspective essentially centres in the notion of caring. More recent theorists in the care-ethics camp, while not necessarily giving up the claim of a unique female ethics experience or point of view, have gone on to address general issues of dependency and justice in their speculations,[70] thereby moving beyond issues that are unique to women's position, to consider issues of general interpersonal dependence in society. This has found reflection in connection with structuring long-term care for dependent patients.

Others have distanced themselves from the original care orientation. Susan Sherwin, in particular,[71] has voiced the concern that the care perspective merely reinforces the traditional "patriarchal" view of women's characters as distinctively different from men's—which in itself would turn biology into destiny, reduce moral discourse between the sexes into crossed monologues and turn the resolution of ethical claims into a matter of power differentials.[72] Feminist theorists in this camp argue that a principled approach to ethics in general, and to bioethics in particular, is not completely wrong but merely incomplete, because it provides only a limited and truncated view of ethics and ethical situations. They advocate that as long as these principles are formulated in non-exclusionary terms that reflect the relational context of individual lives, they are an appropriate part of an ethical framework.

Another development in feminist ethics follows this line but strikes out in a different direction. In order to overcome what they regard as the limitations of a pure care-oriented approach, a number of feminist theorists have incorporated what they consider some of the insights of virtue ethics into what still remains a care-centred philosophy. In the health care field, they have attempted to develop—and are continuing to develop—a bioethics that draws on both traditions.[73]

Still others have moved more towards the deontological camp in their attempt to expand on the care perspective. More specifically, they have attempted to combine deontological insights centred in the idea of justice with the ethics of care, with particular emphasis on insurance coverage, research and female representation on policy-making bodies as specific issues.[74] There has also been a movement to incorporate the Principle of Autonomy into feminist health care ethics under the rubrics of self-trust[75] and self-improvement, with a special focus on health care structures and health care delivery.[76] In much of the latter, the emphasis has been on issues in reproductive ethics.[77]

Some of the issues raised by feminist theorists will be discussed in subsequent chapters, particularly in Chapter 3 (which deals with the physician–patient relationship), Chapter 4 (which deals with informed consent), Chapter 6 (which, among other things, deals with representative inclusion in experimental protocols), Chapter 8 (which deals with abortion) and Chapters 11 and 12, which deal with reproductive rights and the issue of biotechnologies (including ectogenesis) respectively. The question that may legitimately be asked, however, is whether a feminist approach is uniquely qualified to deal with these issues and whether it is necessary to switch to a feminist perspective when dealing with power relationships (as in informed consent), with due representation in research and in access to health care, and when dealing with abortion and the reproductive technologies. Arguably, a properly developed deontological ethics can also deal appropriately with these issues, and the fact that contemporary feminist theorists have found it necessary to include deontological and virtue ethics considerations in their attempts to develop a full-fledged bioethics suggests that, while a feminist perspective adds important elements to bioethical considerations, it need not be treated as an independent ethical theory in its own right.

Virtue Ethics

Virtue ethics, as its name indicates, is based on the concept of virtue. As one of the most noted modern proponents of the theory has put it, a morally upright person is one who performs the right kinds of acts because he or she possesses a certain kind of character:

namely, a virtuous character. This virtuous character is one that allows the individual to realize those characteristics and qualities that define human beings as human beings.[78]

Virtue ethics shares several important traits with other ethical approaches. Like feminist ethics, it rejects the position that ethics is fundamentally concerned with duties and rights.[79] Instead, it argues that the fundamental concern of ethics is the development of a virtuous character, which in turn is intimately related to the notion of a happy life.[80] It is similar to deontological ethics in that it rejects the thesis that the greatest good for the greatest number is the ultimate aim of ethical action. At the same time, it has a certain similarity to teleological ethics in its central insistence that we should foster the attainment of a virtuous character or disposition.[81]

So far as virtue ethics is concerned, the virtues that find their most obvious expression in health care are those of compassion and care. This is not surprising, since these *other-directed* virtues have been synonymous with health care since its very beginning. This is also what makes virtue ethics so attractive to hands-on caregivers, such as physicians and nurses. However, virtue ethics also maintains that health care provides the opportunity for *self-directed* virtues, such as courage and forbearance. Consequently, it also has something to recommend it from the patient's perspective. *Social* virtues, such as justice and beneficence, have also emerged as important in recent discussions. These are virtues that find ready acceptance from the perspective of society as a whole.[82]

Virtue ethics as a theory has ancient philosophical roots, going back to Plato and above all Aristotle in the Western world and has equally ancient roots in the Asian world in Daoist and Buddhist ethics. In contrast to deontological and utilitarian theories, virtue ethics maintains that one cannot produce a universal and globally binding set of principles that can be understood (and that can be followed) by all people.[83] They maintain that experience is a crucial element in ethical decision-making and that virtuous dispositions, rather than mere adherence to rules, lead to ethically much more appropriate actions.

The reason—so goes the argument—is that virtue is a character trait or disposition that grounds how people will view the world and how they will act. The virtuous person, therefore, has an overall perspective or mindset that is structured by such considerations as veracity, honesty and compassion, where these will condition both the nature of a given action as well as the perceived need for the action itself without, however, functioning as absolute and inviolable determinants. Instead, this mindset results in a functionally balanced approach to any given situation. Moreover, these virtues, as part of the structuring determinants of the mind, are not confined in their effects to purely rational deliberations but will also influence the emotional life of virtuous persons and how they situate themselves in the world. This does not mean that fully virtuous persons will not experience contrary emotions, feelings or desires that pull against what reason tells them would be the virtuous thing to do. Rather, the integrated nature of their personality will allow them to overcome such conflicting internal forces.[84] Such a fully virtuous disposition, however, is rare.[85]

Incomplete integration of virtuous disposition is one way in which someone can fall short of being completely virtuous; another is a lack of practical insight.[86] That is to say, if generosity, honesty and courage may be considered parts of a virtuous personality, these character traits can be carried to an extreme—for instance, by someone being too generous, too honest or too courageous. The fault here lies not with the virtuous disposition itself, but with the lack of insight into the situations as they actually obtain. The exercise of any specific virtuous disposition, therefore, is always subject to the conditions at hand, and due regard must always be paid to what would be reasonable limits under the circumstances that obtain. This comes only with experience—which is why, as traditionally understood, people who lack experience (such as children) are not wholly virtuous even though they may have virtuous traits. It also explains why a fully virtuous disposition can be inculcated only through training and experience. Moreover, only virtuous traits that are exercised within an overall conception of what is a genuinely worthwhile life—of a life that leads to true happiness or *eudaemonia* in keeping with human nature—have true ethical value. Since, according to modern virtue theorists, human nature involves intellectual as well as social elements, all modern virtue ethicists agree that a human life devoted solely to physical pleasures or material goods is a wasted life.[87]

An immediate consequence of this is that from a virtue ethics perspective, health care that is devoted solely to alleviating physical ailments or producing only physical healthy human beings is only partially virtuous at best. At both the policy and the hands-on level, an appropriately structured health care system will seek to advance both physical and spiritual well-being, and will try to do so in a way that leads not merely to advancing virtuous dispositions but also to maximizing the chances of producing healthy and fully virtuous persons and a morally good life for all. Such a life will be responsive to changing conditions and will make due adjustments in individual actions within the overall determinants of a happy life.[88]

For instance, virtue ethics will not give a hard and fixed answer to the question of whether it is ethical to have an abortion but rather will consider whether a policy on abortion that sets hard and fast answers as a matter of principle is compatible with developing (and maintaining) a fully human outlook and disposition. From a virtue ethics perspective, therefore, to structure the debate in terms of rights and duties is to ignore the entire moral character of human actions.[89] As one noted virtue ethics theorist put it, "*nothing* follows from this supposition about the morality of abortion . . . once it is noted . . . that in exercising a moral right I can do something cruel, or callous, or selfish, light-minded, self-righteous, stupid, inconsiderate, disloyal, dishonest—that is, act viciously."[90] Moreover, the status of the human fetus—which is sometimes treated as the decisive issue in the abortion debate—is considered relevant only insofar as it figures in the question of what a virtuous person in her particular situation, embedded in a social context that has more than biological ramifications, would do in the case of an unwanted pregnancy.[91]

Virtue ethics theory would also not approach the issue of euthanasia and assisted suicide in terms of rights and duties. Instead, it would focus on such matters as compassion, beneficence and empathy. Therefore, rather than assuming that autonomy would carry the day, a virtue ethics approach would argue that the question of euthanasia (and assisted suicide) must be framed in terms of the consonance of such actions with a virtuous disposition centred in self-realization of the individual as a human being, i.e., centred in the notion of *eudaemonia*.[92]

While virtue ethics has an ancient lineage, it has only recently seen a resurgence of popularity—at least in the academic setting. There are several reasons why it is currently not one of the main themes in actual health care policy-making or at the hands-on level of primary care—with the possible exception of palliative care. *First*, there is the meta-ethical problem of justifying the claim that particular virtues are basic and in fact genuine, and determining which vision of human nature is correct.

Second, there is the general conviction that different cultures embody different virtues, and therefore that cultural relativism is a challenge. In a multicultural society such as Canada, it is difficult to see what set of virtues all parties to the social contract would agree on. To fall back on the claim that these virtues can be identified by looking at what is good for human nature is to assume that all parties would agree on what human nature really is. So far, there has been no agreement on that score. In reply, virtue theorists have argued that it is just as much a problem for the other ethical approaches, and that the putative cultural variation in character traits regarded as virtues is no greater—indeed markedly less—than the cultural variation in rules of conduct. As well, they would say, different cultures have different ideas about what constitutes happiness or welfare. In fact, some virtue theorists have even claimed that when properly decoded and understood, virtues are in fact not culture relative at all.[93]

Third, there is the problem that virtue ethics as currently structured seems to provide no readily apparent conflict resolution mechanism when virtue considerations confront competing claims. Health care professionals are increasingly faced with limited resources, which means that they are faced with conflicting demands for materials, personnel and time. Conflict resolution mechanisms are particularly important for dealing with such situations, because not to decide is in fact to decide; therefore, a rational and equitable decision must be made. Further, since health care measures frequently have a threshold level of effectiveness, a shared or cooperative approach will not be effective for any of the parties concerned and, in fact, may harm all of them to some degree. In cases like these, it is unclear which virtue would provide an answer—or should prevail—or how the view of a eudaemonic life would provide an answer.

THE STRUCTURE OF ETHICAL JUSTIFICATION

Before concluding this chapter on ethical theory, a brief word about the structure of ethical justification. All of us are concerned that our ethical decisions be above reproach. Unfortunately, there is no way to guarantee that. The best one can do is to think clearly, try to make sure not to confuse legal considerations with ethical ones, and keep psychological convictions and personal values distinct from ethical principles. Here it is useful to keep in mind two points that have already been mentioned: *First*, what people take to be true is not necessarily the same as what is true, nor is the depth of a conviction a reliable guide to the truth of what is believed. *Second*, that which leads someone to accept a certain statement or to adopt a particular decision is not necessarily the same as that which justifies this position in the first place.

Although these facts are trivial and commonplace, they are frequently overlooked. However, not distinguishing between them constitutes confusion between the *psychology of ethical decision-making* and the *ethical justification or acceptability of a given decision*. The actual process of ethical decision-making, of course, is a matter of psychology. It involves psychological, personal and cultural variables. How this occurs may be a function of the culture in which the individual has been raised, the social pressures that are being brought to bear on the person—or even the individual's hormonal[94] or blood-sugar levels.[95]

But even if the psychological process is the most reasonable one in the world, it is different from ethical justification. An ethical claim is justified if, and only if, it is derivable from basic principles by the application of facts. And here it does not matter whether one is moving within a utilitarian or a deontological framework. If a particular ethical claim cannot be traced back to a fundamental principle in this way, it may feel right, but it will lack moral justification. The following diagram (Figure 1.1) shows this relationship in graphic terms.

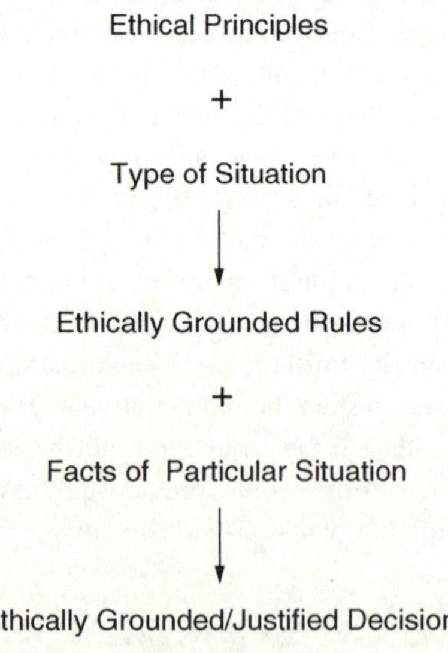

Figure 1.1 Structure of Ethical Justification

CONCLUSION

Health care consists in the delivery of health-oriented services to persons. Whether this care is delivered on a privatized basis—like a commodity that can be bought and sold in the marketplace—or as a socialized service that belongs to members of the community as a matter of right, and whether one is dealing with public health measures or with intensive care treatment, ultimately it is the individual person who is central. Likewise, when there is scarcity, it is the individual person's rights that have to be balanced against the competing rights of others. Therefore, there is a congenial fit between the person-oriented perspective of a deontological approach and the *raison d'être* of health care itself. At the same time, modern health is impossible without research, formalized administrative structures and budgets that make such hands-on care possible. Therefore, utilitarian considerations also have their place. The chapters that follow will look at the implications of this in greater detail, beginning with the role played by codes of medical ethics.

Further Readings

Brandt, R.B. *Morality, Utilitarianism, and Rights* (Cambridge, U.K.: Cambridge University Press, 1992).

Frankena, W.K. *Ethics* (Englewood Cliffs, NY: Prentice Hall, 1973).

Hursthouse, R. *On Virtue Ethics* (Oxford: Oxford University Press, 1999).

McIntyre, A. *After Virtue*, 2nd ed. (Notre Dame, IN: University of Notre Dame Press, 1984).

Noddings, N. *Caring: A Feminist Approach to Ethics and Moral Education* (Berkeley: University of California Press, 1984).

Rawls, J. *A Theory of Justice* (Cambridge, MA: Harvard University Press, 1999).

Sherwin, S. *No Longer Patient: Feminist Ethics and Health Care* (Philadelphia: Temple University Press, 1992).

Singer, P. *A Companion to Ethics* (Oxford: Blackwell, 1993).

Tong, R. *Feminist Thought: A More Comprehensive Introduction*, 3rd ed. (Boulder, CO: Westview Press, 2009).

Endnotes

1. Universal Declaration of Human Rights, available at www.wunrn.com/reference/pdf/univ_dec_hum_right.pdf

2. International Criminal Court, accessed 3 Jun 2011 at www.icc-cpi.int/Menus/ICC/About+the+Court/

3. See J.L. Mackie, *Ethics: Inventing Right and Wrong* (New York: Viking Press, 1977).

4. World Medical Association, International Code of Medical Ethics, accessed 2 Jun 2011 at www.wma.net/en/30publications/10policies/c8/index.html.pdf?print-media-type&footer-right=[page]/[toPage]

5. Canadian Medical Association, CMA Code of Ethics (Update 2004), accessed 2 Jun 2011 at http://policybase.cma.ca/PolicyPDF/PD04-06.pdf

6. See Chapter 6 in A.J. Ayer, *Language, Truth and Logic* (London: Gollanz, 1948).

7. See C.L. Stevenson, *Ethics and Language* (New Haven: Yale University Press, 1944).

8. See R.M. Hare, *The Language of Morals* (Oxford: Oxford University Press, 1952).

9. This would be similar to saying "It's raining but I don't believe it!" and is called Moore's paradox. Moore's paradox hinges on the difference between an assertion and an epistemic attitude about what is asserted. For a collection of essays that attempt to analyze Moore's paradox, see M.S. Green and J.N. Williams (eds.), *Moore's Paradox: New Essays on Belief, Rationality and the First Person* (New York: Oxford University Press, 2007).

10. For a philosophical statement of relativism and its implications for multiculturalism and justice, etc., see W. Kymlicka, *Multicultural Citizenship* (Oxford: Clarendon Press, 1995); C. Taylor, *Philosophy and the Human Sciences: Philosophical Papers 2*, especially Chapter 1 (Cambridge, U.K.: Cambridge University Press, 1985); M. Walzer, *Spheres of Justice* (Oxford: Blackwell, 1983), Chapter 8; and I.M. Young, *Justice and the Politics of Difference* (Princeton: Princeton University Press, 1990), Chapter 4.

11. World Health Organization, "Female genital mutilation," Fact sheet N°24 (February 2010), accessed 2 Jun 2011 at www.who.int/mediacentre/factsheets/fs241/en/

12. For a discussion of the ethics of female circumcision, see E.-H.W. Kluge, "Female Genital Mutilation, Cultural Values and Ethics," *Journal of Obstetrics and Gynaecology* 16.2 (1996): 2611–2618.

13. L. Kohlberg, *The Philosophy of Moral Development* (New York: Harper & Row, 1981). See also A. Colby, L. Kohlberg, B. Speicher-Dubin, A. Hewer, D. Candee, J. Gibbs and C. Power, *The Measurement of Moral Judgment* (Cambridge, U.K.: Cambridge University Press, 1987).

14. See E. Turiel, *The Culture of Morality: Social Development, Context, and Conflict* (Cambridge, U.K.: Cambridge University Press, 2002).

15. L. Katz (ed.), *Evolutionary Origins of Morality: Cross-Disciplinary Perspectives* (Exeter, U.K.: Imprint Academic, 2000); K.B. MacDonald, "Sociobiology and the Cognitive-Developmental Tradition on Moral Development Research" in *Sociobiological Perspectives on Human Development*, ed. K.B. MacDonald (Springer Verlag, 1988), 140–167; and M. Ruse, "Evolutionary Ethics: A Phoenix Arisen" in Paul Thompson, *Issues in Evolutionary Ethics* (Albany: State University of New York, 1995).

16. International Criminal Court, accessed 3 Jun 2011 at www.icc-cpi.int/Menus/ICC/About+the+Court/

17. Plato, *The Republic*, Book I.

18. O. O'Neill, "Practical Principles and Practical Judgment," *The Hastings Center Report* 31.4 (2001): 15–23; C. Hodgkinson, *Administrative Philosophy* (Oxford: Pergamon, 1996); E.-H.W. Kluge, "Competence, Capacity and Informed Consent: Beyond the Cognitive-Competence Model," *Canadian Journal on Aging* 243 (2004): 85–94.

19. Saudi Arabia has no formal penal code but follows Sharia law, which prescribes flogging and stoning (as well as judicial amputation) for certain offences.

20. Republic of Yemen, Penal Code 1994 (no. 12/1994), Articles 263 and 264.

21. The classic statement of ethical non-naturalism is in G.E. Moore, *Principia Ethica* (Cambridge, U.K.: Cambridge University Press, 1903). For more contemporary discussions, see A. Gibbard, "Normative Concepts and Recognitional Concepts," *Philosophy and Phenomenological Research* 64 (2002): 151–162 and M. Huemer, *Ethical Intuitionism* (New York: Palgrave Macmillan, 2005). For a critique, see C. Pigden, "Naturalism" in P. Singer (ed.), *A Companion to Ethics* (Oxford: Blackwell, 1993), 421–431.

22. Moore used the term *intuition*. By this he meant that an intellectual effort is necessary for one to become aware of moral properties or facts. For another classic statement of this, see H.A. Prichard, "Does Moral Philosophy Rest on a Mistake?" *Mind*, N.S., (1912) Vol. 21. This position in many ways resembles the moral sense position of Francis Hutcheson in *An Essay on the Nature and Conduct of the Passions and Affections, with Illustrations on the Moral Sense*, available online at http://files.libertyfund.org/files/885/0150_LFeBk.pdf

23. For a discussion of naturalism, see C.R. Pigden, "Naturalism" in *A Companion to Ethics*, ed. P. Singer (Oxford: Blackwell, 1993), 421–431.

24. S. Blackburn, *Essays in Quasi-Realism* (Oxford and New York: Oxford University Press, 1993). See also E.-H.W. Kluge, "Non-naturalism Revisited: Rights/Obligations as Emergent Entities." *Grazer Philosophische Studien* 30 (1987): 139–144.

25. For an introductory discussion of deontic logic, see P. McNamara, "Deontic Logic" in *The Stanford Encyclopedia of Philosophy* (Fall 2010 Edition), ed. E.N. Zalta, accessed at http://plato.stanford.edu/archives/fall2010/entries/logic-deontic/. For a classic article on the subject, see von G.H. Wright, "Deontic Logic," *Mind* 60 (1951): 1–15. For a useful collection of articles, see R. Hilpinen, *Deontic Logic: Introductory and Systematic Readings* (Dordrecht: D. Reidel, 1970).

26. Strictly speaking, this is not true. A branch of ethics called descriptive ethics involves the comparative analysis of distinct ethical systems as held by different societies or by people at different stages of their moral development. However, descriptive (as opposed to normative) ethics is generally considered a social or psychological discipline.

27. For a classic statement of a religiously based natural law theory, see Thomas Aquinas, *Summa Theologica* IaIIae, 91, 94, et pass.; for a secular version, see H. Grotius, *The Rights of War and Peace*, ed. R. Tuck (Indianapolis: Liberty Fund, 2005) and S. Pufendorf, *On the Duty of Man and Citizen according to Natural Law*, ed. J. Tully, trans. M. Silverthorne (Cambridge, U.K.: Cambridge University Press, 1991).

28. Strictly speaking, this is not quite true. See preceding note. The so-called natural law tradition maintains that there are certain laws—the *ius gentium*—which apply to all people and are grounded in the nature of humanity itself. This finds its earliest expression in the writings of the Stoics and entered Roman jurisprudence through Cicero and Seneca. In the Middle Ages, it was combined with a Christian perspective by St. Thomas Aquinas and others. In the 16th and 17th centuries it was modified and systematized by Grotius, Montesquieu, Rousseau, Spinoza, Pufendorf and Wolff on the Continent, and in the English-speaking world by thinkers such as Locke, Adams, Paine and Jefferson. In 1998, the power of the International Criminal Court was ratified in the Rome Statute by 120 nations; see Rome Statute, available at www.icc-cpi.int/NR/rdonlyres/0D8024D3-87EA-4E6A-8A27-05B987C38689/0/RomeStatuteEng.pdf

29. K. Becker, M. Becker and J.H. Schwarz, *String Theory and M-Theory: A Modern Introduction* (Cambridge, U.K.: Cambridge University Press, 2006).

30. C. Rovelli, *Quantum Gravity* (Cambridge, U.K.: Cambridge University Press, 2004).

31. Different theories fall under the heading of utilitarianism—and in fact, utilitarianism is itself a species of teleological ethics, of which communitarianism is another example.

32. Cf. D. Callahan, *Medical Goals in an Aging Society* (New York: Simon & Schuster, 1987).

33. Cf. J. Rawls, *A Theory of Justice* (Cambridge, MA: Harvard University Press, 1971).

34. See Chapter I, "Of the Principle of Utility," in J. Bentham, *An Introduction to the Principles of Morals and Legislation*.

35. See R.G. Frey, "Introduction: Utilitarianism and Persons" in *Utility and Rights*, ed. R.G. Frey (Oxford: Blackwell, 1985), 3–19.

36. R.B. Brandt, *Ethical Theory* (Englewood Cliffs, NJ: Prentice Hall, 1959), 380–391.

37. Brandt, op. cit., 253–258 and 396–405.

38. See Frey, op. cit., 18; see also H.L.A. Hart, "Between Utility and Rights" in *The Idea of Freedom*, ed. A. Ryan (Oxford: Oxford University Press, 1979). For an opposing view, see P. Singer, *Practical Ethics* (Cambridge, U.K.: Cambridge University Press, 1979).

39. Immanuel Kant, *Foundations of the Metaphysics of Morals* (New York: Bobbs-Merrill, 1959), 422.

40. Loc. cit.

41. Compare A.J. Paton, *The Categorical Imperative: A Study in Kant's Moral Philosophy* (London: Hutchinson, 1947).

42. Cf. Paton, op. cit., Chapter XIV.

43. For a similar point, see S. Bok, *Lying: Word Choice in Public and Private Life* (New York: Pantheon Books, 1978), Chapter 4.

44. W.D. Ross, *The Right and the Good* (Oxford: Clarendon Press, 1938).

45. J. Rawls, *A Theory of Justice* (rev. ed.), (Cambridge, MA: Belknap Press of Harvard University Press, 1999).

46. Deontological theories also differ in the orientation of their principles. Quality-oriented approaches maintain that certain moral qualities have intrinsic value. The justice-oriented perspective of Rawls is a good example. Person-oriented approaches, as their name suggests, find their focus in the concept of persons as beings of ultimate and incommensurable value. The Kantian system is here representative. It is therefore not surprising that this sort of approach places a strong emphasis on personal autonomy. For a modern restatement of Kant's person-focused deontological ethics, see A. Gewirth, *Reason and Morality* (Chicago: University of Chicago Press, 1978).

47. See T. Beauchamp and J. Childress, *Principles of Biomedical Ethics* (Oxford: Oxford University Press, 2001), 357.

48. Mr. Justice Oliver Wendell Holmes, giving the unanimous majority judgment in Schenck v. United States, 249 U.S. 47 (1919).

49. Available at http://policybase.cma.ca/PolicyPDF/PD04-06.pdf

50. L. Edelstein, *The Hippocratic Oath: Text, Translation, and Interpretation* (Baltimore: Johns Hopkins Press, 1943).

51. K.R. Sherbourne, H.M. Earl, L. Whitehead, S.J. Jefferies and N.G. Burnet, "Blood Transfusion Requirements for Patients with Sarcomas Undergoing Combined Radio- and Chemotherapy," *Sarcoma* 9.3–4 (Sep–Dec 2005): 119–125.

52. In some ways, this parallels the question of how to resolve conflict when using the Kantian categorical imperative.

53. G.A. Soper, "The Work of a Chronic Typhoid Germ Distributor," *Journal of the American Medical Association* 48 (1907): 2019–2022.

54. This example is based on a Vancouver case related to the author by the attending physician.

55. For the classic case that established this as a principle in common law, see Taylor v. Caldwell [1863] EWHC J1 (QB).

56. G.P. Smith, "Utility and the Principle of Medical Futility: Safeguarding Autonomy and the Prohibition Against Cruel and Unusual Punishment," *Journal of Contemporary Health Law and Policy* 12 (1996): 1–39.

57. Hippocrates, "Art," in *Ethics in Medicine: Historical Perspectives and Contemporary Concerns*, ed. S.J. Reiser, A.J. Dyck, and W.J. Curran (Cambridge, MA: MIT Press, 1977): 6. For more discussion, see N. Jecker, "Knowing When to Stop: The Limits of Medicine," *The Hastings Center Report* 21.3 (1999): 5–8. See also L.J. Schneiderman, N. Jecker, A.R. Jonsen, "Medical Futility: Its Meaning and Ethical Implications," *Ann Intern Med* 112.12 (1990): 949–954. For a critical discussion of the notion, see J.P. Burns, R.D. Truog, "Futility: A Concept in Evolution," *Chest* 132.6 (2007): 1987–1993 and R.D. Truog, A.S. Brett and J. Frader, "The Problem with Futility," *N Engl J Med* 326 (1992): 1550–1564. For formal recognition of this notion by a professional medical association, see "Medical Futility in End-of-Life Care: Report of the Council on Ethical and Judicial Affairs," *JAMA* 281 (1999): 937–941.

58. N. Noddings, "Feminist Fears in Ethics," *Journal of Social Philosophy* (Fall/Winter 1990), reprinted in D.T. Goldberg, *Ethical Theory and Social Issues*, 2nd ed. (Orlando, FL: Holt Rhinehart and Winston, Inc., 1990), 215–225, at 223.

59. N. Noddings, *Caring: A Feminist Approach to Ethics and Moral Education* (Berkeley: University of California Press, 1984).

60. C.J. Gilligan, *In a Different Voice* (Cambridge, MA: Harvard University Press, 1982); J. Grimshaw, *Philosophy and Feminist Thinking* (Minneapolis: University of Minnesota Press, 1989); N. Noddings, *Caring: A Feminist Approach to Ethics and Moral Education* (Berkeley: University of California Press, 1984); S. Sherwin, *No Longer Patient: Feminist Ethics and Health Care* (Philadelphia: Temple University Press, 1992); R. Tong, *Feminine and Feminist Ethics* (Belmont, CA: Wadsworth, 1993).

61. A. Baier, "What Do Women Want in a Moral Theory?" *Nous* 19 (March 1985): 53–56.

62. See S. Sherwin, *No Longer Patient* at 13.

63. G.J. Annas, "Pregnant Women as Fetal Containers," *The Hastings Center Report* 16.6 (1986): 13–14; K.E. Maier, "Pregnant Women: Fetal Containers or People with Rights?" *Affilia* 4.2 (1989): 8–20; L.M. Purdy, "Are Pregnant Women Fetal Containers?" *Bioethics* 4 (1990): 273–291.

64. V. Merton, "The Exclusion of Pregnant, Pregnable, and Once-Pregnable People (A.K.A. Women) from Biomedical Research," *American Journal of Law and Medicine* XIX.4 (1993): 369–451.

65. See N. Noddings, *Caring: A Feminist Approach to Ethics and Moral Education* (Berkeley: University of California Press, 1984).

66. A. Jaggar, "Feminism and the Objects of Justice" in *Social and Political Philosophy: Contemporary Perspectives*, ed. J.P. Sterba (London: Routledge, 2001), 251–269.

67. For example, H.L. Nelson, "Feminist Bioethics: Where We've Been, Where We're Going," *Metaphilosophy* 31.5 (2000): 492–508; H.L. Nelson, *Damaged Identities, Narrative Repair* (Ithaca, NY: Cornell University Press, 2001).

68. C.J. Gilligan, *In a Different Voice* (Cambridge, MA: Harvard University Press, 1982).

69. C.J. Gilligan, *Mapping the Moral Domain: A Contribution of Women's Thinking to Psychological Theory and Education* (Cambridge, MA: Harvard University Press, 1989).

70. S. Ruddick, "Maternal Thinking" in *Mothering: Essays in Feminist Theory*, ed. J. Trebilcot (Totowa, NJ: Rowman and Allanheld, 1989), 213–230; E.F. Kittay, *Love's Labor: Essays on Women, Equality, and Dependency* (New York: Routledge, 1999); and E.F. Kittay and E.K. Feder, *The Subject of Care: Feminist Perspectives on Dependency* (Lanham, MD: Rowman & Littlefield, 2003).

71. Op. cit.

72. For an application of her theoretical considerations to medicine and bioethics, see S. Sherwin, "Whither Bioethics? How Feminism Can Help Reorient Bioethics," *International Journal of Feminist Approaches to Bioethics* 1.1 (2008): 7–27. See also S. Sherwin, "Abortion Through a Feminist Ethics Lense," *Dialogue* 30.3 (1991): 327–342.

73. S. Dodds, "Depending on Care: Recognition of Vulnerability and the Social Contribution of Care Provision," *Bioethics* 21.9 (2007): 500–510; R. Groenhout, *Connected Lives: Human Nature and the Ethics of Care* (Lanham, MD: Rowman & Littlefield, 2004).

74. See special issues of *Hypatia* devoted to this subject: 16.4 (2001) and 17.3 (2002).

75. For example, S. Goering, "Postnatal Reproductive Autonomy: Promoting Relational Autonomy and Self-Trust in New Parents," *Bioethics* 23.1 (2009): 9–19; and C. McLeod, *Self-Trust and Reproductive Autonomy* (Cambridge, MA: MIT Press, 2002).

76. C. Mackenzie and N. Stoljar (eds.), *Relational Autonomy: Feminist Perspectives on Autonomy, Agency, and the Social Self* (New York: Oxford University Press, 2000).

77. See J. Gupta, *New Reproductive Technologies, Women's Health and Autonomy: Freedom or Dependency?* (New Delhi and Thousand Oaks: Sage Publications, 2000); R. Kukla, *Mass Hysteria: Medicine, Culture, and Mothers' Bodies* (Lanham. MD: Rowman & Littlefield, 2005); K. Harwood, *The Infertility Treadmill: Feminist Ethics, Personal Choice, and the Use of Reproductive Technologies* (Chapel Hill: University of North Carolina Press, 2007).

78. A. MacIntyre, *After Virtue: A Study in Moral Theory* (Notre Dame, IN: Notre Dame University Press, 1984).

79. G.E.M. Anscombe, "Modern Moral Philosophy," *Philosophy* 33 (1958): 1–19.

80. MacIntyre, *After Virtue: A Study in Moral Theory*. For a classic statement, see Aristotle, *Nicomachean Ethics*. For an attempt to apply it in the health care setting, see R.J. Christie and C.B. Hoffmaster, *Ethical Issues in Family Medicine* (New York and London: Oxford University Press, 1986).

81. MacIntyre, op. cit. at 155 ff.

82. See R.J. Christie and C.B. Hoffmaster, *Ethical Issues in Family Medicine* (New York and Oxford: Oxford University Press, 1985).

83. For classic statements of this stance, see E.L. Pincoffs, "Quandary Ethics," *Mind* 80 (1971): 552–571, and J. McDowell, "Virtue and Reason," *Monist* 62 (1979): 331–350. For a later restatement of a similar stance, see R. Hursthouse, *On Virtue Ethics* (Oxford: Oxford University Press, 1999).

84. See P. Foot, *Virtues and Vices* (Oxford: Blackwell, 1978), 11 ff.

85. N. Athanassoulis, "A Response to Harman: Virtue Ethics and Character Traits," *Proceedings of the Aristotelian Society* (New Series) 100 (2000): 215–221.

86. The roots of this are in Aristotle's concept of phronesis. See *Nicomachean Ethics*, Book 6.

87. P. Foot, *Virtues and Vices* (Oxford: Blackwell, 1978); R. Hursthouse, *On Virtue Ethics* (Oxford: Oxford University Press, 1999); A. MacIntyre, *After Virtue*, 2nd ed. (London: Duckworth, 1985); and M.C. Nussbaum, *Frontiers of Justice* (Cambridge, MA: Harvard University Press, 2006).

88. C. Swanton, *Virtue Ethics: A Pluralistic View* (Oxford: Oxford University Press, 2003).

89. See R. Hursthouse, "Virtue Theory and Abortion," *Philosophy & Public Affairs* 20.3 (1991): 223–246.

90. Hursthouse, op. cit., at 235.

91. Loc. cit., at 238.

92. L. van Zyl, *Death and Compassion: A Virtue-Based Approach to Euthanasia* (Farnham, U.K.: Ashgate, 2000).

93. M. Nussbaum, "Non-Relative Virtues: An Aristotelian Approach," in *Midwest Studies in Philosophy Vol. XIII, Ethical Theory: Character and Virtue*, ed. P.A. French, T. Uehling, Jr. and H. Wettstein (Notre Dame, IN: University of Notre Dame Press, 1988), 32–53.

94. G.A. van Wingen, L. Ossewaarde, T. Bäckström, E.J. Hermans and G. Fernández, "Gonadal Hormone Regulation of the Emotion Circuitry in Humans," *Neuroscience* 24 Apr 2011, Epub ahead of print; J.C. Dreher, P.J. Schmidt, P. Kohn, D. Furman, D. Rubinow and K.F. Berman, "Menstrual Cycle Phase Modulates Reward-Related Neural Function in Women," *Proc Natl Acad Sci USA* 104.7 (13 Feb 2007): 2465–2470.

95. C.N. DeWall, T. Deckman, M.T. Gailliot, and B.J. Bushman, "Sweetened Blood Cools Hot Tempers: Physiological Self-Control and Aggression," *Aggressive Behavior* 37:1 (Jan–Feb 2011): 73–80.

Chapter 2
Codes of Ethics and the Medical Profession

In Canada, as in most other countries, access to formalized health care is through licensed health care professionals such as physicians, nurses and registered therapists. How these professionals interact with the health care system and their patients is strongly influenced by their respective codes of ethics. This chapter, whose focus is the Code of Ethics of the Canadian Medical Association, takes a look at codes of ethics—where they come from, their legal status and their ethical basis. It lays the groundwork for the next chapter, which deals with various models of the physician–patient relationship.

Questions to Keep in Mind While Reading this Chapter:

1. What is the difference between medical ethos, medical protocol and medical ethics?
2. What is the basis of a code of medical ethics, and from what does it derive its binding power?
3. What are the limits of a code of medical ethics?
4. Why should a code of ethics for the profession of medicine include statements of rights as well as statements of duties?
5. What are the implications of medicine as a professional service monopoly?

INTRODUCTION

In an ideal world, people would make ethical decisions based on careful deliberation, after first getting the clearest possible grasp of the facts and then applying ethical principles. Real life is not like that. Real people—and in particular health care professionals such as physicians, who often have to make decisions with far-reaching implications on a moment's notice—simply do not have the time. Nor do they have the training. That is why in real life, physicians follow codes of conduct or, as they are more usually called, codes of ethics.

There is nothing wrong with this. Codes of ethics, if they are properly constructed, are developed by applying ethical principles to the types of situations physicians are likely to encounter in actual practice and deriving rules or clauses in that way. In actuality, codes of medical ethics were not developed that way. To focus on Canada: In 1867—the year of Confederation—the Canadian Medical Association (CMA) was incorporated as the national professional association of physicians in Canada. Its mandate was to represent and advocate for the interests of Canadian physicians and their patients. The Committee on Ethics was one of the CMA's statutory committees, and its first task was to draft a Code of Ethics.[1] This Code was drafted on an historical basis. It drew on a long series of codes stretching back to the very beginning of medical practice but placed special emphasis on the Hippocratic Oath and on Percival's Code of Ethics—which latter was the first code of medical ethics for the English-speaking world.

One of the interesting things about this CMA Code was that, like Percival's Code, it lacked any religious elements. In this, it continued a trend that had begun in the 19th century. Prior to then, the physician–patient relationship had a quasi-religious dimension, and the codes that guided physicians' behaviour reflected this. Thus, we find it in the Code of Imhotep[2] in ancient Egypt, in the injunctions of the Charaka school of medicine in ancient India[3] and in the Huangdi medical tradition of China.[4] The Oath of Hippocrates itself was no exception[5]—neither were Galen's ethical writings[6] which, together with the Hippocratic Oath, dominated European medicine during the Middle Ages. The quasi-religious dimension was also an integral aspect of medical cultures in the Arabic and the Jewish world during the same time period.[7] The 9th-century C.E. Code of Ethics of al-Ruhawi[8] (the first known textbook devoted specifically to medical ethics) and the 12th-century C.E. Code of Ethics of Maimonides (which went under the title "Oath and Prayer of Maimonides"[9]) leave no doubt on that score.

THE CURRENT CMA CODE

The original CMA Code of Ethics was adopted in 1868. It has since been revised several times—eighteen times, to be exact.[10] This is not surprising: Codes of ethics are supposed to keep abreast of changing social and legal conditions. Nor is it unusual: Other medical associations—for example, the American Medical Association (AMA), the British Medical Association and the Royal Dutch Medical Association—have also revised their codes several times, as has the World Medical Association (WMA),[11] which is the global association of medical associations.

The current CMA Code (it was last revised in 2004) falls into five sections. They deal with what are called fundamental responsibilities, responsibilities to patients, responsibilities to society, responsibilities to the profession and responsibilities to oneself.

Fundamental Responsibilities

The fundamental responsibilities—ten are listed—function as overarching principles that govern all aspects of a physician's professional behaviour. The most important of these are probably the first four: to consider first the well-being of the patient, to treat patients with the respect that is due to them as persons, not to abandon patients when cure is no longer possible but give them appropriate assistance and support, and to keep in mind the well-being of society. Other general injunctions include not being influenced by interests that could undermine the physician's integrity as a medical practitioner and to engage in lifelong learning. The last is probably of special relevance for modern physicians, since it is estimated that medical knowledge doubles every seven years.[12]

Responsibilities to Patients

The section dealing with responsibilities to patients is divided into general responsibilities, responsibilities when initiating or dissolving a physician–patient relationship, communicating and decision-making, privacy and confidentiality, and research and experimentation.

The general responsibilities centre in such issues as size of fees, conflict of interest and the duty to disclose personal values if these should depart from standard Canadian values or in any way interfere with physicians' interactions with their patients.

Duties that come under the rubric of initiating or dissolving a physician–patient relationship include the duty to come to the assistance of anyone who requires medical care without discriminating for medically irrelevant reasons such as ethnicity or nationality, religion or political orientation; and the duty not to dissolve a physician–patient relationship until the patient has been "given sufficient notice" that the physician intends to terminate the relationship or another physician has assumed the care of the patient. This section also enjoins physicians not to provide therapy to their significant others except in "minor emergencies" and when no other physician is readily available.

Probably the most important clause under the heading "Communication, Decision Making and Consent" is that physicians should respect their patients' decision-making authority—as the Code puts it, an ethical physician should respect the patient's "right to accept or reject any treatment or intervention," including those that sustain or save life—and that physicians must disclose all information that is relevant for a patient's decision-making, so that the decision that the patient ultimately makes is properly informed. The latter two clauses are relatively recent additions to the Code. They reflect a shift in perspective that began in the 1980 with *Reibl v. Hughes* and was reaffirmed by the courts in 1990 with *Malette v. Shulman*.

Responsibilities to Society

The section titled "Responsibilities to Society" has also undergone some changes. Unlike some previous versions, it now acknowledges that physicians have a duty to "promote equitable access to health care resources" and to use health care resources prudently. These became matters of professional concern only after the *Canada Health Act* came into force and health care became an individual right and a social responsibility. (See Chapter 9.)

Responsibilities to the Profession

The various clauses under "Responsibilities to the Profession" include injunctions that deal with the willingness to engage in peer review (to ensure quality of service), the duty to report the unprofessional conduct of colleagues (which includes substance abuse and abuse of patients), the duty to share therapeutic discoveries and the duty to engage in continuing medical education. Although the Code still enjoins physicians from engaging in commercial advertising—in this it differs from the stance adopted by the AMA and the WMA—it now makes an exception in the case of advertising one's own services.

Responsibilities to Oneself

The category of duties to oneself acknowledges that physicians are human beings and as such may encounter personal problems that could imperil their own well-being—which in turn may interfere with how well they can fulfill their role as physicians. It therefore enjoins physicians to seek personal help as necessary and appropriate.

Discussion

All of this would be of purely historical interest were it not for the fact that most Canadian provinces and territories have legislation that directly or indirectly identifies the CMA Code as delineating the ethical standards that society may reasonably expect from Canadian physicians.

That is to say, the medical licensing bodies of the various Canadian provinces—which are creatures of their respective provincial legislatures—have either adopted the CMA Code outright (British Columbia and Nova Scotia fall into this category) or in a slightly amended version (Saskatchewan and Manitoba are examples). This, in turn would not necessarily be very interesting were it not for three things: *First*, the Code was developed by the CMA independently of input from the rest of society, essentially on the basis of the experiences and perspectives of the CMA's membership. This suggests that in the eyes of the licensing bodies, the technical expertise of physicians as physicians and the fact that they have joined the CMA (which is a private corporation) makes them the appropriate individuals to decide what constitutes ethically acceptable medical behaviour.

Second, the CMA Code differs from the codes of other health care professions such as nursing and physiotherapy not simply in its specifics but also in what it cites as its basis. This encourages the assumption that the ethical standards of the various health care professions are grounded in distinct principles that are unique to each profession.

Third, since the CMA Code differs from the codes that have been adopted by medical associations in other countries, it suggests that in the eyes of Canadian medicine, the ethical principles that govern the conduct of physicians differ on the basis of nationality.

All three points may be questioned. The first involves the *fallacy of expertise*—the fallacy of assuming that expertise in one area translates into expertise in another unrelated area; the second involves the *fallacy of uniqueness*—the fallacy of assuming that something of special interest should be treated as though it were ethically unique; and the third involves the *fallacy of nationality*—the fallacy of assuming that what is ethically right or wrong depends on nationality and therefore differs from nation to nation.

However, to show why these are (potentially dangerous) fallacies, and to connect the discussion with what has been outlined in the preceding chapter, we shall proceed somewhat circuitously and begin with the question of what a code of ethics is really supposed to be.

THE ETHICAL STATUS OF CODES OF ETHICS

A code of ethics can be construed either as a statement of ethos, as a quasi-legal document, as a statement of the unique ethics that governs a profession or as a statement of role-specific rules that are derived from the ethical principles that apply to all people.

Codes as Statements of Ethos

The word *ethos* may be defined as "the prevalent tone of sentiment of a people or community."[13] Therefore, if a code of ethics is understood in this sense, it reflects the way the profession thinks about ethical issues.

This is a fairly common understanding. However, it is not at all clear that it is valid. If it were correct, then a profession that wanted to develop a code of ethics would be wasting its time if it deliberated about how ethical principles applied to different types of professional situations. That would provide no real clue about the "underlying sentiment" that informed the beliefs of its members. The right thing to do would be to conduct an opinion poll.

More importantly, however, a code construed along these lines would lack ethical binding power. As Socrates pointed out long ago, the fact that people agree on certain ethical rules does not show that the rules are valid. Of course, they may be—but that would be coincidence. Agreement itself is no guarantee of anything except agreement—and there are many historical examples of agreed-upon rules that were ethically simply wrong.

Moreover, purely pragmatically speaking, such a *modus operandi* would saddle the profession with the rather onerous task of having to continually update its code—not, however, because the profession had come to appreciate that its previous opinions were ethically mistaken but because the members had changed their attitudes and perspectives. This would make a code of ethics subject to the changing winds of politics and of personal persuasion and would leave the individual professionals on ever-shifting moral ground. It would therefore be of limited use at best.

Of course, understanding a code this way would have one tremendous advantage: The profession would never have to worry about ethical problems at all. If something struck it as morally wrong, it could make it morally right simply by having its members change their minds.

Codes as Quasi-Legal Documents

All of these problems would disappear if a code were construed as a quasi-legal document. It would then be a statement of the professionals' judicial rights and duties, and it would be in force just as long as the relevant legislation specifically mentioned the code.

This would certainly validate the use of codes by licensing and disciplinary bodies when they conduct disciplinary hearings, and justify the courts taking notice of codes when they adjudicate whether a legal breach of professional obligation has occurred. It would also explain why the courts are generally reluctant to overturn the decisions of disciplinary tribunals.

However, the problem with this interpretation is that it confuses function with content. On this understanding *anything* could be ethically mandated, just as long as it was in the code and the code was sanctioned by the appropriate legislative and licensing bodies. Sanctions, however, even when legally grounded, do not add ethical weight to anything. They merely add an element of coercion.

Codes as Statements of the Unique Ethics that Governs a Profession

Understanding a code as a statement of the unique ethics that governs a profession avoids all of these issues. However, it would be based on two assumptions: *first*, that professions are ethically distinct from all other types of activities and therefore subject to distinct principles, and *second*, that these principles are unique to each profession.

The first assumption contains a grain of truth. Professional–client interactions are fiduciary in nature. This means that professionals have a duty to do their best for their clients, and clients may trust that the professionals will do only what is in the client's best interests. (This is certainly not the case with business ventures.)

Moreover, as will be discussed more fully in a moment, professions usually have a service provider monopoly. This gives them rights and duties that non-professionals don't have.

Finally, professionals have a level of expertise that is not shared by others. Ethically, this puts professionals into a special position because, as a matter of general principle (based in Fidelity), the greater someone's understanding, training and expertise, the more he or she is presumed capable of exercising judgment and of producing positive outcomes in matters that involve that person's areas of competence. That is why licensed professionals are held to higher standards than other persons. The legitimacy of these expectations is further heightened by the fact that professionals give themselves out as having an elevated level of expertise simply by presenting themselves as professionals.

However—and this brings us back to the second assumption that underlies this interpretation of what a code of ethics is—this merely shows that professions and their members are subject to distinctive ethical *rules*. It does not show that they are subject to ethically unique *principles*.

Codes as Statements of Role-Specific Rules Derived from General Ethical Principles

Which of course means that the fourth way of understanding a code of ethics is the correct one: The clauses of a properly constructed code of ethics are merely the results of applying the ethical principles that apply to everyone to the types of situations that the professionals are likely to encounter in their professional lives. Figure 2.1 illustrates this relationship.

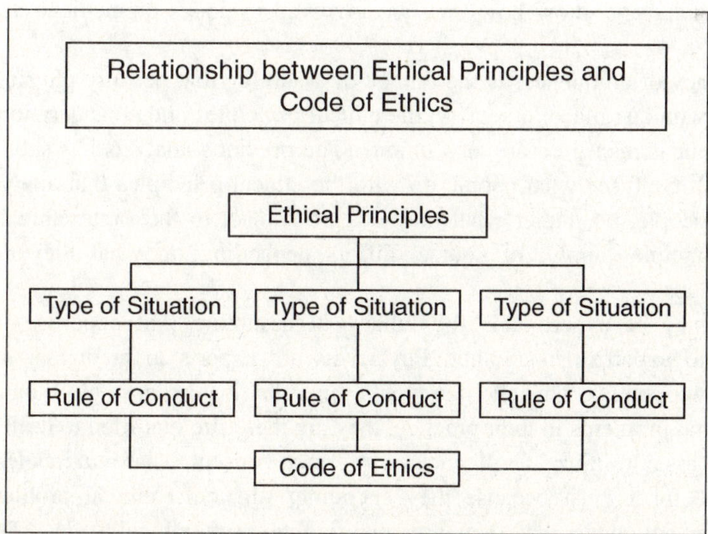

Figure 2.1 Relationship between Ethical Principles and Code of Ethics

Therefore, strictly speaking, there is no need for codes of professional ethics. However, from a pragmatic perspective they are very useful. They spell out what the general ethical principles that apply to everyone mean when they are applied to the types of situations that the professionals encounter in their practice. In that sense, they save time, promote consistency among members of the profession and serve as a handy standard against which society can measure their actions. Practically speaking, therefore, codes of professional ethics are invaluable.

The question to ask at this juncture is whether the CMA Code follows this pattern. However, to answer that question would require a clause-by-clause analysis to see whether each can be derived from ethical principles in the way indicated. While that might be interesting, it would be relevant only as long as the Code did not change—which is anybody's guess, given that it has already changed eighteen times. Moreover, such an analysis would give very little insight into what really should be in a code of medical ethics, and why. It would be more useful—and certainly more constructive—to give a brief sketch of what a code of ethics for the medical profession might look like if it were actually developed wholly on the basis of the nature of medicine itself and the fundamental principles that were identified in the preceding chapter on ethics. What follows is such an attempt.

Three Fallacies

However, before actually sketching such a model code, we should really go back for a moment to the three fallacies that were mentioned a little while ago (the *fallacy of uniqueness*, the *fallacy of expertise* and the *fallacy of nationality*), indicate why they are fallacies and show how they are involved in codes of medical ethics as they currently exist.

The fallacy of uniqueness is the fallacy of assuming that because physicians occupy an essentially unique place in society, the ethical principles and considerations by which their behaviour is measured are also unique. The previous analysis has shown why that is a fallacy. It confuses what people do with the ethical principles that apply to them as people. All people, no matter what they do, are subject to the same ethical principles. How the principles apply, of course, differs depending on what they do; but that is another issue.

The fallacy of expertise is the fallacy of assuming that expertise in one area translates into expertise in another. Physicians are experts in medicine; they are not experts in law or ethics. Thus, no one would think that just because physicians encounter (difficult) legal problems in their practice, they are therefore qualified to draft legal codes dealing with assault, injury, negligence or informed consent. That requires legal training. By the same token, just because they encounter (difficult) ethical problems in their practice does not mean that they are qualified to draft ethical codes. That requires training in ethics.

Finally, the fallacy of nationality is the fallacy of assuming that what is ethically appropriate differs from nation to nation, and that the medical associations of different countries should therefore have different codes of medical ethics. This essentially amounts to ethical relativism, and it confuses tradition and ethos with ethics. Of course, codes of medical ethics could legitimately differ from one country to another if the types of problems that physicians typically encountered in the respective countries were different. But this does not mean that their *ethics*—their *ethics as physicians*—would be any different. It merely means that it would be pointless to include such clauses in their codes of ethics.

A MODEL CODE OF ETHICS FOR PHYSICIANS

Some Preliminary Considerations

A code of ethics must walk a fine line between generality and specificity. To be practically useful, it must be sufficiently free of specifics to allow application to the whole array of situations that typically characterize medicine in that setting. At the same time, it must be specific enough to provide guidance in actual situations.

Moreover, a code of ethics should not confuse ethical and legal considerations. The two are not necessarily the same. For example, the laws of some countries allow prisoners to be subjected to interrogation techniques and corporal punishment that necessitate the assistance of physicians[14] but which, according to Amnesty International and the Convention for the Protection of Human Rights and Fundamental Freedoms of the Council of Europe, amount to torture. Waterboarding, flogging and the judicial amputation of hands or feet are some examples. No ethical person should be involved in this, and that includes physicians. However, if a code of medical ethics were to stipulate that physicians should follow the law, this would mean that they had a duty to assist in such practices. If the law is referenced at all, it should be only with the stipulation that the law should be ethically defensible on its own terms.

To reiterate, codes of medical ethics should include only clauses that derive from the role that physicians play as physicians. This gives rise to at least seven general themes. Two of them may be expressed as rights and five as obligations.

Duties or Obligations

1. Physicians have an obligation to promote their patients' health potential to the greatest degree possible under the circumstances. Health care does not take place in a vacuum. Lack of resources may constrain the range of interventions that are open to physicians or that they can recommend. For instance, sophisticated diagnostic equipment such as CAT scanners or MRIs may not exist in a small rural community; surgical or psychiatric interventions that are possible in one setting may not be available in a particular location, and so on. Similarly, one physician may be trained in oncology, another in gynecology and a third in otolaryngology, yet none of them may be competent to perform a pediatric bowel resection. The context—and that includes the physician's training—limits what can reasonably be expected from a physician. Consequently there may be cases in which it is simply impossible for physicians to provide patients with the care or the resources that are necessary to attain their full health potential. If physicians do the best they can within the limits of their training and the resources that are available, that is ethically sufficient. The fact that something is theoretically possible—or even possible in other locations—does not mean that it becomes a duty for these physicians here and now.

Of course, the expertise or resources that are unavailable in one setting may be available or accessible in another. For instance, the surgical or diagnostic techniques mentioned a moment ago may not be available in a small rural community but may be accessible from that community by Medivac or through telemedicine. Similarly, it may be possible for a physician who is not an oncologist to refer a patient to someone who is because the health care system has made provisions for referring patients. Under these circumstances, transferring or referring the patient would be ethically mandated by the Principle of Fidelity.

Moreover, not all patients have the same health potential. Clearly an anemic octogenarian with a broken femur does not have the same potential for recovery as an athletic young Olympic sprinter with a femur fracture who is otherwise in the prime of health. Therefore, physicians cannot be expected to achieve the same outcomes for all patients. All that the Principle of Fidelity entails is that they have a duty to do the best they can. They do not have a duty to produce ideal outcomes or even the same outcome.

Finally, maximizing a patient's health potential is not like changing the oil on a car. It involves active participation on the part of the patient—which in turn means that the patient must know what to do. Of course, with modern technology such as the Web, patients have access to a lot of that information. However, much of what is on the Web is misleading or downright false, and even when it is correct it really needs to be explained and interpreted by someone knowledgeable. Physicians are uniquely placed in that regard. Moreover, while Canada is one of the most "wired" countries in the world, not all Canadians have Web access or even access to libraries and other sources of medical information. Finally, all of the information that is thus available has to be interpreted in terms of the specific condition of the individual patient. Therefore, the physician's duty to maximize a patient's health potential also includes the duty to educate.

These considerations can be captured under four subheadings. Physicians have

(a) a duty to do the best one can within the limits of one's training and expertise,

(b) a duty to make appropriate use of all available resources,

(c) a duty to refer when this is appropriate and

(d) a duty to educate.

2. Physicians have an obligation to respect their patients as persons.

Patient Decision-Making Promoting a patient's health potential to the greatest degree possible is not the same as making decisions for the patient. As will be explained in greater detail in the next two chapters (see Chapter 3, "The Health Care Professional–Patient Relationship" and Chapter 4, "Informed Consent") the decision-making role unequivocally belongs to the patients themselves. The ethical reason that underlies this, of course, is the Principle of Autonomy and Respect for Persons, and it is appropriate to highlight this in a code of ethics.

At the same time, not all patients have decision-making capacity—an issue whose ethical implications will be explored in Chapter 5. This means that ethical physicians will accord the same respect to decisions made by patients' duly empowered substitute decision-makers as to those made by the patients themselves. And since rational decision-making is impossible without appropriate and adequate information, the Principle also mandates that physicians should provide their patients (or their substitutes) with such information. This includes access to the patients' own records, since the information contained in them will be instrumental for rational decision-making.

Finally, as autonomous individuals, patients may decide not to have someone else make decisions for them in the eventuality of their own incapacity, but instead may wish to record ahead of time what form their care should take. Physicians who respect their patients as persons should therefore be open to exploring advance directives with them.

Since these are considerations that frequently arise in medical practice, a physician's duties would be appropriately captured as follows:

(a) a duty to respect the decision-making rights of patients,

(b) a duty to extend the same decision-making rights to duly empowered substitute decision-makers as to the patients themselves,

(c) a duty to facilitate patient or substitute decision-making by providing appropriate and adequate information, including patients' health records and

(d) a duty to explore and respect advance directives with patients if the latter are so inclined.

Patient Values However, respect for patients as persons has deeper implications than just patient decision-making—implications that derive from the fact that both physicians and patients are persons and hold values that condition their world views and influence their decision-making. It is therefore possible that patients' values may conflict with the values of their physicians, and *vice versa*, and that physicians may be tempted to use their greater position of power—something that will be discussed further in the next chapter— to influence their patients' decision-making; or, alternatively, to withhold particular medical services if providing these services conflicts with their own values.

Both of these are ethically indefensible—the one absolutely, the other under certain conditions. It is absolutely indefensible for physicians to force patients' decision-making along the lines of their own values—or simply to adopt a paternalistic stance and make the decisions in line with their own and not the patients' values. That not only would contradict the duties just mentioned, it would also be to treat patients as objects.

At the same time, because physicians are persons, they have just as much right to their values and beliefs as their patients. If there are reasonable grounds to suspect that a physician's values might in any way interfere with his or her ability to practise or with patients' autonomous decision-making, the ethically appropriate procedure would be to alert patients to this fact at the inception of the physician–patient relationship and give them the opportunity to decide whether or not to continue as patients of this physician. In this way, what would otherwise be ethically indefensible becomes ethically defensible, because it respects both physicians and patients as persons.

Of course, there may be occasions when a patient has no choice but to continue with the physician in question, even though the physician has clearly stated her values and has indicated her misgivings. For example, a patient in an outlying community who requires an abortion or needs birth control medication may not have the opportunity to find another physician. The possibility of this sort of situation arising was specifically recognized in the case of *R. v. Morgentaler*—albeit in a different connection. (The Court found that travelling long distances from rural communities to facilities where abortions could be performed constituted an undue burden and potentially violated section 7 (Security of the Person) of the *Charter of Rights and Freedoms*.[15] For more on this, see Chapter 9.) In cases like these, ethical physicians have no choice but to go against their own values and provide what would otherwise be considered medically appropriate. While this might be thought to violate the personhood of the physicians themselves, for reasons that will be explained a little further on, this is not actually the case.

Again, the duties of physicians can be summarized as follows:

(a) a duty to respect their patients' values,

(b) a duty to disclose their own values if these are likely to interfere with the care they provide for patients and to give patients sufficient opportunity to find another physician and

(c) a duty to provide medically appropriate care to patients when no other physician is reasonably available, even if such care violates their own values.

Confidentiality The duty of confidentiality is grounded in the fact that patients interact with physicians not as private individuals but in their capacity as professionals. The access that physicians thus have to patients and to information about them is predicated on this professional context, and on the assumption that the physicians' use of that access and of that information will be limited to their professional capacity only. This allows physicians to use whatever patient information is relevant and to communicate it to appropriate others when that becomes necessary in the conduct of their professional role—for instance, when consulting.[16] However, such communication must always be as protective of patient privacy as is consistent with the conditions under which the physician–patient relationship was established. This means, for example, that if it is possible to consult without revealing the patient's identity, there lies an obligation to do so. However, under no circumstances may a physician use information provided by a patient for private gain or divulge patient information in an identifiable form without the express permission of the patient.[17]

Of course, there are exceptions to this. However, they are very limited. They tend to involve situations in which physicians become privy to information that leads them to believe that in their professional opinion a patient's condition or actions or both, etc., constitute a clear and present danger to others, or that they may otherwise violate or threaten to violate the rights of others in an ethically unacceptable fashion. For instance, if a patient discloses the intent to kill another person and the physician is professionally convinced that this is not a mere ideation but constitutes a realistic threat, then confidentiality must be breached.[18] Similarly, if a patient has a communicable disease that would seriously imperil other persons—open tuberculosis, HIV/AIDS and similar diseases are good examples—there lies a duty to breach confidentiality to the relevant authorities. The legal concept of "reportable diseases" is based on this.

Likewise, a physician may allow patient confidentiality to be breached for legitimate health planning and research purposes, as well as for quality assurance. This is grounded in the Principle of Impossibility. It is impossible to plan and maintain a health care system without data about the incidence and prevalence of health conditions, the efficacy of treatments, outcomes, side effects, costs, etc. Likewise, quality assurance requires patient data. Of course, if such data can be anonymized or de-identified this should be done, but that may not always be possible. Therefore, the acknowledgement of such exceptions has an appropriate place in a code of ethics.

Furthermore, confidentiality in the strict sense of the term must also be breached by physicians when their patients are incompetent and a medical decision has to be made by a substitute decision-maker. Here the relevant information must be passed on to the latter. Moreover, confidentiality may also be breached when other health care professionals are appropriately involved in the treatment of a patient and require the relevant information. There are still other occasions when confidentiality may be breached: for example, if patients direct that information about them may be disclosed to identified third parties such as next-of-kin or insurance agencies. However, we shall leave further discussion of this topic to the chapter on informed consent.

The preceding duties of physicians can be summarized as follows:

(a) a duty to protect and keep confidential patient information unless doing so is likely to seriously imperil the well-being of third parties,

(b) a duty to allow access to patient data by duly authorized third parties for health planning, research or quality assurance purposes,

(c) a duty to provide substitute decision-makers with the same level of patient data as the patients themselves and

(d) a duty not to use patient-relevant information for personal purposes.

Equality Finally, equality of service is ethically mandated as a matter of professional obligation.

That is to say, the Principle of Equality, as one of the fundamental ethical principles, should govern all human interaction, professional or otherwise. Therefore, physicians should not discriminate on the basis of medically irrelevant things such as religion, ethnic extraction or sexual orientation. Age and sex/gender, of course, may constitute legitimate grounds because they may involve special medical issues that the physician is not trained to treat. At the same time, the seriousness of a particular medical condition such as infection status would not be a medically relevant reason for refusing care.

Such matters are relatively clear. However, equality may present a special problem when different patients compete for the services of the same physician or for the same limited medical resources. The temptation here is to resolve the problem along utilitarian lines by trying to calculate the greatest good for the greatest number and act on that basis. This, however, would reduce patients to objective quantities with merely calculative value. That is ethically unacceptable. Physicians should try to find a solution by balancing the patients' competing rights relative to each other and under the circumstances that obtain. This may not always be easy. Some indications of how it may be achieved will be presented in Chapters 9 and 10.

These physicians' duties can be summarized as follows:

(a) a duty not to discriminate on the basis of medically irrelevant factors,

(b) a duty not to discriminate on the basis of medical condition unless treatment or care do not fall into the area of the physician's competence,

(c) a duty not to allow utilitarian considerations to influence medical decision-making and

(d) a duty to balance competing patient rights solely on the basis of ethically relevant criteria.

3. Physicians owe a duty of care to their patients.

Physicians owe a duty of care to their patients. On the surface this is obvious—but it holds two ambiguities: Who counts as a patient, and what constitutes care?

To resolve these ambiguities, let us begin with the fact that it is impossible for a physician to provide health care for an unlimited number of patients at any given point in time. The Principle of Impossibility simply rules it out. However, a physician can provide care to a potentially open-ended number of patients, one after the other. One must further distinguish between the duty of care that is owed by a physician in an institutional setting from the duty of care that is owed by a physician in private practice—which in turn is different from the duty of care that is owed by a physician in private life when encountering someone who needs medical attention. All of these give different answers to who counts as a patient.

Physicians who work in institutional settings such as hospitals or walk-in clinics have no say over who will count as their patients. The more or less automatically operating institutional determinants (which stamp the setting as institutional) identify who is their patient and who is not. In this sense, then, physicians who work in institutional settings such as hospitals—for instance, a hospitalist or an anesthesiologist— or in walk-in clinics have an open-ended duty of care to anyone who meets the criteria of patienthood as defined by the institutional structure. The latter, then, are their patients.

Things are different in the non-institutional professional context. Physicians here have some choice about whom to take as a patient.[19] As long as the reasons for refusing to accept someone as patient are not unacceptably discriminatory—the preceding discussion gave some indication of what would count as discriminatory in this sense— and as long as the refusal itself does not contravene the conditions of service access tacitly contained in the establishment of medicine as a service provider monopoly (about which more later), physicians have a right of refusal that is as firmly entrenched as that of any other professional. Therefore, according to this interpretation, only those who are accepted by a physician count as his or her patients.

Therefore, when it is said that physicians owe a duty of care to their patients, this is not a duty that is owed to anybody and everybody. It is a duty owed only to those who fulfill the relevant criteria of patienthood. Of course, once someone is a patient, a physician cannot simply get rid of the patient when it becomes inconvenient to provide care, ignore the needs of the patient when other interests intervene or otherwise not do one's best.

And this brings the second ambiguity into focus: What constitutes care? Care is not the same as cure. There is an old Roman saying that for centuries coloured the general perception of what one could expect from physicians. *Medicus curat, natura sanat!* which means "The physician cures, nature heals!" According to this perception, the physician's role was to cure. If a physician could not provide a cure, it was time to turn the patient over to care providers—who were not members of the medical profession but next-of-kin or religious persons such as monks and nuns, and who specialized in doing charitable work.

Of course, such a view of medicine was entirely unrealistic. Medicine, whether historically or in modern times, could not possibly have duty to cure. Whether an intervention is curative depends on factors that lie largely outside of the physician's control. All a physician can do is maximize the chances of cure, not guarantee it. Moreover, this bifurcation of roles between physicians and other caregivers eroded as medicine matured, because it became clear that the medications and interventions that physicians could provide were effective not simply in curing but also in alleviating pain and suffering when cure was not possible. As medicine became a licensed profession, the prescriptions of these medications and the use of these interventions became a matter of legal medical prerogative. This meant that the ambit of medical practice was extended beyond trying to cure and began to encompass care in this latter sense of the term.

It is in this extended sense, then, that a physician's duty of care must be understood. It is a duty to deal with the patient as a person, not simply as a symptom, condition or disease, and to provide whatever medical assistance is in the power of the medical professional to give in order to alleviate pain and suffering. This is appropriately captured by clause 4 of the CMA Code of Ethics: "Provide for appropriate care for your patient, even when cure is no longer possible, including physical comfort and spiritual and psychosocial support."

At the same time, the duty of care has limits. Physicians are not identical with their profession. They are persons, and as such have a right to their own private lives. This limits the extent of a physician's duty to accept patients and to provide services on a round-the-clock basis—as does the fact that a physician may not be competent to provide the type of care a particular patient needs. Thus, an oncologist does not have a duty to provide psychiatric care, and a dermatologist does not have a duty to deal with cardiac patients.

Furthermore, all other things being equal, the fact that physicians are persons also guarantees them the right to terminate the physician–patient relationship if the fiduciary nature of that relationship is violated by a patient. This would be the case, for example, if a patient consistently lied about medically relevant matters or was abusive. In such cases, a physician's duty extends only to informing the patient that continuation of the physician–patient relationship will be impossible under the circumstances, and to giving the patient a reasonable amount of time to find another physician. With the increasing availability of walk-in medical services, this would not violate a physician's duty of care.

Likewise if (as was mentioned above) there is a fundamental opposition between a physician's values and those of a patient and this interferes with the physician's ability to provide what otherwise would be considered appropriate or relevant care, the physician may terminate the relationship—again allowing the patient sufficient time to find another physician.[20]

However, all of these considerations are conditioned by one important factor: emergency. In an emergency, the physician's expertise and training impose a duty to act even when the individual who needs medical attention is not his or her patient. This duty is rooted in the Principle of Beneficence and non-Malfeasance—specifically, a physician who deliberately refrains from appropriate action in an emergency situation becomes responsible for the foreseeable outcome of that failure—as well as in the fact that medicine is a service provider monopoly. This is not merely a matter of ethics[21] but also of case law,[22] and is even enshrined in some provincial legislation.[23] The exceptive condition, of course, is if providing such assistance entails undue danger to the physician—where the notion of danger is defined in other than medical terms. Thus, while a physician does not have a duty to rush into a burning building to provide medical emergency services, he or she does have a duty to provide emergency services to an HIV-seropositive person who is in danger of exsanguinating.

The preceding considerations can be summarized in the following subclauses:

(a) a duty to provide patient care in the best way possible consistent with resources and training,

(b) a duty to provide palliative care as and when appropriate,

(c) a duty not to terminate a physician–patient relationship except for medically or ethically appropriate reasons,

(d) a duty not to terminate a physician–patient relationship unless appropriate steps have been taken to allow the patient to receive care from another physician and

(e) a duty to provide emergency medical assistance to anyone if it is possible to do so without undue danger to oneself.

4. Physicians have a professional obligation towards society. This obligation has three roots: the social cost of educating physicians, their social indebtedness for the development of their knowledge and skills, and the fact of professional monopoly.

To begin with education: Medical education is expensive and most medical students accumulate a heavy educational debt burden, mostly in terms of tuition fees.[24] However, tuition fees cover only a fraction of the total cost of their education,[25] which is heavily subsidized by society. Nor do the services they provide during internship and residency— for which they get paid—constitute anything like an adequate recompense. The Principle of Equality and Justice therefore entails that anyone who receives a medical education has a moral duty to provide some sort of return once they are licensed. This might take several forms—for instance, by providing a certain amount of free medical service for society (the way lawyers do when they provide *pro bono* services for indigent clients), by adjusting fee schedules or by setting up practice for a certain number of years in underserviced areas. It was this understanding of the ethical implications of subsidizing medical education (and of establishing medicine as a monopoly) that underlay British Columbia's (unsuccessful) attempt to enforce this in the 1980s.[26]

However, even if physicians paid fully for their own education, or even if one argued that despite the subsidization of medical studies, medicine was no different from other professions, there is still the fact that the knowledge and skills they have acquired in becoming physicians have a social component that is unlike what is involved in other disciplines. It is not simply that medical knowledge has been developed over millennia in a process of mutual cooperation with other professions such as biochemistry, physics and engineering. Its very existence depends on society. Without humans as experimental subjects, medicine could never have been developed. (For more on research and experimentation, see Chapter 6, "Research Using Human Subjects.")

Then there is the fact that medicine is a service monopoly. This is not a necessary or inevitable state of affairs. Other societies and other times—even our own society in the past—have handled things differently. Rather, it is the result of a conscious and deliberate decision on the part of our society. There were several reasons for this decision. One, of course, was to control the number of physicians and to make it economically attractive for people to enter the profession.[27]

Another was to try to guarantee standardization and quality of medical services. Historically, this figured most prominently in the health care acts and legislations in Canada in the *Act of 1818* in Upper Canada and was re-emphasized in the Flexner Report of 1910. All other things being equal, standardization and service quality has remained the strongest reason why society has persisted in retaining the monopolistic status of the profession in this way.

Whatever the reason, the fact of monopoly entails three consequences that affect both the profession and individual physicians themselves: quality, ubiquity and universality. As to quality, it means that the profession has a duty to ensure that the standards of medical education and practice are the best possible and to ensure, as medical knowledge changes, that these changes are incorporated into the professional standards. Individual physicians, in turn, have an obligation to engage in continuing medical education and to adjust their practice according to current standards.

As to ubiquity, unless the profession assists society in making medical services available to all areas of the country, it would be creating a service vacuum that could not legally be filled by anyone else. Therefore, everyone's right to health care—for more on this, see Chapter 9—would not be met equally. As service provider monopoly holder, therefore, the profession has an ethical obligation to avoid such a situation.

Similarly, with respect to universality, the profession has a duty to set up an appropriate framework within which necessary medical services are provided to everyone who needs it; and individual physicians, by joining this service provider monopoly, accept the responsibility of treating affected persons insofar as treatment falls into their area of competence.[28]

To sum up, the profession of medicine has a collective duty to ensure that necessary medical services are available to all who need it, and individual physicians have

(a) a duty to repay their society for their education and knowledge by practising for a reasonable amount of time in underserviced areas,

(b) a duty to provide the medical services they are qualified to provide without discrimination and

(c) a duty to ensure that the quality of care they provide is current.

5. Physicians have an obligation of professional integrity. To explain what professional integrity for physicians involves, it may be useful to begin with a brief look at the notion of professional integrity itself and its relationship to codes of ethics.

Professional integrity is concerned with the way an individual acts as a professional. As such, it is distinct from the way someone acts as a private person, and an individual's integrity as a private person is relevant to considerations of the individual's professional integrity only insofar as there is a genuine connection between the two. Likewise, professional integrity should not be confused with loyalty to a professional association. Professional associations are private corporations whose mandate is to advance the fortunes of their members, and their rules are on a par with the rules of any private club or corporation. While adherence to these may be a condition of membership in the association, it cannot be an ethical requirement in the sense that it grows out of the nature of the profession itself.

Therefore, it would be inappropriate for a code of medical ethics to include matters that relate to the lives of physicians as private persons except insofar as these affect their functioning as professionals.[29] In other words, matters of professional integrity include only issues that centre in how physicians should conduct themselves as physicians. Included here are competence, power relationships with patients and the reporting of inappropriate behaviour by their colleagues.

Competence Physicians, by presenting themselves as physicians, give themselves out as qualified and competent in the areas in which they practise. Therefore, a practising physician who is unqualified in what he or she does or who lacks competence is guilty of professional misrepresentation. This constitutes a lack of professional integrity.

However, *competence* is a relative term. Someone is competent only relative to a particular standard or measure. In medicine, this is known as the standard of clinical practice. This standard changes as medical knowledge and techniques change. Consequently the duty of competence also includes the duty to engage in continuing medical education.[30] By implication, practising physicians who do not keep current lack professional integrity.

At the same time, competence includes more than having and maintaining technical abilities. It also includes realizing the limits of one's professional capabilities. Integrity-as-competence, therefore, also entails a duty to realize the limits of one's professional capacity, to act only within those limits, to consult when those limits are likely to be reached and to refer when the limits are likely to be overstepped.

Furthermore, competence is also affected by the conditions under which professional skills are employed. This includes the work environment—the actual working context—and the mental and physical conditions of the professionals themselves. If either of these interfere with a professional's ability to meet current standards of care, that professional will be acting incompetently. Specific to medicine, this means that except in emergencies when any medical help is better than none, physicians should not provide medical services when they are too tired[31] or otherwise personally incapable of working competently. It will be obvious that physicians also have the further duty to try to make sure that conditions that impair their capacity to function competently do not obtain in the first place. A code of medical ethics, therefore, should contain an appropriate clause that highlights these considerations.

Abuse of Patients Physicians have privileged access to the bodies and minds of patients. Moreover, patients seek out physicians because they have needs that only physicians can satisfy. This places patients in a vulnerable position. To take advantage of this privileged access or of the power differential that is inherent in this dependence relationship contravenes the Principle of Fidelity. Professional integrity therefore entails that physicians should not abuse this privileged access or this power, whether that be for personal reasons—for instance, to gain sexual favours[32]—or to coerce patients into making decisions they would not otherwise make.

Reporting Inappropriate Professional Actions While this duty may also be listed under Responsibilities to Society, it is probably more appropriately classed as falling under Integrity. The reason lies in the fact that someone who becomes aware of unethical or injurious behaviour and takes no steps to deal with or prevent it is in fact condoning that behaviour. That says something about the individual's moral stance. Further, —and this will be discussed more fully when dealing with euthanasia in Chapter 7—someone who allows harm to occur when it is possible to prevent that harm thereby becomes co-responsible for that harm. The first demonstrates one's lack of integrity as a professional; the second constitutes a violation of the Principle of non-Malfeasance.

Specific to medicine, then, physicians sometimes become aware that the level of treatment provided by a medical colleague is not up to current standards and possibly injurious, or that the colleague has acted in an otherwise inappropriate fashion—such as taking advantage of a patient in a sexual manner, acting abusively or in a discriminatory manner, or being impaired when delivering medical care. Not to report such a state of affairs to the appropriate licensing authority would be to deliberately treat an unacceptable situation as though it were acceptable—a clear violation of the Principle of Integrity—and to allow preventable harm to occur—a violation of the Principle of non-Malfeasance. Physicians therefore, as a matter of professional integrity, have an obligation to report a colleague when they become aware of such a situation.[33]

Professional integrity, therefore, entails that physicians have

(a) a duty to have and maintain competence in their area of practice,

(b) a duty to practise medicine only under material or personal conditions that do not compromise the quality of their action, except in emergencies when no other appropriately qualified caregiver is reasonably available,

(c) a duty not to abuse the trust placed in them by their patients and

(d) a duty to report inappropriate actions of colleagues to the relevant licensing authorities who should function in an open and transparent way.

Rights

As a matter of general principle, no obligation is without a corresponding right. Minimally, an obligation entails a right to whatever is instrumental to meeting that obligation. Therefore, if physicians have certain duties that derive from their status as professionals, then they also have rights to whatever is instrumentally necessary for fulfilling those duties.

6. Physicians have the right to adequate information and authority to allow them to fulfill their professional duties. This right needs little discussion. It is merely an instance of the Principle of Impossibility: One cannot have an obligation to do the impossible. (See Chapter 1.) If physicians need certain information to fulfill their role as physicians—for instance, whether a patient is an IV drug user—then they also have a right to that information. Otherwise, they cannot make a proper diagnosis or prescribe appropriate treatment. Therefore, if patients deliberately withhold relevant information, the standard of care that could normally be expected of a physician as a matter of fiduciary obligation is reduced to a commensurate degree.

Similarly, once a patient has given informed consent to a particular course of treatment (see Chapter 4, for more on informed consent), the physician must have the authority to manage the details of that treatment insofar as it involves the medically safe delivery of care. Anything else would be to force the physician to violate the Principle of Fidelity and to act in a professionally inappropriate manner. For instance, the debriding of burns involves certain techniques without which this cannot be accomplished safely. Here, once the patient (or duly empowered substitute decision-maker) has given consent to debriding, how it is performed, what instruments are used, etc., fall within the competence of the physician and are not a matter of patient choice. Similarly, if a woman has agreed to a C-section for medically appropriate reasons—placenta previa with an os overlap greater than 5 percent at 35 weeks gestation[34]—she cannot choose the type of incision. What type of incision is performed depends on what is medically safe because, again, a physician cannot ethically be expected to become an agent of harm by performing surgery that leads to downstream complications. That would violate not only the Principle of Fidelity but also the Principle of non-Malfeasance.

However, like any right, this right has limits. For instance—to continue with the above example—suppose the patient has agreed to a C-section on the understanding that blood or blood products will not be used; however, because of an unexpectedly heavy blood loss it becomes necessary to transfuse the patient to save her life. The physician may not do what is medically appropriate and give blood even though that would normally be a matter of medical decision-making, because to do so would violate the parameters within which the original consent was given. (For more on this, see "The Doctrine of Emergency" in Chapter 4.) Therefore, the right of a physician to make technical medical decisions is always constrained within the limits of patient values and consent. (For more on this, see Chapter 4.)

Finally, physicians have a right to count on patient cooperation. That is to say, as was pointed out above when discussing the duty to respect patient autonomy (and as will be discussed more fully in Chapter 4), patients have the right to accept or reject any intervention. Moreover, physicians have a duty, rooted in Fidelity, to act in the best interests of their patients. However, there are times when this right and this duty intersect in a problematic manner. Specifically, this occurs when physicians do the best they can but patients refuse to follow medical advice or to adhere to regimens they have otherwise agreed to, not because they are incapable of doing so—for instance, because of mental problems or addiction—but simply because they do not feel like it. Yet, at the same time, the patients insist that the physicians continue to act as their physicians. In such cases, physicians cannot fulfill their duty. If physicians have done the best they can to remedy such situations by counselling their patients, etc., they have the right to terminate the physician–patient relationship, after giving due notice, and to recommend that the patient seek out another physician.

Therefore, physicians have a right

(a) to adequate information to allow them to act in a professionally appropriate manner,

(b) to decide on the technical nature of the therapy they deliver insofar as this does not violate the fundamental values of the patient,

(c) to expect patient cooperation with the treatment provided and

(d) to terminate a physician–patient relationship if continuation of that relationship does not allow them to practise in a medically appropriate manner, where such termination should be preceded by sufficient notice and counselling.

7. Physicians have the right to working conditions that are adequate to allow them to fulfill their professional duties. The Principle of Impossibility entails that one cannot have a duty to do the impossible. In medicine, what is possible is sometimes a function of the resources that are available and the conditions under which the physicians have to practise. For physicians to be forced to practise under conditions that do not allow them to meet current professional standards commensurate with patients' needs would be to force them to act unprofessionally. While such situations might arise when resources are limited—the matter will be discussed more fully in Chapters 9 and 10, when we deal with the right to health care and with resource allocation— and such resource limitation is not the result of necessity but other factors, physicians have a right to take appropriate action. (What form that action may ethically take will be discussed separately below.)

No special argument is required to show that the concept of working conditions does not include working conditions that are personally pleasant or that would make the work easier than would normally be expected, and so on. The only thing it means is that when conditions are such that physicians cannot fulfill their professional duties, even with the best of intentions, without becoming morally guilty—working overly long hours when this is not strictly necessary was already mentioned in this regard—then the strength of the relevant duties is reduced to a commensurate degree.

Moreover, the notion does not extend to private contractual conditions such as fringe benefits, pension plans and the like. These are an entirely different matter. They are irrelevant insofar as a physician's ability to function in a professionally competent manner is concerned. Therefore, although physicians do have a right to fair and equitable recompense for their work, this matter has no place in a code of ethics, as it does not concern itself with physicians *as physicians*. It will also be clear that emergency conditions may also constitute exceptions. But that has already been touched on above.

These rights, therefore, insofar as they are appropriately placed in a code of medical ethics, can be summarized into two points. Physicians have a right

(a) to working conditions that allow them to deliver adequate and competent patient care and

(b) to see that the standards to which their professional actions are held are commensurate with their working conditions.

WITHDRAWAL OF SERVICE: PHYSICIANS, THE MEDICAL PROFESSION AND SOCIETY

Finally, a few words about the relationship between individual physicians, the profession of medicine and society.

As was mentioned under 6 and 7 above, there may be occasions when the conditions under which physicians are forced to practise compromise their ability to deliver competent care. Unsanitary working conditions, dangerously outmoded or malfunctioning equipment and facilities, insufficient staffing or unduly lengthy working hours are cases in point. Likewise, physicians may feel that the recompense they receive for their work is not proportional to the work they do or the level of their responsibility. For these and other reasons, physicians may feel that they have the right to withhold their services—i.e., to go on strike—in order to press for changes. Is that ethically appropriate?

The question is really misstated as it stands, because it combines two reasons for going on strike that are not on a par. One is a matter of ethics that derives from the nature of medicine as a profession; the other is a matter of ethics that is grounded in economics. The former is properly an issue that touches physicians *as physicians*; the latter touches physicians only as wage earners. The real question, insofar as physicians *as physicians* are concerned, is whether physicians may ever use a strike as a tool, no matter what the reason.

At this juncture, the fiduciary duty that individual physicians have towards their patients intersects with the monopolistic position of medicine as a profession. A physician who withholds care from his or her patients must take appropriate steps to allow those patients to find another physician. At the same time, if the profession as a whole withdraws its services, no one else may legally step in to fill the breach. Therefore, if all physicians withdraw their services, there will be no one to take over the fiduciary duty of the individual physician because, given the monopolistic position of the profession, no one else will be able to provide medical care.

A possible solution to this difficulty lies in distinguishing between the obligations of the individual physician and the obligations of the profession. Individual physicians have the right to withdraw services if this occurs within the parameters outlined above. The obligation to ensure that some physicians are available to provide necessary care, however, which grows out of the profession's monopolistic position, does not allow the profession to sanction a total withdrawal of medical services, no matter what the reason. This means that the profession as a whole has a duty to ensure that a sufficient number of its members are available to provide necessary medical care if physicians go on strike. How it does that is a matter between the profession and its members—but here it should be remembered that in becoming a member of the profession, the individual physician also accepts the conditions that characterize the profession itself. Therefore, the duty to provide necessary services is a distributive duty that to some degree touches everyone who becomes a member of the medical profession.

At first glance, requiring the profession to provide continuity of medically necessary services may seem unrealistic, because it would appear to undermine any chance of success that a job action might have. Arguably, if those physicians who are designated to provide the relevant services really do their job properly, those against whom the action was directed would not feel constrained to consider the demands of the striking group seriously. Furthermore, the fact that a certain minimum level of health care would be maintained would not guarantee that the health status of individual patients would be preserved. Finally, the physician–patient relationship of individual physicians would still seem to be violated by this move.

These are, of course, serious considerations, but they do not militate against the right of the profession to withdraw its services under the conditions that we have indicated. Instead, they point to one further condition: Hand in hand with the obligation of the profession to provide minimum service goes the right of the profession to ask for binding arbitration through a third party who is mutually agreeable to both sides. Not to recognize a right to binding arbitration is to place the profession of medicine into an untenable position. Physicians would be faced with the stark option of either ceasing to be physicians or accepting whatever society sends their way. And that would be unfair.

It is also important to remember that the peculiar position in which the profession finds itself is the result of the service monopoly that was conferred on it by society. Of course, that monopoly places an obligation on the profession—but it also imposes a duty on society: the duty, namely, to deal fairly with the profession, not to hold it to ransom and to make it possible for members of the profession to act in a competent manner. Society has remedies to enforce its part of the monopoly bargain on the profession. Equality and justice demand that the profession also have some way of having its demands heard and adjudicated. The only way to do that is through binding arbitration.

CONCLUSION

The discussion in this chapter has sketched some of the major ethical parameters that condition the relationship between the profession of medicine, individual physicians and society, and how this relates to a code of medical ethics. Several important points should emerge from all this. One is that the relationship between medicine, society and individual physicians is not a simple one-way affair. It involves rights and duties on both sides. Second, this relationship is grounded in fundamental ethical principles that are the same for all sides; and that what differs is how these principles express themselves. This, in turn, is a function of those features of the profession that uniquely identify it in the social context in which it is embedded. Since society consists of individual persons and the profession of medicine is constituted of individual physicians, the relationship between individual physicians and their patients moves to centre stage. Therefore, a code of medical ethics, when properly constructed, will provide guidance for physicians in this regard—but it can provide only guidance, not answers to specific questions. The reason is that a code of medical ethics is merely a collection of general rules derived by applying fundamental ethical principles to the types of situations that physicians are likely to encounter. How these rules apply depends on the specifics of the situation—and that cannot be determined ahead of time. That is why a code of medical ethics may be of help to physicians in orienting their practice, but it cannot take the place of ethical reasoning and ethics education.

There remains one further question that may reasonably be asked in connection with the medical profession and its code of ethics. A code of medical ethics purports to set the framework within which physicians can orient their professional behaviour towards patients and society. In that sense it is—or, given the above, at least claims to be—morally authoritative. However, the medical profession, through various associations such as the CMA and the WMA, sometimes adopts policies and makes pronouncements that deal not with the practice of medicine but the with activities of persons who are not medical professionals. Implicated here are policies and pronouncements on such activities as boxing, smoking and the like. Moreover, these policies are frequently announced with an air of moral authority mimicking that of the clauses in a code of ethics. Does the profession have the mandate to make such policies and pronouncements, and are the policies really morally authoritative?

A full discussion of what is at stake here requires an in-depth analysis of the role of professions as social institutions in general, and of medicine in particular. It therefore transcends the bounds of this text. This much, however, can legitimately be said: Professions are authoritative in their respective fields of expertise, and are therefore qualified to make statements about activities insofar as these have implications for the work the professionals perform as professionals. However, whether the activities that lead to the engagement of the professionals in their professional capacity have a particular moral status, or whether they should be allowed or forbidden, is not a question of how the relevant professional expertise should be exercised. It is a question of whether the activity that leads to their engagement as professionals should be controlled by society. And that—as will become clear from the discussions in Chapters 3 and 4— is a question of how, whether and to what degree society wishes to control the behaviour of its members. Therefore, while the medical profession has the right—and indeed the duty—to point out that particular types of activities such as boxing, soccer, basketball or hockey carry medical risk,[35] it does not have a mandate (or, arguably, the expertise) to present its pronouncements as morally authoritative.

Further Readings

Antoniou, S.A., G.A. Antoniou, F.A. Granderath, A. Mavroforou, A.D. Giannoukas and A.I. Antoniou. "Reflections of the Hippocratic Oath in Modern Medicine." *World J Surg.* 34.12 (Dec 2010): 3075–3079.

Canadian Medical Association. Code of Ethics (Update 2004), available at http://policybase.cma.ca/PolicyPDF/PD04-06.pdf

Lakhan, S.E., E. Hamlat, T. McNamee and C. Laird. "Time for a Unified Approach to Medical Ethics." *Philosophy, Ethics, and Humanities in Medicine* 4.13 (Sep 2009).

O'Connor, M.J. "Can We Prevent Doctors Being Complicit in Torture? Breaking the 'Serpent's Egg.'" *Law Med.* 17.3 (Dec 2009): 426–438.

World Medical Association. *An International Code of Medical Ethics*, adopted by the 3rd General Assembly of the World Medical Association, London, England, October 1949 and amended at the 57th WMA General Assembly, Pilanesberg, South Africa, October 2006, available at www.wma.net/en/30publications/10policies/c8/

Endnotes

1. H.E. MacDermott, *History of the Canadian Medical Association, 1867–1921.* (Toronto: C.M.A. Murray, 1958). See also R. Hamoway, *Canadian Medicine: A Study in Restricted Entry* (Vancouver: The Fraser Institute, 1984).

2. A.C. Pickett, "The Oath of Imhotep: In Recognition of African Contributions to Western Medicine," *J Natl Med Assoc.* 84.7 (Jul 1992): 636–637.

3. C. Chakraberty, *An Interpretation of Ancient Hindu Medicine*, 2 vols. (Calcutta: Cosmo Publications, 2010).

4. B.S. McDougall and A. Hansson, *Chinese Concepts of Privacy* (Leiden, Boston and Tokyo: Brill, 2002).

5. L. Edelstein, *The Hippocratic Oath* (Baltimore: Johns Hopkins Press, 1923).

6. T.J. Drizis, "Medical Ethics in a Writing of Galen," *Acta Med Hist Adriat* 6.2 (Fall 2008): 333–336.

7. Prayer of Maimonides, available at www.ketubotbynaomi.com/prayer_of_maimonides.html

8. Al-Ruhawi, "Adab Al-Tabib: the Conduct of a Physician," discussed in M. Levey, "Medical Ethics of Medieval Islam with Special Reference to Al-Ruhawi's Practical Ethics of the Physician," *Transactions of the American Philosophical Society*, Vol. 57, Part 3 (1967). See also S. Aksoy, "The Religious Tradition of Ishaq ibn Ali Al-Ruhawi: The Author of the First Medical Ethics Book in Islamic Medicine," *Journal of the International Society for the History of Islamic Medicine* 3.5 (2004): 9–11. For another Arabic example, see Al-Razi (Razes), *The Spiritual Physick of Rhazes*, trans. A. Arberry (London: John Murray, 1950).

9. Oath and Prayer of Maimonides, available at www.library.dal.ca/kellogg/Bioethics/codes/maimonides.htm

10. A.K. Brownell and E. Brownell, "The Canadian Medical Association Code of Ethics 1868 to 1996: A Primer for Medical Educators," *Ann R Coll Physicians Surg Can* 35.4 (Jun 2002): 240–243.

11. World Medical Association, International Code of Medical Ethics, available at www.wma.net/en/30publications/10policies/c8/index.html

12. L.L. Weed, "New Connections Between Medical Knowledge and Patient Care," *British Medical Journal* 315 (26 July 1997): 231–235.

13. *Oxford English Dictionary.*

14. Cf. British Medical Association, *Medicine Betrayed: The Participation of Doctors in Human Rights Abuses* (BMA: London, 1992), available at http://books.google.com/books?id=bMTu_olfVsIC&printsec=frontcover#v=onepage&q&f=true

15. R. v. Morgentaler, [1988] 1 S.C.R. 30, 63 O.R. (2d.) 281, 26 O.A.C. 1, 44 D.L.R. (4th) 385, 82 N.R. 1, 3 C.C.C. (3rd)449, 62 C.R. (3rd) 1, 31 C.R.R.

16. This of course assumes that the patient or substitute decision-maker has given informed consent to consultation.

17. Cf. CMA Code, clauses 21–37.

18. See L.E. Ferris, H. Barkun, J. Carlisle, B. Hoffman, C. Katz and M. Silverman, "Defining the Physician's Duty to Warn: Consensus Statement of Ontario's Medical Expert Panel on Duty to Inform," *CMAJ* 158 (1998): 1473–1479. This duty was originally affirmed by the courts in the U.S. case of Tarasoff v. Regents of the University of California, 17 Cal. 3d 425, 551 P.2d 334, 131 Cal. Rptr. 14 (Cal. 1976). It was followed in Canada in Wenden v. Trikha, Royal Alexandra Hospital and Yaltho (1993), 14 CCLT (2d) 225 (Alta. CA) and Smith v. Jones (1999), 169 Dominion Law Reports (4th) 385 (SCC).

19. Cf. CMA Code, clause 17.

20. Cf. CMA Code, clauses 12 and 19.

21. Cf. CMA Code, clause 18.

22. Egedebo v. Windermere District Hospital Association [1991] B.C.J. No. 2381 (S.C.) affirmed (1993) 78 B.C.L.R (2d) 63 (C.A.).

23. E.g., Alberta (R.S.A. 2000, c. A-20, s. 21(1)(d)) and Quebec Charter of Human Rights and Freedoms, R.S.Q. c. C-12, art. 2.

24. The debt load ranges from $30,000 in Quebec to up to $70,000 in the rest of Canada. S. Merani, S. Abdulla, J.C. Kwong, L. Rosella, D.L. Streiner, I.L. Johnson and I.A. Dhalla, "Increasing Tuition Fees in a Country with Two Different Models of Medical Education," *Med Educ* 44.6 (Jun 2010): 577–586.

25. Medical tuition fees for in-province students range from $3,000 to $20,000, whereas the tuition fees for out-of-province students range from $21,000 to $85,000. Association of Faculties of Medicine of Canada, "Tuition Fees in Canadian Faculties of Medicine: Session Commencing Fall 2010," accessed 23 May 2011 at www.afmc.ca/pdf/2010-11%20Tuition.pdf

26. Re Mia and Medical Service Commission of British Columbia (1985), 17 D.L.R. (4th) 385 (B.C.S.C.).

27. B.T.B. Chan, "From Perceived Surplus to Perceived Shortage: What Happened to Canada's Physician Workforce in the 1990s?" Canadian Institute of Health Information, 2002, accessed 23 May 2011 at http://secure.cihi.ca/cihiweb/en/downloads/media_05jun2002_background_e.pdf; R.B. Sullivan, M. Watanabe, M.E. Whitcomb and D.A. Kindig, "The Evolution of Divergences in Physician Supply Policy in Canada and the United States," *JAMA* 276.9 (1996): 704–709.

28. The CMA General Council in 1989 refused to accept a motion from the Committee on Ethics that HIV seropositivity is not a reason for refusing medical services. However, clause 17 of the 2004 Code, which states that a physician should "not discriminate against any patient on such grounds as . . . medical condition" can be read as implying a change in this stance and as acknowledging a duty to treat even seriously infectious patients.

29. Cf. M. Bayles, *Professional Ethics* (Englewood Cliffs, NJ: Prentice Hall, 1985), passim.

30. Cf. CMA Code, clauses 6, 15.

31. V.R. Comondore, J.B. Wenner and N.T. Ayas, "The Impact of Sleep Deprivation in Resident Physicians on Physician and Patient Safety: Is It Time for a Wake-up Call?" *BCMJ* 50.10 (2008): 560–564 ; C.P. Landrigan, J.M. Rothschild, J.W. Cronin, R. Kaushal, E. Burdick, J.T. Katz, C.M. Lilly, P.H. Stone, S.W. Lockley, D.W. Bates and C.A. Czeisler, "Effect of Reducing Interns' Work Hours on Serious Medical Errors in Intensive Care Units," *N Engl J Med* 351.18 (28 Oct 2004): 1838–1848.

32. See Special Task Force on Sexual Abuse of Patients (Ont.), "What about accountability to the patient? Final Report of the Special Task Force on Sexual Abuse of Patients" (Toronto: The Task Force, 2000).

33. E.-H. Kluge, "Reporting on an Impaired Colleague," *Canadian Medical Association Journal* 141 (1989): 973, 1080–1081.

34. SOCG Clinical Practice Guidelines, "Diagnosis and Management of Placenta Previa," accessed 25 May 2011 at www.sogc.org/guidelines/documents/189e-cpg-march2007.pdf

35. J.W. Powell and K.D. Barber-Foss, "Traumatic Brain Injury in High School Athletes," *JAMA* 282.10 (8 Sep 1999): 958–963.

SAMPLE CASES

1. Dr. R. Santas was working in the emergency department of S. Hospital when a military police escort brought in a man in severe shock. He had broken facial bones, broken ribs and crushed testicles. The man also had a ruptured spleen, cranial injuries and a severed left thumb. If the man was not treated immediately, he would probably die. Dr. S was told to treat the patient, because the patient held important information about the activities of the communist party in Greece—information that was vital to an attempt to stabilize the country. Dr. S. knew that if he acted as he had been trained, he could save the man's life, but the man would be tortured further. On the other hand, he felt that as physician, the Hippocratic Oath gave him no choice but to provide all necessary and available medical care.

2. Dr. M., who had taken some courses in substance abuse disorders when in medical school and had since had some experience in the field, was offered the position of medical director of the newly funded supervised injection site for drug addicts in W. She was thrilled at the opportunity to prevent real harm for homeless addicted persons. However, she was beginning to have some doubts as to whether making it safer for drug addicts to satisfy their addiction was really consistent with her role as a physician, since it merely facilitated addiction rather than curing it. Should she structure the facility's protocol to require addiction treatment? Was that even realistic, since the clients were so in the grip of their addiction that they would agree to almost anything and then revert?

3. In 1961, the Saskatchewan College of Physicians and Surgeons informed the Saskatchewan government that if the Saskatchewan Medical Care Insurance Bill was passed by the Saskatchewan legislature and became law, the College would refuse to cooperate with the scheme. The bill essentially provided that all Saskatchewan residents would be covered by provincial health insurance and that physicians could no longer bill their patients privately but had to bill the provincial government. On July 1, 1962, when the bill became law, most physicians withdrew their services.

They maintained that such an insurance scheme interfered with the physician–patient relationship and violated the rights of physicians as individuals and professionals. The Medical Care Insurance Commission brought in physicians from Britain and encouraged physicians from the U.S. and other parts of Canada to provide emergency services in Saskatchewan.

Chapter 3
The Health Care Professional–Patient Relationship

Whether health care is construed as a right or as a commodity, health care professionals are the gatekeepers to formalized health care. This makes how health professionals view their role very important, because how they view it determines how they interact with those who want access to the system. Several different perspectives of this role have evolved over the years. Some give more power to the professionals, some less; some construe the professional–patient relationship in purely contractual terms, others see it as fiduciary in nature, and still others introduce an element of friendship into the picture, in contrast to those who view health care professionals as disinterested purveyors of sophisticated services—essentially as agents for hire. And so on.

This chapter introduces several of the more common models and analyzes their tenability in the context of contemporary health care. Because physicians have traditionally been (and continue to be) the primary gatekeepers, the focus will be on the physician–patient relationship. The resurgence of midwifery is changing this picture to some degree, as is the emergence of nurse practitioners. However, with due alteration of detail, the considerations that apply to the relationship between physicians and their patients also apply to all other health care professionals.

Questions to Keep in Mind While Reading this Chapter:

1. What are some models of the physician–patient relationship? How have they evolved over the years, and which one is currently seen as ethically the most appropriate? Why?

2. How does a particular model of the professional–patient relationship affect health care decision-making at the level of hands-on care?

3. Does the model of the professional–patient relationship have legal implications?

INTRODUCTION

Historically, people who fell ill were treated either by knowledgeable family members, by neighbours or by significant others. When their condition exceeded the latter's knowledge, resources or expertise, they were treated by people who had received specialized health care training and who fulfilled a more or less clearly defined social role. Herbalists, shamans, witch doctors and, as time went on, physicians and nurses fell into this latter category. From a purely systems-oriented perspective, therefore, health care was traditionally provided either as a matter of kindness or as a more or less professional service.

When health care was provided as a kindness, it was not subject to ethical or legal rules and regulations; however, when it was provided as a service, ethical norms and legal regulations did apply. These were usually captured either in codes of ethics or in legal provisions—or both. (See Chapter 2.)[1]

As we saw in the preceding chapter, the first known code of medical ethics came from ancient Egypt: the *Advice* of Imhotep, who was chief minister to King Djoser and lived in the 3rd millennium B.C.E. It combined medical advice with ethical admonitions on how to treat patients.[2] The Code of Hammurabi (ca. 1700 B.C.E.) contains the first known example of legal provisions. It not only stipulated the fees that physicians could charge for their services but also set out the punishments to which they were liable if they made a mistake.[3] Well-known later codes are the Hippocratic Oath (ca. 4th century B.C.E.), the Code of Ethics of al-Ruhawi (9th century C.E.)—which is in the first known textbook devoted specifically to medical ethics[4]—and the Prayer of Maimonides (12th century C.E.). Still other examples of codes are found in Chinese medical texts from the 4th century B.C.E.,[5] as well as in Indian texts on Ayurvedic medicine from the 5th century B.C.E.[6] They all contained ethical injunctions that were intended to impress on physicians the importance of respectful behaviour and ethical deportment.

The fact that ethics played an important role in medicine from its very beginnings is really not surprising. As will be explained further in Chapter 9, the concepts of wellness and illness are inextricably linked to our understanding of what it is to be a human person. That is why, as medical practice became formalized and involved advanced professional training, philosophical theories of personhood became integral to medical science. This is clearly illustrated by Ayurvedic medicine, which was based on the philosophical Hindu conceptions of personhood that are contained in the *Bhagavad Gita*, by Chinese medicine which was predicated on the Taoist philosophy of Yin and Yang,[7] and by the fact that Pythagoreanism and Greek philosophy were integral to the Hippocratic tradition. As Galen said, "The best physician is also a philosopher."[8]

Not unexpectedly, therefore, this association between medicine and philosophy entailed that the ethical standards of the relevant philosophical views would guide the practice of medicine itself. One of the best (and historically most influential) examples of this is Ibn Sina's *Canon on Medicine*, which served as a major formative text of medical knowledge for the European and Islamic world for over five hundred years. It had an Aristotelian philosophical basis, and its virtue-ethics orientation shaped the perspective of people such as Thomas Percival, whose 1803 *Code of Ethics* was the first textbook on medical ethics published in the English-speaking world and was adopted as the official Code of Ethics of the American Medical Association in 1847.[9]

But there is more to the story. Medicine as a profession is a formalized attempt to diagnose and deal with the causes of human sickness and ill health. By its very nature, therefore, it is also closely linked to the dominant scientific world view of its time. For most of the past two thousand years, the dominant scientific perspective of the Islamic and Western world was Aristotelian in nature. It construed human beings not merely as biological organisms but as political animals—which is to say, as biological beings who by their very nature must be embedded in a society, because they achieve their full potential only in a social context. To be embedded in a social context, however, is to be embedded in a web of ethical relations. This meant that according to Aristotelian philosophy human beings were ethical as well as material/biological beings. This in turn meant that scientific health care (which is to say, medicine within the Aristotelian framework) when it was properly conducted, could not focus solely on the material needs of human bodies but had to acknowledge the social—and with it the ethical—aspects of human beings as persons. It was only natural, therefore, that the conduct of physicians should be guided by the ethical considerations that were integral to the Aristotelian world view that underlay their discipline. While these considerations were often coloured by religious elements—the Prayer of Maimonides and *The Ethics of the Physician* of al-Ruhawi are cases in point—the basic ethical tenets that derived from the philosophical perspective remained.

The dominant Aristotelian perspective on science was gradually replaced by the mechanistic causal perspective that is characteristic of modern science. Similarly, the Aristotelian ethical world view, with or without religious colouration, was gradually replaced by the two major competing ethical systems that were discussed in Chapter 1, namely, deontological and utilitarian ethics.

Not surprisingly, utilitarianism, with its emphasis on the greatest amount of good for the greatest number of people and its tendency to make individual rights functionally dependent on the good of the majority, did not establish itself at the level of hands-on medical care. Instead, in part because of its calculative efficiency and in part because of the relative ease with which it could deal with groups of populations, it became the dominant perspective at the level of health care policy. (See Chapters 1, 2 and 10.) By contrast, deontological ethics, with its emphasis on the rights of the individual, was more congenial to hands-on care. Moreover, it had the advantage of being compatible—at least superficially—with the traditional Aristotelian ethical approach that focused more on individual persons and that had shaped historical codes of ethics for so long. It therefore gradually became the dominant ethical perspective for hands-on health care.

This evolution in ethical perspective triggered a corresponding evolution in the understanding of the physician–patient relationship. This is not to say that with the rise of scientific medicine, the patient suddenly emerged as autonomous decision-maker. The process was gradual. In the beginning, the prestige of physicians as scientifically trained and medically sophisticated practitioners—and above all the increasing success of the causal model of medicine itself—exerted a dominant effect on the ethics of the physician–patient relationship. While the rights of the patient as decision-maker gradually increased in importance, it was initially felt that the patient's best interests could be served properly only if the patient acceded to the technical expertise of the physician and accepted the dominance of the physician as decision-maker. This resulted in what has since been called a paternalistic view of the physician–patient relationship, with the friendship model as a somewhat more anemic variant. The picture changed only with the increasing overall social insistence on an autonomy-centred ethics. When this development combined with a gradual increase in the medical sophistication of patients themselves, it resulted in a fundamental shift in decision-maker authority. The patient became the ultimate decision-maker in matters of health care, and the physician became the service-providing professional who was an expert in his or her field, but who had to defer to patient values. These developments were reflected in a corresponding shift in the orientation of medical codes of ethics from paternalism to a fiduciary perspective.

However, these developments were not uniform. Different perceptions of how to operationalize the basic deontological understanding of the patient as person gave rise to different models of the physician–patient relationship even after the abandonment of the Aristotelian perspective. Moreover, the development of specialized medical technologies and a corresponding institutionalization of health care, combined with an associated rise in the cost of health care services themselves, also affected the picture. This meant that non-medical factors supplemented the purely medical parameters that had previously dominated the equation and gave rise to still different models of the physician–patient relationship. The contractual and agency models respectively were implicated in this regard.

The fiduciary model was the final outcome of these developments, and it ultimately became the standard model of contemporary medical practice. However, while contemporary health care law and contemporary codes of medical ethics generally have a fiduciary orientation—as does the Code of Ethics of the Canadian Medical Association[10]—the various models that have just been mentioned can still be encountered in hands-on medical practice. This does not mean that they all are considered ethically acceptable or, for that matter, that they are all legally defensible. Thus, a paternalistic approach would encounter serious difficulties with respect to informed consent, as would the friendship model—at least in the Canadian setting; and the contractual approach would contradict the view that health care is a right and not a commodity—a perspective that, as we shall see in Chapter 9, is characteristic of Canadian society. Nevertheless, the fact that they still structure medical practice—and indeed the fact that they have made something of a resurgence[11]—makes it appropriate to consider them more closely. What follows, then, briefly sketches the various models, discusses their advantages and disadvantages, places them into the Canadian legal context and ultimately shows why the fiduciary model is to be preferred.[12]

However, before doing so it may be useful to briefly highlight some of the ethically relevant features of the physician–patient encounter, because they give some indication why certain ethical considerations are deemed so important to the physician–patient relationship.

1. Medicine is a service provider monopoly. This means that with but a few exceptions—licensed psychologists, dentists and nurse practitioners constitute partial exceptions—licensed physicians are the only ones who, by law, are allowed to practise medicine, to provide medical care that involves surgery and drug prescription, and to generally function as gatekeepers to the health care system as a whole.

2. The physician is in a position of technical expertise and on that basis recommends treatment to the patient. The patient generally lacks such expertise and is dependent on the physician's advice and services. In other words, in an intuitively clear sense there exists a dependence and power relationship between the patient and the physician.

3. The patient usually has some degree of emotional or psychological concern connected with the reason for seeking medical help.

4. The patient claims a right to health care, whereas the physician has a professionally acquired obligation to provide relevant services.[13]

5. A decision has to be made on the direction that the medical services shall take, whereby this decision is made on the basis of the information that is presented to the patient by the physician, and whereby this decision is ultimately functionally determined by the patient's values. (For further discussion of this, see Chapter 4, "Informed Consent.")

With this in mind, let us now turn to the various models of the physician–patient relationship that were mentioned above.

MODELS OF PHYSICIAN–PATIENT RELATIONSHIPS

One of the most important ethical issues that arises with the inception of a physician–patient relationship is that of control. The physician is a member of a monopolistic profession with knowledge and services for sale; the patient is a person with a need. Not surprisingly, therefore, the nature and direction of the physician–patient relationship, its quality and the very fabric of the physician–patient interaction will be heavily influenced by the physician's technical knowledge and by the physician's judgment about which treatment is appropriate, and why. In other words, viewed from a process perspective, it is the physician who controls the interaction. The ethical question, therefore, is how that control should be structured in keeping with the fundamental ethical principles that underlie health care itself. The various models of the physician–patient relationship referred to above all give different answers.

The Paternalistic Model[14]

The most traditional model is the paternalistic model.[15] Its name derives from the fact that in ancient Rome the head of the household, who was called *pater familias*, had ultimate decision-making power over all members of the household. In the physician–patient context, then, paternalism gives ultimate decision-making power to the physician. It is reflected in Percival's *Medical Ethics*,[16] in which the physician is exhorted to make decisions for the patient by blending "firmness with kindness."

This model has by no means disappeared from contemporary practice. The clearest case of paternalism is when the physician simply informs the patient that a particular treatment or intervention is required and, without asking the patient's permission, goes ahead and treats the patient. However, it need not be that blatant. For example, the paternalistic model also underlies the oncologist's decision not to inform a patient about drugs that are not covered by the health care provider[17] or a family physician's decision to fake a diagnosis or to provide a false or misleading certificate because the physician fears that not doing so will harm the patient.[18] Paternalism may be still more covert, as for example when physicians give socially correct answers to patients' questions without really addressing the core of the patients' queries,[19] or when they do not disclose to their patients the existence of clinical trials for their particular conditions because they believe that participation in the trials would not be in the patients' best interests.[20]

To repeat, a paternalistic model of the physician–patient relationship construes the physician's role not simply as that of technical expert but also as that of ultimate decision-maker. However, it is important to note that this stance is not based on some kind of power trip. It derives from the belief that physicians have a duty to do what is in their patients' best interests and that, because of their training and expertise, they are best placed to determine what that really is.

The Agency Model

If the paternalistic model of the physician–patient relationship stands at one end of the control spectrum, the agency model stands at the other.[21] Under this model, the physician is simply a technical expert who does what the patient asks. Here, the patient is in complete control over what will happen, and the physician's personal ethical or valuational scruples count for nothing, nor do his or her professional concerns. Even when what the patient wants is against the physician's better judgment, the physician goes ahead and does it anyway. Examples here would include situations in which the physician prescribes a drug requested by the patient not because it is the appropriate drug but because the patient has learned about it on the Internet and specifically requests it; or when the physician performs needless surgery—for instance, (extreme) cosmetic enhancement surgery—simply because the patient asks for it. Another example along these lines—with the added complication of a cultural variable—would be a physician performing an infibulation on a young girl because her mother has demanded it.[22]

The Contractual Model

The contractual model sees the relationship between physicians and their patients as defined by the terms of the contract between them.[23] In a way, it is similar to the agency model. In other words, it agrees with the agency model insofar as the services that are provided by the physician are determined by a contract, where what is covered by the contract—and hence what services will be provided—is purely a matter of what the patient asks for and what the patient can afford.

However, it differs from the agency model in that under this model there is no obligation for the physician to accept the terms of such a contract in the first place. Moreover, under an agency model there is some expectation that when unforeseen problems arise and the patient is not in a position to make a decision, the physician will provide the appropriate services in line with the values that were initially indicated by the patient. Under a contractual model, however, when unforeseen circumstances arise, the physician has no obligation to provide anything except emergency care. In all other cases, the physician has the right to adhere to the letter of the contract. This would mean, for example, that if the patient suffered from pneumonia but was not in any immediate danger, and if treatment of pneumonia was not covered in the contract, the physician could refuse to treat the patient. Or, if a patient needed a kidney and transplantation was not covered in the contract, the physician would have no duty to refer the patient for transplantation. The contractual model tends to structure the relationship between physicians and patients in health maintenance organizations (HMOs) and in institutions that are funded by private medical insurance providers.

The Friendship Model

The friendship model has a lot in common with the paternalistic model. However, it differs in that it assumes that the physician has an obligation to take a personal interest in the welfare of the patient. In other words, as the name implies, under this model the physician is the patient's friend. Therefore the physician may argue with the patient when he or she does not agree with the patient's choice and may use emotional pressure to persuade the patient to accept (or reject) a particular line of treatment. Under this model it would also be perfectly legitimate for the physician to withhold information from the patient—or at least to "manage" it; or for the physician to make a decision for the patient rather than allowing the patient to make a wrong decision or become exposed to what the physician feels would be too great a burden; and so on. But as is the case among friends, there will always be a readiness to account for what the physician has done, and a readiness to defer to the patient, should he or she insist.[24]

The Fiduciary Model

Under the fiduciary model—the name comes from the Latin word for trust—trust is the dominant theme. Both physician and patient trust each other. The physician trusts that the patient will be truthful and will act in a responsible manner and cooperate as patient, and the patient trusts that the physician will always act in the patient's best interests. The model acknowledges the existence of a physician–patient power differential but treats the patient's values as the determining factors in the direction of any health care intervention. Moreover, rather than seeing the physician merely as a technical expert it respects the physician as a person with values and rights.[25] Among other things, this means that the physician need not do what is against his or her values—for instance, in matters such as abortion[26]—and may terminate the physician–patient relationship if it becomes too difficult for the physician to sustain.[27]

DISCUSSION

If one looks at these models—and others are possible, but these are the more common ones[28]—one can see that some are ethically more appropriate than others.

The Paternalistic Model

The paternalistic model compromises the patient's right to self-determination too much and therefore violates the Principle of Autonomy. It assumes that expertise in a particular technical modality—in this case, medicine—confers authority over whether that expertise should be employed in the first place and in what direction, and in so doing commits what has sometimes been called the fallacy of expertise. (For further discussion of this, see Chapter 4, "Informed Consent.") In other words, while it is appropriate to acknowledge the physician's expertise and legal authority in matters of prescribing or providing medical services—in fact, all Canadian provinces and territories have legislation that essentially restricts the practice of medicine to licensed physicians[29]—this does not give physicians ultimate decision-making authority. What should be done is not simply a function of what is medically appropriate or feasible but also a matter of values: of *patient* values. That is why, as will be discussed further in the next chapter, it is essentially a matter of informed patient consent.

Moreover, by making the physician the decision-maker—whereby this decision has to be made in the best interests of the patient—the model places a tremendous psychological burden on the physician. It requires that the physician be knowledgeable about each and every patient, since otherwise the physician could not make a decision that was in the patient's best interest. Given contemporary health care with walk-in clinics and medical practices that exceed two thousand patients, this is hardly possible even with the best of record keeping and with the use of searchable electronic medical records.

Finally, while the model was historically dominant for many decades, even in tradition-oriented countries such as Japan, where health care decision-making traditionally lay entirely in the hands of physicians, the physician–patient relationship is changing. In the middle of the 20th century, the Japanese courts, acknowledging cultural changes that had occurred since World War II, ruled that informed consent for treatment had to be sought from either the patients themselves or, if the physician thought that this might be unduly stressful for the patient, the patient's immediate family.[30] In other words, the traditional physician-knows-best and physician-decides perspective that had dominated Japanese health care for so long is slowly being replaced. China also appears to be moving towards a less paternalistic model because it legally recognized the physician's duty to obtain informed consent.[31] This has implications both for physicians who immigrate from Japan and China to Canada as well as for immigrants from those countries who seek out Canadian physicians. It can no longer be assumed that the traditional paternalistic perception of the physician–patient relationship that was once characteristic of those cultures still holds sway.

The Agency Model

The agency model fails for exactly the opposite reason from the paternalistic model. Instead of underplaying the patient's autonomy and overplaying the authority of the physician, it overplays the authority of the patient and underplays the physician's autonomy. Although patients have ultimate decision-making power in matters of health care—something the CMA Code of Ethics acknowledges very clearly when it states that the competent patient "has the right . . . to accept or reject any medical care recommended"[32]—this does not mean that physicians lose all decision-making autonomy in matters that affect their practices or that conflict with their personal or with accepted social ethics. Physicians still retain their integrity both as persons and as professionals.

The model also ignores the fact that physicians have obligations towards third parties and towards society, whereby these obligations derive from the nature of medicine and from the fact of professionalism itself. These come into play when the condition of a patient constitutes a threat to another person or when acceding to the health care request of a patient would, in the physician's professional judgment, lead to medical harm that could not be justified in terms of legitimate ethical values. An example of the first would be the duty to warn appropriate others when the patient constitutes a psychiatric threat,[33] or the duty to breach patient confidentiality when the patient has a serious communicable disease and contact tracing is necessary to prevent its spread.[34] An example of the second would be the refusal to perform an infibulation on a patient even though infibulation may be part of the patient's cultural heritage.[35]

The Contractual Model

The contractual model is correct in that it accepts the patient as ultimate decision-maker, but it errs in that it neglects the fiduciary aspect of the physician–patient relationship. Thus, while the physician's role has contractual elements, it is not defined by the letters of a contract. The model might be appropriate if health care were a commodity. However, as will be argued in Chapter 9, ethically speaking, that is not the case. The fact that, ethically speaking, health care is a right entails that whoever is instrumentally involved in fulfilling that right has a duty to do whatever is necessary (and ethically appropriate). That, however, cannot be spelled out in a contract. No contract can specify the various exigencies that might arise. Patients have to trust that their physicians will do what is in their best interest—whatever that may be—within the value boundaries that are set by the patients. Physicians who practise in the U.S. and within the contractual frameworks of privately insured health services or of HMOs encounter serious professional and ethical difficulties on this very issue, precisely because they feel that, operating within a purely contractual environment, they cannot fulfill their fiduciary obligations towards their patients.[36]

The Friendship Model

As to the friendship model, it connotes an element of personal concern on the part of physicians. It seems to turn the clock back to "the good old days" when physicians had small patient pools, knew most of their patients "from cradle to grave," and believed that they not only knew what their patients wanted but were also justified in acting on that assumption because of the personal relationship that existed between them and their patients.

However, irrespective of whether this view of the physician–patient relationship is historically correct, the model is really quite unrealistic. *First* of all, there are good data which show that physicians really do not know their patients' values very well.[37] *Second,* whether we like it or not, the profit motive in medicine is a fact. While physicians may be motivated by zeal to help their patients, they are also motivated by economic considerations. To put it simply, they charge for their services, and they charge at rates that are bargained for very seriously and very determinedly by their professional associations.[38] However, friendship is not something that is for sale. Therefore, while a physician may also be a patient's friend—a point to which we shall return in a moment—the relationship of friendship is incidental to the interaction between physician and patient as physician and patient.[39]

Furthermore, friends are emotionally involved with each other. If there is no emotional involvement, then there is no friendship. However, it would be unrealistic to expect physicians who have over two thousand patients, or who fill in when on call or who take over a locum or work out of a walk-in clinic to have an emotional stake in the welfare of their patients. They do not know them well enough for that. Moreover, like all human undertakings, medicine has its failures—and sooner or later all patients die. When a friend undergoes a reversal of fortune, we are emotionally swept along and suffer; and when a friend dies, we are deeply affected. To require physicians to operate on a friendship model would be to require that they be assailed by emotional turmoil every time something similar happens to their patients. That way lies burnout.

Finally, the friendship model is inappropriate because it maximizes the possibility of medical mistakes. Because friends are emotionally involved with each other, physicians may not deal with patients who are also friends as objectively as they should and may make mistakes that they would otherwise not make. That is why contemporary codes of ethics state that physicians should not treat their significant others except in emergencies when no other health care professional is available.[40] Moreover, friends also tend to steer each other in the direction they think is best or to manage information if they think their friends would make inappropriate choices. They may even make choices for them if they think that these would be in their friends' best interest. In other words, friends tend to adopt a somewhat of paternalistic approach out of sheer friendship. For reasons that have already been pointed out, paternalism is inappropriate in the physician–patient setting.

The Fiduciary Model

The fiduciary model is the gold standard of the physician–patient relationship. It is a model of balance and trust. It is a model of balance because it gives appropriate weight to the interests of both parties.[41] The autonomy of patients is balanced against the expertise of physicians and their role as professionals. More specifically, in a fiduciary model, the control that physicians exercise over the physician–patient encounter from a process perspective—control that uniquely belongs to them because of their legal position, their professional decision-making authority and their training and expertise—is structured around doing what is in their patients' best interests and in keeping with the physicians' professional judgment (whereby what is in the patients' best interests is determined by the patients' values and not by the physicians' professional standards).[42]

The fiduciary model is also a model of trust. While the patient trusts that the physician will act in the patient's best interests, the physician trusts that the patient will tell the truth, will be forthcoming and will withhold nothing that the physician needs to know in a professional capacity—and will cooperate with the physician's endeavours. If these conditions are not met, then the physician has the right to review and perhaps even to end the relationship unilaterally.[43] Of course, there are situations in which this last is not an option, for example, when there is no other physician who can (or will) take on the patient. Here the obligation to provide care for the patient remains—but not on the original terms. The physician then has the right to practise defensive medicine and need no longer practise on a basis of trust.

The fiduciary model is strongly deontological in orientation. For this reason, it also constitutes an appropriate foundation for the doctrine of informed consent—which is based on the principle of patient autonomy and has become integral to health care since the middle of the 20th century. However, patient autonomy under the fiduciary model is autonomy that is conditioned by trust. In this sense it differs from patient autonomy under the agency and the contractual models. Under the latter two models, patient autonomy is subject to the condition of *caveat emptor*: "let the buyer beware." According to them, the physician has no obligation to ensure that the patient has fully understood the issues or has explored the ins and outs of a particular decision. By contrast, patient autonomy under the fiduciary model is autonomy that is fostered by the physician's best efforts to ensure that the patient really understands all relevant options and that these options will really meet the health care needs of the patient as person.

EMERGING ISSUES

The preceding discussion has been based on the traditional pattern of the physician–patient encounter in which physicians and patients are in direct contact with each other. Increasingly, however, this pattern of direct contact is being replaced by a pattern of indirect contact, whereby physician and patient interact with each other only through electronic media. Telehealth (sometimes also called e-medicine) is a good example of this. In telehealth, physicians use email to communicate with their patients, to give them advice or to order drug prescriptions, etc., and either use indwelling electronic telemetry to determine patients' status and diagnose their conditions, or have patients take their own clinical measurements and report these to a central data clearing house, where a physician will interpret the data and make appropriate medical decisions.

Telehealth departs from the traditional pattern not simply because it introduces into the relationship an element of distance that did not previously exist in the physician–patient encounter, but also because by reading diagnostic results from a monitor or by taking blood-sugar levels, blood-pressure readings, etc., and communicating these to a physician, the patient is becoming an active participant in the diagnostic process that was formerly solely the purview of the physician. Telehealth has also seen the advent of medical outsourcing, whereby patient data that are acquired in one location by specialized diagnostic or laboratory equipment on the orders of one physician are sent electronically to another location to be read and evaluated by another physician or specialist who is never in contact with the patient, and who then makes suggestions for treatment of the patient.[44] It may even extend to providing surgical interventions either through consultation or through the use of robotic devices that are steered from a distant control facility,[45] and to providing mental health services.[46]

It is clear that the fiduciary model of the physician–patient relationship still applies in these cases. That is not the problem. The problem is how the model should be construed under these circumstances. The fact that in many of these patterns of interaction the patient becomes integral to the physician's professional activity in a way that was not the case in traditional hands-on medicine adds a new parameter to the equation. The patient, so to speak, becomes an active participant in and contributor to the diagnostic and consultative process itself.[47] This is even the case when the physician—who is generally part of an impersonal institutional network—consults electronically with the patient. The fact that the physician never really encounters the patient, or encounters the patient second-hand, as it were, raises the question of whether the fiduciary model has to be adjusted to incorporate a more contractual element.

Moreover, with exception of uncooperative patients or a conflict of personal values, the fiduciary model of the physician–patient relationship enjoins physicians not to abandon their patients.[48] However, the literature suggests that patients may view the use of telehealth ambivalently in this respect. While some have reported an increased sense of care and involvement,[49] others have reported a feeling of distancing[50] and an impression of abandonment.[51] The perceived shift from a person-centred to a technology-focused relationship may also impact ambivalently on autonomy and respect as perceived by the patient. The patient may feel compromised as a decision-maker, feeling like a mere cog in an impersonal and machine-like process over which he or she has no control.[52] This raises the question of whether the fiduciary nature of the professional–patient relationship may be compromised by the very modality itself.

No clear way has emerged of how to understand the fiduciary model of the physician–patient relationship in this newer approach to physician–patient interaction. Two CMA policy statements—"Physician Guidelines for Online Communication with Patients"[53] and "Guiding Principles for Physician Electronic Medical Records (EMR) Adoption in Ambulatory Clinical Practice"[54]—have attempted to provide guidance in this regard; however, they are far from complete and do not cover all aspects of such practice. Some additional guidance had originally been provided by the World Medical Association's "Statement on Home Medical Monitoring, 'Tele-Medicine' and Medical Ethics." Unfortunately, that Statement was rescinded in 2006.[55] Various other attempts have been made to draft codes and practice guidelines; however, so far none has achieved wide acceptance.[56] Therefore, while it is generally agreed that physicians always have a fiduciary obligation towards their patients, no matter what their pattern of interaction, it remains far from clear how that should be spelled out in the modern telehealth setting.

CONCLUSION

The health care environment is one of the most delicate and most intimate of all human settings. Certainly this is true for patients. They have to not only expose themselves in a physical sense to receive treatment, but also be forthcoming, open and truthful for the treatment to be appropriate and effective. By thus opening up, patients become vulnerable. This vulnerability is frequently increased by the patients' compromised health status. Furthermore, patients are almost invariably driven by a mix of motivations and feelings: the desire to receive help, the drive to remain independent and the wish to retain autonomy, etc. These tend to complicate the picture.

From the side of the health care professional, there is an equally strong and complicated mix of driving forces. There is the desire to do what is best for the patient, the interest in the disease process itself, considerations of professional duty mixed with personal values and perception, and so on.

As was pointed out at the beginning of this chapter, in most cases physicians are in a dominant position to shape the relationship, not only because of their training and expertise but also because of their legal position as gatekeeper to the health care system. Consequently, physicians have a fundamental responsibility to ensure that the nature of the physician–patient relationship remains ethically appropriate. This means that they have a duty to structure this relationship deontologically—which is to say, they have a duty to structure it not around calculations of effectiveness and efficiency, or of the greatest good for the greatest number or by considerations of what will advance their professional position or that of the profession, but by concern for the patient as a person. If physicians lose sight of this, then the physician–patient relationship becomes a relationship between a vendor and a consumer, and what makes it a uniquely fiduciary relationship disappears.

Further Readings

Andereck, W.S. "Commodified Care." *Cambridge Quarterly of Healthcare Ethics* 16 (2007): 398–406.

Canadian Medical Association. CMA Code of Ethics (Update 2004), available at http://policybase.cma.ca/PolicyPDF/PD04-06.pdf

Childress, J.I., and M. Siegler. "Metaphors and Models of Doctor–Patient Relationships: Their Implication for Autonomy." *Theoretical Medicine* 5 (1984): 17–30.

Dworkin, G. "Paternalism." *The Monist* 56 (Jan 1972).

Emanuel, E.J., and L.L. Emanuel. "Four Models of the Physician–Patient Relationship." *Journal of the American Medical Association* 267.17 (1992): 221–226.

Gerber, B.S., and A.R. Eiser. "The Patient–Physician Relationship in the Internet Age: Future Prospects and the Research Agenda." *Journal of Medical Internet Research* 3.2 (2001), accessed 21 Mar 2011 at www.jmir.org/2001/2/e15/

Masters, R. "Is Contract an Adequate Basis for Medical Ethics?" *Hastings Center Report* 5 (Dec 1975).

Sandman, L., and C. Munthe. "Shared Decision Making, Paternalism and Patient Choice." *Health Care Analysis* 18.1 (2010): 60–84.

Veatch, R.M. "Models for Ethical Medicine in a Revolutionary Age." *Hastings Center Report* 2 (June 1972): 5–7.

Endnotes

1. For a good introduction to the history of medical ethics, see A.R. Jonsen, *A Short History of Medical Ethics* (Oxford: Oxford University Press, 2000).

2. J.H. Breasted, *The Edwin Smith Surgical Papyrus*, published in facsimile and hieroglyphic transliteration with translation and commentary in two volumes. University of Chicago Oriental Institute publications, v. 3–4 (Chicago: University of Chicago Press, 1991).

3. "The Code of Hammurabi," translated by L.W. King (2005), accessed 21 Feb 2011 at http://avalon.law.yale.edu/ancient/hamframe.asp: 214–224.

4. Al-Ruhawi, "Adab Al-Tabib, the Conduct of a Physician," discussed in M. Levey, "Medical Ethics of Medieval Islam with Special Reference to Al-Ruhawi's Practical Ethics of the Physician," *Transactions of the American Philosophical Society*, Vol. 57, Part 3 (1967).

5. *The Yellow Emperor's Classic of Internal Medicine*, translated by I. Weith (Berkeley and Los Angeles: University of California Press, 2002), Chapters 1–34.

6. P.N. Desai, "Medical Ethics in India," *Journal of Medicine and Philosophy* 13.3 (1988): 231–255.

7. M. Porkert, *The Theoretical Foundations of Chinese Medicine* (Cambridge and London: MIT Press, 1974).

8. T.J. Drizis, "Medical Ethics in a Writing of Galen," *Acta Medico-Historica Adriatica* 6 (2008): 333–336.

9. W.J. Thomas, "Informed Consent, the Placebo Effect, and the Revenge of Thomas Percival," *Journal of Legal Medicine* 22.3 (2001): 313–348.

10. Canadian Medical Association, Code of Ethics (Update 2004), available at http://policybase.cma.ca/PolicyPDF/PD04-06.pdf

11. J.C. Callahan, "Paternalism and Voluntariness," *Canadian Journal of Philosophy* 16.2 (1986): 199–220; G. Dworkin, *The Theory and Practice of Autonomy* (Cambridge: Cambridge University Press, 1988). See also D. Callahan, "When Self-Determination Runs Amok," *Hastings Center Report* (March/April 1992): 52–55.

12. The classic discussion of the various models is by R.M. Veatch, "Models for Ethical Medicine in a Revolutionary Age," *Hastings Center Report* 2 (June 1972) 5–7; J.I. Childress and M. Siegler, "Metaphors and Models of Doctor–Patient Relationships: Their Implication for Autonomy," *Theoretical Medicine* 5 (1984): 17–30; E.J. Emanuel, *The Ends of Human Life: Medical Ethics in a Liberal Polity* (Cambridge: Harvard University Press, 1991). For a somewhat mitigated position on patient autonomy, see A.I. Tauber, *Patient Autonomy and the Ethics of Responsibility* (Cambridge: MIT Press, 2005).

13. E.I. Picard and G.B. Robertson, *Legal Liability of Doctors and Hospitals in Canada*, 4th ed. (Toronto: Carswell, 2007). See also C.A. Kent, *Medical Ethics: The State of the Law* (Toronto: LexisNexis-Butterworths, 2005).

14. G.C. Graber, "On Paternalism in Health Care," in *Contemporary Issues in Biomedical Ethics*, ed. J.W. Davis, B. Hoffmaster and S. Shorten (Clifton, NJ: Humana Press, 1981); A. Buchanan "Medical Paternalism," *Philosophy and Public Affairs* 7 (1978): 370–390; J. Ellin, "Comments on 'Paternalism in Health Care'" in *Contemporary Issues in Biomedical Ethics* (see ref. above); B. Gert and C.M. Culver, "Paternalistic Behaviour," *Philosophy and Public Affairs* 6 (1976): 45–47; G. Dworkin, "Paternalism," *The Monist* 56 (Jan 1972); J. Feinberg, *Social Philosophy* (Englewood Cliffs, NJ: Prentice Hall, 1973), 52; J.C. Callahan, "Paternalism and Voluntariness," *Canadian Journal of Philosophy* 16.2 (1986): 199–220; H.T. Engelhardt, Jr., *The Foundations of Bioethics* (New York: Oxford University Press, 1986), 252–262; W. Glannon, *Biomedical Ethics* (New York and Oxford: Oxford University Press, 2005), Chapter 2.

15. It is sometimes also called the priestly model because priests were sometimes seen as gatekeepers to spiritual health. For a good discussion of the role of paternalism in health care, see J.F. Childress, *Who Should Decide? Paternalism in Health Care* (New York: Oxford University Press, 1982).

16. T. Percival, *Medical Ethics: Or a Code of Institutes and Precepts, Adapted to the Professional Conduct of Physicians and Surgeons* (London: Russell and Bickerstaff, 1803), newly edited by C.D. Leake as *Percival's Medical Ethics* (Huntington, NY: Krieger, 1975).

17. T. Dare, M. Findlay, P. Browett et. al., "Paternalism in Practice: Informing Patients about Expensive Unsubsidised Drugs," *Journal of Medical Ethics* 36.5 (May 2010): 260–264.

18. G. Helgesson and N. Lynöe, "Should Physicians Fake Diagnoses to Help Their Patients?" *Journal of Medical Ethics* 34.2 (Mar 2008): 133–136.

19. N. Lynöe, N. Juth and G. Helgesson, "How to Reveal Disguised Paternalism," *Medicine, Health Care and Philosophy* 13.1 (Feb 2010): 59–65. See also C. Gavaghan, "'You Can't Handle the Truth': Medical Paternalism and Prenatal Alcohol Use," *Journal of Medical Ethics* 35.5 (May 2009): 300–303.

20. L.A. Jansen and S. Wall, "Paternalism and Fairness in Clinical Research," *Bioethics* 23.3 (Mar 2009): 172–182.

21. See E.J. Emanuel and L.L. Emanuel. "Four Models of the Physician–Patient Relationship," *Journal of the American Medical Association* 267.17 (1992): 221–226. The Emanuels call it the "Informative Model."

22. This example involves the further ethical complication of substitute decision-making, which is discussed in Chapter 5. The example itself is based the author's experience as Director of Ethics and Legal Affairs of the CMA.

23. See Veatch, *supra*. See also R. Masters, "Is Contract an Adequate Basis for Medical Ethics?" *Hastings Center Report* 5 (Dec 1975) 24–28; and R. May, "Code and Covenant or Philanthropy and Contract?" in *Ethics in Medicine: Historical Perspectives and Contemporary Concerns*, ed. S.J. Reiser, A.J. Dyck and W.J. Curran (Cambridge, MA: MIT Press, 1977), 65–76.

24. For an analogous discussion, but under the rubric of "deliberative model," see Emanuel and Emanuel, op. cit., *supra*.

25. For recent legal developments in Canada that essentially constitute a legal endorsement of this model, see E.I. Picard and G.B. Robertson, *Legal Liability of Doctors and Hospitals in Canada*, 4th ed. (Toronto: Thomson-Carswell, 2007), 4–15. See also C.A. Kent, *Medical Ethics: The State of the Law* (Markham, ON: LexisNexis, 2005), 12–15.

26. CMA Code of Ethics (Update 2004) clause 12, available at http://policybase.cma.ca/PolicyPDF/PD04-06.pdf

27. Ibid., clause 19.

28. E.g., see E.J. Emanuel and L.L. Emanuel, "Four Models of the Physician–Patient Relationship," *JAMA* 267.17 (1992): 221–226. But see also G. Clarke, R. Hall and G. Rosencrance, "Physician–Patient Relations: No More Models," *The American Journal of Bioethics* 4.2 (2004): 16–19.

29. The relevant legislation is variously called the *Health Professions Act* (British Columbia), *Regulated Health Professions Act* (Ontario), *Medical Act* (Nova Scotia), etc.

30. A. Akabayashi and B.T. Slingsby, "Informed Consent Revisited: Japan and the U.S." *The American Journal of Bioethics* 6.1 (2006): 9–14; Y. Tejima, "Recent Developments in the Informed Consent Law in Japan," *Kobe University Law Review* 36.1 (2002): 45–59.

31. O. Döring, "China's Struggle for Practical Regulations in Medical Ethics," *Nature Reviews* 4 (2003): 233–239.

32. CMA Code of Ethics, clause 24.

33. The U.S. case of Tarasoff v. The Regents of the University of California (17 Cal. Rep., 3rd. 425 [1976]) is instructive. See also CMA Code of Ethics, clause 35.

34. Cf. CMA Code of Ethics, clauses 35 and 42.

35. Infibulation of persons under eighteen years of age for non-medical reasons is also a criminal offence in Canada. See *Criminal Code* of Canada R.S., 1985, c. C-46, s. 268.

36. For a discussion of some of these issues, see M.H. Savitz et al., "Ethical Differences between Socialized and HMO Systems," *Mt. Sinai Journal of Medicine* 71.6 (Nov 2004): 392–400.

37. A.B. Seckler et al., "Substituted Judgment: How Accurate Are Proxy Decisions?" *Annals of Internal Medicine* 115.2 (1991): 92–98; The SUPPORT Principal Investigators, "A Controlled Trial to Improve Care for Seriously Ill Hospitalized Patients: The Study to Understand Prognoses and Preferences for Outcomes and Risks of Treatments (SUPPORT)," *JAMA* 274 (1995): 1591–1598.

38. J. Lomas, C. Charles and J. Greb, "The Price of Peace. The Structure and Process of Physician Fee Negotiations in Canada," *Centre for Health Economics and Policy Analysis (CHEPA)*, McMaster University, Hamilton; accessed 17 Mar 2011 at http://ideas.repec.org/p/hpa/wpaper/199217.html#provider

39. W.S. Andereck, "Commodified Care," *Cambridge Quarterly of Healthcare Ethics* 16 (2007): 398–406.

40. CMA Code of Ethics, clause 20.

41. For a different evaluation, see A. Chinen, "Modes of Understanding and Mindfulness of Clinical Medicine," *Theoretical Medicine* 9.1 (Feb 1988): 45–72, who advocates a mix of formal, hermeneutic and pragmatic modes. The formal approach, which is that of Veatch, is here presented as focusing too much on the structure of obligations without giving due weight to the attitudinal aspects of the physician–patient relationship. It is said to "objectify" the individuals. This, so it is argued, is counterbalanced by a hermeneutic element, which involves a "subjectification" of the value systems and a "being-with" of both parties. Since a purely hermeneutic relationship is said to run the danger of paternalism, Chinen suggests that there should be an initial attempt to establish a "congruence" of values, and that this should then be applied in a pragmatic sense.

42. Cf. R. Veatch, *The Physician–Patient Relation: The Patient as Partner* (Bloomington: Indiana University Press, 1991). See also R. Tong, *New Perspectives in Health Care Ethics* (Upper Saddle River, NJ: Pearson Prentice Hall, 2007), Chapter 3.

43. See CMA Code of Ethics, clauses 17 and 19.

44. M. Clarke and J. Barnett, "Teleoncology Uptake in British Columbia," *Stud Health Technol Inform* 164 (2011): 399–404.

45. R.D. Bucholz, K.A. Laycock and L. McDurmont, "Operating Room Integration and Telehealth," *Acta Neurochir Suppl.* 109 (2011): 223–237; S. Shivji et al., "Pediatric Surgery Telehealth: Patient and Clinician Satisfaction," *Pediatr Surg Int* (18 Jan 2011).

46. M.L. Wendel, D.F. Brossart, T.R. Elliott, C. McCord, and M.A. Diaz. "Use of Technology to Increase Access to Mental Health Services in a Rural Texas Community." *Fam Community Health* 34.2 (Apr–Jun 2011): 134–140.

47. See K. Tran et al., *Home Telehealth for Chronic Disease Management* [Technology report number 113] (Ottawa: Canadian Agency for Drugs and Technologies in Health, 2008).

48. E.I. Picard and G.B. Robertson, *Legal Liability of Doctors and Hospitals in Canada* (Toronto: Carswell, 2007).

49. M.M. Bujnowska-Fedak et al., "System of Telemedicine Services Designed for Family Doctors' Practices," *Telemedicine Journal & E-Health* 6.4 (2000): 449–452.

50. L. Jarvis and B. Stanberry, "Teleradiology: Threat or Opportunity?" *Clin Radiol* 60.8 (2005): 840–845.

51. E.E. Hogue, "Legalities in Home Care: Telehealth and Risk Management in Home Health," *Home Healthc Nurs* 21.10 (2003): 699–701.

52. J. Liaschenko, "Ethics and the Geography of the Nurse–Patient Relationship: Spatial Vulnerable and Gendered Space," *Sch Inq Nurs Pract* 11.1 (1997): 45–59. While this article deals with nursing, with due alteration of detail the same points apply to medical practice. G. Hindricks et al., "Telemedizin in der Kardiologie: was bringt die Telekardiologie für Patient und Arzt?" *Deutsches Ärzteblatt* 105.4 (2008): A156.

53. Canadian Medical Association. Physician guidelines for online communication with patients. In: CMA Policy [database online]. Ottawa: CMA, 2005. PD05-03, accessed 21 Mar 2011 at http://policybase.cma.ca/dbtw-wpd/PolicyPDF/PD05-03.pdf

54. Canadian Medical Association. Guiding principles for physician electronic medical records (EMR) adoption in ambulatory clinical practice. In: CMA Policy [database online]. Ottawa: CMA, 2008. PD08-05, accessed 21 Mar 2011 at www.cma.ca/multimedia/CMA/Content_Images/Inside_cma/HIT/HIT_meeting/deliverables/EMR_Guiding_Principles_CMA_Policy.pdf

55. World Medical Association, World Medical Association statement on Home Medical Monitoring, "Tele-Medicine" and Medical Ethics. Adopted by the 44th World Medical Assembly, Marbella, Spain, September 1992. Rescinded at the WMA General Assembly, Pilanesberg, South Africa, 2006. Geneva (CH): WMA, 2006, accessed 11 Apr 2008 at www.wma.net/e/policy/h22.htm

56. K.V. Iserson, "Telemedicine: A Proposal for an Ethical Code," *Cambridge Quarterly of Healthcare Ethics* 9.3 (2000): 404–406.

SAMPLE CASES

1. A young woman who is a heroin addict is admitted to hospital with what is diagnosed as an infected tricuspid valve. She is treated with antibiotics and the infection clears up. Three years later, she again presents with an infected tricuspid valve but now needs a valve replacement. She is given a valve replacement and agrees to methadone therapy to deal with her addiction. Two years later, she is admitted to hospital in heart failure—again with an infected tricuspid and again requiring a replacement. There is evidence that she is still suffering from heroin addiction, and it is probable that she contracted the infection from IV heroin use. The infection is currently being controlled—but not cured—by antibiotics. She continues to inject heroin/methadone though the IV tubing while in hospital. She has received counselling about the dangers and problems associated with continued drug use in general and her current position in particular. She has left the hospital on occasion and has returned with evidence of drug use in her urine. The physician in charge of her case is frustrated because of her lack of cooperation and wishes to withdraw from the case.

2. Mrs. B. has been on dialysis for several years and has become increasingly unhappy with her situation. She is not a candidate for transplantation, since she has already had two transplants, both of which have been rejected. Although she has conscientiously adhered to her dietary and lifestyle restrictions, she has voiced dissatisfaction with her situation on many occasions. "Life like this is just not worth living!" One day, while in hospital with pneumonia, she announces that she no longer wishes to be dialyzed; that she "has had it." Her physician tells her that this is "just your uremia talking," and that she will feel better and see her situation differently once she has been dialyzed. She orders dialysis. Mrs. B. is an extremely compliant patient and does not challenge the order.

Chapter 4
Informed Consent

The focus of this chapter is the notion of informed consent and its role in health care decision-making. It sketches several current models of informed consent, evaluates them critically in light of the ethical and legal considerations that arise in actual practice and then explores some of the implications for health care professionals, patients and significant others. Other topics that will be considered include truth telling and the use of placebos.

Questions to Keep in Mind While Reading this Chapter:

1. What is the ethical basis of requiring informed patient consent for health care?

2. Are there exceptions to a physician's duty to obtain informed consent to health care interventions? How does the concept of therapeutic privilege enter here? The Doctrine of Emergency?

3. Which of the three standard approaches to informed consent is ethically the more preferable in the Canadian setting? Why?

4. What is the difference between standards of disclosure and standards of comprehension? Why is this difference important?

5. Is it ever ethical to give placebos?

INTRODUCTION

One of the conclusions to be drawn from the preceding chapters is that all other things being equal, the right to make health care decisions that affect a patient fundamentally belong to that patient. As will become clear in a moment, however, ethics and law have not always agreed on this point—or at least not to the same degree. While the ethical basis that informed this right always lay in the Principle of Autonomy, its legal reflection was a gradual process that began with the general recognition that everyone had the right to be free from personal contract without consent in ordinary situations;[1] but this did not fully extend to the health care context until 1980 with the leading case of *Reibl v. Hughes.*[2] And even then, it took some time for the law to embrace the principle that the right to accept or reject a health care intervention was not tied to age but to competence[3]—which the law calls capacity—that people had the right to prepare advance directives in anticipation of becoming incompetent and that these directives would be binding on health care professionals even if that meant that the individual in question would die.[4]

As was said above, ethically speaking, the right to informed consent is rooted in the Principle of Autonomy: Everyone has the right to self-determination, subject only to the equal and competing rights of others.[5] Clearly, this means that unless a patient (or a duly empowered substitute decision-maker: see Chapter 5, "Substitute Decision-Making") has consented to health care, treating the patient will constitute a violation of the patient's autonomy irrespective of whether the treatment involves physical or mental health care services. Therefore, the phrase "informed consent" is really short for "informed consent or refusal." This was already established in law in the 1935 case of *Mulloy v. Hop Sang*,[6] in which a physician was found guilty of battery for amputating a patient's hand against the patient's express instruction, even though this was medically necessary and he saved the patient's life.

The reason Dr. Mulloy was found guilty of battery is that battery consists of intentionally and voluntarily coming into contact with someone without their consent, whereby that contact is either harmful or offensive to that person. Clearly, amputation requires contact, and as became clear during the trial, this contact occurred without consent and was found "offensive" to Mr. Sang, who valued the integrity of his person. The fact that Dr. Mulloy probably saved Mr. Sang's life was irrelevant. It would have been relevant only if there had been an overriding duty for physicians to save their patients' lives at all costs, irrespective of what the patients wanted. That, however, is not the case, as should already be clear from the discussion of paternalism in the preceding chapter and as will be discussed more fully in Chapter 7, "The Ethics of Deliberate Death," when we deal with the case of *Malette v. Shulman* and the case of *Nancy B. v. Hôtel-Dieu de Quebec* below.

At the same time, Dr. Mulloy would not have been guilty of negligence if he had not amputated Mr. Sang's hand and Mr. Sang had died because, in contrast to battery, negligence involves three standards that must conjointly be met: There must be a duty to act, the failure to act must result in a loss for the person to whom the duty is owed, and the person who has the duty must have shown wanton disregard for the life or safety of the affected person. Since there was no duty to save Mr. Sang's life against his wishes, there would have been no negligence if Dr. Mulloy had followed Mr. Sang's wishes and Mr. Sang had died.

The issue of the physician's duty to use life-saving treatment against the wishes of the patient was again examined by the courts in *Nancy B. v. Hôtel-Dieu de Québec*,[7] and the court agreed—as one would have expected on the basis of the Principle of Autonomy— that even though Ms. B. was ventilator dependent as a result of Guillain-Barré syndrome, she had the right to request that physicians discontinue her life support.[8] One could hope for no stronger expression of this acceptance of autonomy than the Supreme Court's assertion in the 2003 case of *Starson v. Swayze* that "[t]he right to refuse unwanted medical treatment is fundamental to a person's dignity and autonomy."[9] Of course, this assumes that the patients are competent when they reject treatment, because only competent patients can exercise their autonomy in the proper sense of that term. That matter will be explored further in Chapter 5, which deals with substitute decision-making.

This fundamental acceptance of patient autonomy with respect to consent is also recognized by professional medical associations such as the World Medical Association, which states that "a physician shall respect a competent patient's right to accept or refuse treatment,"[10] and by the Canadian Medical Association, which in its Code of Ethics states that an ethical physician should "respect the right of a competent patient to accept or reject any medical care recommended."[11]

However, it is impossible for patients to exercise this right if they either do not have adequate and appropriate information about the choices that are open to them or do not understand them. Even then, patients cannot make a reasonable decision unless they also know their own medical condition. Without such knowledge, their decision-making is essentially blind and cannot be reasonable, because what is reasonable very much depends on the individual's health status.

Finally, patients cannot make rational decisions unless they are competent. If patients are incompetent, their decision-making may be informed, but it will lack ethical validity. Therefore, when patients are incompetent, duly empowered substitute decision-makers must make the relevant decisions for them, lest the patients lose their right to autonomy because of their disability. This would constitute a violation of the Principle of Equality. Of course, it is a nice question how someone who cannot exercise their right to self-determination can still preserve their right to autonomy through a substitute decision-maker who makes their decisions for them. However, this chapter will not deal with this issue. That is the topic of the next chapter, which deals specifically with substitute decision-making. The focus of this chapter are the conditions that must be met for something to count as informed consent. The chapter will simply assume competence on the part of patients. This is not entirely gratuitous. It is the default position in health care decision-making. It is assumed as a matter of course that patients are competent. And while this is a rebuttable presumption, anyone who questions a patient's competence must have reasonable grounds to suppose the contrary.

As an aside—albeit an important one—it does not matter why the patient is competent, i.e., whether the patient is competent through medication without which the patient would be clinically certifiable, or without medication and, so to speak, naturally. The test is whether the patient is competent at all. This is why, in the case of *Starson v. Swayze*, already referred to above, the court found that although the patient was competent only when heavily medicated, because he was then competent, he could then refuse psychotropic medication even though this meant that he would be institutionalized.

PATIENTS AND THEIR MEDICAL RECORDS

As was said a moment ago, the capacity to act as autonomous decision-makers avails patients nothing if the conditions that are necessary for exercising that capacity are not met. Therefore, if one assumes competence, then it is absolutely essential for patients to know what their health status is. Without that knowledge, their decision-making will be blind. However, this information is contained in their medical records. Therefore, it follows that in order for patients to be able to make informed decisions about their health care, they must have access to their medical records.

Several concerns have traditionally been raised against allowing patients access to their own records. One centres in the patients' ability to understand what is in those records. Unless the patients are trained in medicine, they will not understand what is in them and may either make a wrong decision or jump to unwarranted conclusions—which may be just as dangerous.

A second concern is that if litigiously inclined patients had unrestricted access to their records they might be tempted to go "fault fishing." That is to say, medical records contain assessments, diagnoses, prescriptions, etc., that have been made by the physicians who interacted with the patients. Therefore, the records are not only about the patients themselves but also contain information about what might be called a physician's pattern of practice. Unrestricted patient access to medical records would therefore open the door to litigation by any patient who was dissatisfied with a particular outcome or treatment, and physicians would have no defence against this, because their own words could then be used against them.

It has also been argued that patients do not have a right to access their medical records because these belong to the physicians, not the patients. Of course, the patients do provide the basis for what is in the records, because without the patients there would be nothing for the physicians to record. However, what is in the records—the diagnoses, prognoses, prescriptions, etc.—is the work of the physicians. It is the application of their training, expertise and understanding to the problems and issues that are presented to them by their patients. The records are the product of the physicians' work, and as such belong to them. Therefore, access to them should be only at the physicians' discretion.

Finally, it is sometimes argued that patient records often contain information about third parties—i.e., about people other than the patients themselves. To let patients have unrestricted access to their records would thus be to allow them access to information to which they have no right. For instance, medical records may contain information not only about the blood group of a particular patient but also about the blood group of that person's father—for instance, when a patient who has leukemia has to undergo chemotherapy, which might require blood transfusions, but it turns out that the father who volunteered to be a blood donor has a blood group that is incompatible with that of the patient. If the patient had unrestricted access to his or her record, paternity issues might arise and have serious family repercussions. Therefore, access to patient records must always be at the discretion of physicians, precisely to avoid such unfortunate situations.

Patient Ignorance and Failure to Understand

None of these arguments, however, stand up to closer examination. For instance, the argument that patients should not have access to their records because they might misunderstand what is in them and make inappropriate or misguided decisions is easily countered. All physicians have to do to avoid this is offer to go over the records with their patients to make sure that they understand them.

In other words, one may readily accept the premise that patients are not as well qualified as physicians to understand what is in their records, and one may also grant that when patients don't really understand what is in their records they are likely to make inappropriate and misguided health care decisions. However, rather than showing that patients should not have access to their records, what this shows is that physicians should explain the significance of what is in the records and assist patients in gaining an appropriate understanding. In fact, arguably, this is mandated by physicians' fiduciary obligation towards their patients. After all, making informed and reasonable decisions is in the patients' best interests. Presumably, that is why the CMA Code of Ethics states that ethical physicians will provide their patients with the information that they need in order to be able to make informed decisions about their medical care, and that they will "answer their questions to the best of [their] ability."[12]

Patient Records and Litigation

The argument that allowing patients unrestricted access to their records would open the door to fault fishing and litigation is based on two assumptions: *first*, that if patients had access to their records they would in fact be likely to go fault fishing; and *second*, that physicians should be protected against patients finding (or trying to find) fault with the treatment they have received from their physicians either with respect to the manner of that treatment or with respect to its outcome.

Both of these assumptions may be questioned. As to the claim that patients will go fault fishing, the available data indicate quite the contrary. Rather than resulting in increased litigation, patients' access to their records results in increased patient engagement with the health care process and increased patient satisfaction.[13]

As to the assumption that physicians should be protected against patients finding fault with their treatment, it is unclear how one would defend such a position. It certainly does not follow from the fiduciary nature of the physician–patient relationship. The fact that patients are entitled to trust that physicians will act in the patients' best interests does not mean that patients do not have the right to see whether this has in fact occurred. Moreover, it should always be remembered that, in the interest of quality assurance, physicians are subject to checks by provincial medical licensing authorities to see whether their patterns of practice meet and continue to meet appropriate standards. This involves checking the physicians' records inclusive of their patient records. Therefore, there is no presumption that physician records are immune from inspection by appropriate and interested parties. Who could be more appropriate—or more interested—than the subjects of the records themselves?

Ownership of Patient Records

The argument that patient records are the product of the physicians' work and therefore belong to the physicians, not the patients, is equally flawed. Superficially, this stance is justified because, as is generally accepted, everyone is entitled to the fruits of their labour. However, closer consideration shows that acceptance of this principle does not entail that physicians are entitled to claim ownership of the medical records of their patients.

To see why this does not follow, all one needs to do is look at the nature of the physician–patient relationship itself and the condition of its inception. The physician–patient relationship is not simply an encounter between two individuals, one of whom happens to have health care needs and another who happens to have medical qualifications. It is an encounter between two persons, one of whom assumes a professional role— the physician—and another who is the object of the latter's action—namely, the patient. An underlying and generally unstated assumption of this encounter, and of the professional role of the physician, is the understanding that the physician will provide certain services for the patient. Integral to this role is the collection of patient-relative data and the development of a medical record inclusive of diagnosis, prognosis, etc. Outside of this professional role, the physician would not have access to the patient, could not generate patient-relative data and consequently could not produce a medical record. Therefore, the construction of the medical record is predicated on the physician functioning in a professional capacity.

Furthermore, since the physician is paid for this service, it is something that is purchased by the patient.[14] If something is purchased, then whatever is integral to the nature of what is purchased is also part of that purchase. Hence, whatever is produced by the physician in the course of providing the relevant service belongs not to the physician but to the patient who has engaged the physician for that purpose. An integral aspect of providing that service is the production of a patient record. Consequently, the patient record belongs to the patient. And it is the patient who has a dispositionary power over the record, not the physician.[15]

The situation may be likened to that of an artist who produces a work of art on commission, possibly even using materials provided (or paid for) by a client. The artist produces a work of art. However, the artist cannot claim ownership of the work of art thus produced. It belongs to the person who entered into the artist-client relationship with the artist. Likewise, a lawyer may be asked to produce a contract or a will for a particular person. This person will provide the lawyer with data and information. However, again, the lawyer cannot claim a proprietary interest in the contract or the will that he or she produces. In each case, the work of art, the contract or the will, respectively, belong to the client. In other words, they belong to the person who is at the centre of the professional efforts of the professional. The fact that the professional uses her or his professional expertise does not transfer ownership of what is produced using that expertise to the producer. For analogous reasons, then, physicians cannot claim ownership of the patient profiles or records they produce. In fact, proprietary interest in and the right of control over their records lie with the patients.[16]

Therefore, the fact that the patient records are produced by physicians does not establish that they belong to the physicians. Consequently, this cannot be used as a reason for saying that patients have no right of access to their records. There may be reasons why patients should not see their records. In fact, the Doctrine of Therapeutic Privilege, which will be explored in a moment, provides just such a reason. However, that has nothing to do with record ownership. It is based on the physician's fiduciary obligation not to do harm.

Patient Records and Third Parties

Finally, the claim that patients should not have access to their medical records because these may contain third-party information, contains a core of truth. Third-party information is generally privileged. However, this does not entail the blanket conclusion that patients should not have access to their records. All it entails is that those parts of the record that are about third parties should be withheld from the patients. With modern electronic health records, this is relatively easy to do; but even with old-style paper records it does not present much of a problem. But even then, this rule does not apply in all cases. For instance, if the information about third parties is in the record because the patient has divulged it to the physician, there is no reason to withhold it from the patient. No third-party privacy right would be breached by letting the patient see it, because the patient already knows it. After all, that is why the information is in the record in the first place.

The standard rule of thumb, therefore, is that with the exception of therapeutic privilege (which will be discussed later), patients have a right of access to their whole record so as to be able to make informed choices about their health care. This is not merely a matter of ethics. It is also a matter of law. In the leading case of *McInerney v. MacDonald*,[17] the Supreme Court of Canada ruled to the same effect.

INFORMED CONSENT

Since patients have the right to accept or reject any intervention (as is guaranteed by the Principle of Autonomy) and given that they have the right to access their own records, it might seem that this would be sufficient for informed consent. However, this is not quite true. One cannot give informed consent—which is to say, one cannot act as an autonomous person—if one has no options from which to choose. One also cannot make a choice if one is unaware of these options and, equally important, if one does not understand them or their implications. Physicians, therefore, have a duty to take all reasonable steps to ensure that their patients have and understand the available treatment options, so that they can make informed choices. This duty is rooted in the fiduciary nature of the profession.[18] It may be breached only under exceptional circumstances, which will be explored next.

STANDARDS OF DISCLOSURE

This, of course, raises the question of how much information is reasonable. In other words, it raises what has come to be called the issue of appropriate *standard of disclosure*. From a purely conceptual standpoint, there are four possible standards: full, professional, subjective and objective.

Full Disclosure

The standard of full disclosure requires that the patient be provided with all information that has a bearing on the situation in question. From a practical standpoint, however, this presents insuperable problems. No health care professional is aware of all that information. Not only would that require that physicians have access to all possible databases and spend all their time doing research, it would also require that they be fluent in foreign languages such as German, Japanese and Spanish, because not all medical advances are published in English. And even if this were possible, it would be unreasonable, because it would leave no time for physicians to actually practise medicine.

It would also be unrealistic from the patients' perspective, because it would swamp them with information and leave no time for decision-making—to say nothing of the problem of how they are supposed to separate the contextually important from the unimportant. The Principles of Impossibility (no one can have an obligation to do what is impossible) and of Fidelity/best action (if there is a duty to do something, then there is a correlative duty to do it in the best way possible within the limitations of the practical setting) therefore rule out the complete disclosure standard—at least as understood in this sense. Therefore, when one talks about the duty of "complete disclosure," this really refers to the modified objective reasonable person standard that will be discussed in a moment.

Professional Disclosure

The professional standard requires that the physician disclose all and only that information that a similarly placed colleague would disclose under analogous circumstances. This was the traditional standard in Canada. In Canada, it found its most celebrated legal expression in the case of *Kelly v. Hazlett*.[19] In this 1976 Ontario case, the plaintiff had suffered from both crookedness and stiffness of an elbow joint. Her surgeon had proposed to clean out the joint to reduce the stiffness but had advised against an osteotomy to reduce the crookedness. The patient had agreed, but the following day changed her mind and, before being brought into the operating room, persuaded the surgeon to do the osteotomy as well. Under the circumstances, the physician gave her very little information about the possible effects of the osteotomy. The result of the operation was a permanent stiffness of the elbow joint. The judge, in deciding the case, found that the operation itself had been performed with appropriate competence and care and that therefore no cause for action existed on that point. Nevertheless, he found against the surgeon because of lack of adherence to a professional standard of disclosure. As Mr. Justice Morden put it,[20]

> I take it to be the law of this jurisdiction that the duty to disclose the collateral risks inherent in any proposed procedure is substantially a matter of medical judgement, as opposed to being one of absolute and invariable consent unlike the law in some U.S. jurisdictions where the duty is based on a notion of what a reasonable patient might be expected to wish to hear in order to make up his mind.

This was the law for years. However, there are ethical difficulties with a professional standard of disclosure. Because it ties the standard of disclosure to what the medical profession thinks is appropriate, it ignores the status of the patient as an autonomous agent and essentially makes the patient's autonomy subject to the consensus of professional opinion. It therefore confuses technical expertise (which unquestionably belongs to the health care professional) with the right to make a decision (which unquestionably belongs to the patient) because by limiting the information, it limits the patient's decision-making power. In other words, it commits what has been called the fallacy of expertise.[21]

Not surprisingly, therefore, four years later, in 1980 in the leading case of *Reibl v. Hughes*, the Supreme Court of Canada rejected this standard:[22]

> . . . evidence of medical experts of custom or general practice as to the scope of disclosure cannot be decisive, but at most a factor to be considered (when deciding whether a breach of duty of disclosure obtains). *To allow expert medical evidence to determine what risks are material is to hand over to the medical profession the entire question of the scope of the duty of disclosure, including whether there has been a breach of that duty.* [Emphasis added] Expert medical evidence is, of course, relevant to findings as to the risks that reside in or are a result of recommended surgery or other treatment. It will also have a bearing on their materiality, but this is not a question that is to be concluded on the basis of expert medical evidence alone. The issue under consideration is a different issue from that involved where the question is whether the doctor carried out his professional activities by applicable professional standards. *What is under consideration here is the patient's right to know what risks are involved in undergoing or foregoing certain surgery or other treatment.* [Emphasis added]

Subjective Disclosure

These comments may suggest that in the eyes of the Court the subjective standard—which is to say, gearing the physician's duty of disclosure to what the patient wants to know—is the appropriate standard. However, the subjective standard also presents certain problems. To begin with, patients generally are not as expert as physicians. They frequently have no inkling of what information is relevant and what is not. Even worse, quite often patients do not even know where to seek the relevant information and what questions to ask. Even when they use the Internet to expand their understanding, their search is unlikely to result in a truly knowledgeable information base without physician guidance.[23] Therefore, the subjective standard could easily leave patients in a worse position than even the professional standard. That standard, after all, might well require the divulging of information that was not even guessed at by the patients.

The only way to avoid this and save the subjective standard would be to require that physicians adopt a hypothetical stance—i.e., for physicians to reveal what they assume their patients would want to know if they were aware of the relevant parameters. However, this would not really solve the problem either, because it would require that physicians really know their patients. Given modern patient pools of two thousand or more patients, or physicians working in walk-in clinics, etc., that is entirely unrealistic.

Moreover, there is another major difficulty. It is demonstrated quite clearly in the U.S. case of *Canterbury v. Spence*:[24]

> When causality is explored at a post-injury trial with a professedly uninformed patient, the question whether he actually would have turned the treatment down if he had known the risks is purely hypothetical . . . *(Any) answer which the patient supplies hardly represents more than a guess, perhaps tinged by the circumstance that the uncommunicated hazard has in fact materialized*. In our view, this method of dealing with the issue . . . comes in second best. It places the physician in jeopardy of the patient's hindsight and bitterness. It places the fact finder in the position of deciding whether a speculative answer to a hypothetical question is to be credited. It calls for a subjective determination solely on testimony of a patient witness shadowed by the occurrence of an undisclosed risk. [Emphasis added]

In other words, the subjective standard invites retrospective patient re-evaluation in the event of a negative outcome of what they really wanted to know at the time they gave the original consent. Hindsight—particularly after an unfortunate event has occurred—can easily alter one's recollection. The subjective standard therefore puts the physician unfairly at risk. For these reasons, then, the Supreme Court of Canada rejected the subjective standard of disclosure as well.

Objective Reasonable Person Standard

With this in mind, the Supreme Court turned to what is sometimes called the objective reasonable person standard. According to this standard, physicians have an obligation to disclose, *unasked*, what an objective reasonable person would want to know. However, the Court did not leave it at that. It quite correctly distinguished between what an objective reasonable person would want to know and what an objective reasonable person *in the patient's position* would want to know. To quote Chief Justice Laskin:[25]

> I think it is the safer course . . . to consider objectively how far the balance in the risks of surgery or no surgery is in favour of undergoing surgery . . . [The] objective standard would have to be geared to what the average prudent person, *in the patient's particular position*, would agree to or not agree to, if all material or special risks of going ahead with the surgery or foregoing it were made known to him. Far from making the patient's own testimony irrelevant, it is essential . . . that he put his own position forward. [Emphasis added]

In other words, what this judgment says is that Canadian physicians must take into account the position of the particular patient who is to make the decision. This is important for two reasons. *First*, and quite generally, consent is the exercise of decisional autonomy by a particular person on a given occasion. The objective reasonable person, however, is a statistical entity. Linking the standard of disclosure to this statistical entity would be appropriate only if wanting to know more than the average person automatically branded that request as unreasonable. However, this is not necessarily the case. There may be factors in a patient's life that would make such information eminently reasonable even though it might not be reasonable for other patients who are not in that particular position. Exercising decisional autonomy, therefore, both ethically and legally requires paying attention not only to the options that are available but also to the factual embedding of the decision-maker.

Second, even the factual embedding of a decision-maker does not define what constitutes a reasonable amount of information. Decisions involve the application of values to the facts at hand. Canada is a multicultural society whose various subcultures differ from each other in their values, expectations and standards. For instance, what an objective reasonable member of the Nuu-chah-nulth First Nation would want to know when deciding on a treatment for leukemia would probably differ from what an objective reasonable member of the Jehovah's Witness community would want to know, and what an objective reasonable member of the Chinese-Canadian or Iranian-Canadian community would want to know might differ from this in turn—and these might all differ from what the objective reasonable French- or Anglo-Canadian might want to know. Failure to take such differences into account and insisting on a single objective reasonable person standard would be unethical, because it would constitute a *de facto* abrogation of a patient's decision-making autonomy by ignoring the relevant differences of this person from any other. That is why the Supreme Court insisted that the disclosure must be geared to "the patient's particular position." Ethically speaking, this characterizes the Supreme Court's decision as one of the most enlightened in any jurisdiction. It means that the objective reasonable person standard as enunciated in this fashion becomes tinged with a significant element of subjectivity. In a multicultural society such as Canada, this is extremely important.

Unquestionably, this places a tremendous burden on physicians in that it requires them to be at least somewhat familiar with the circumstances and values of their patients. However, that lies in the very nature of the fiduciary nature of the physician–patient relationship. If physicians cannot (or do not) take the time with their patients to explore what (if anything) makes them different from other patients, then they are not acting as physicians but as glorified mechanics. That is why the Supreme Court also said that "What the doctor knows or *should* know that the particular patient deems relevant to a decision whether to undergo prescribed treatment goes equally to his duty of disclosure as do the material risks recognized as a matter of required medical knowledge."[26]

Taking all this into account, therefore, it may perhaps be more appropriate to call the Canadian standard the *modified objective reasonable person standard* to distinguish it from the objective reasonable person standard that exists in the U.S. The reason it is important to emphasize this distinction is that much of the published literature in health care comes from the U.S. Although in many ways the U.S. is multicultural, it does not see itself as a mosaic of cultures, as does Canada, but as a melting pot. It therefore assumes that there is only one reasonable person—namely, the average American—and structures both its ethics and its consent law accordingly. Any legal considerations, therefore, and most discussions of the ethics of consent that originate in the U.S. context should be viewed with extreme caution. With due alteration of detail, similar remarks apply to considerations that originate in the U.K. While the U.K. has moved somewhat in the direction of Canada on this issue,[27] it has not as yet reached the full application of the principle of autonomy as it is found in the Canadian setting.

Another aspect worth mentioning is that the professional's duty of disclosure is not confined to the disclosure of the risks that are attendant on the various procedures presented to the patient. Health care institutions may have cost containment protocols in place and will not provide all available or even all effective interventions, merely those that are insured under the provincial health care plan. However, it may well be the case that the objective reasonable person in the patient's position would have opted for an uninsured procedure—even at the expense of going to a private clinic—if the patient had known about it. Therefore, the modified objective reasonable person standard includes the duty to disclose relevant treatment options, even though they may not be insured or be available in the patient's home province.[28]

An interesting question is whether disclosure during the informed consent process should also include information about the practice profiles of the physician who will perform a particular procedure, or the track record of an institution in which the procedure will be performed. Arguably, a reasonable person would want to know whether a physician has been successfully sued for negligence or whether the success rate of a particular hospital or clinic in which the particular intervention will be performed is significantly lower than that of another institution.

This idea is expressed in the *Declaration of Lisbon*, which states that "the patient has the right to the information necessary to make his/her decisions."[29] One could reasonably argue that the prerequisite for making an informed decision is information not merely about the proposed intervention but also about the outcomes as performed by the physician in question. Much as the medical profession dislikes admitting it, not all physicians are equally proficient. Indeed, it would be a miracle if they were. Physicians, after all, are only human—and human beings differ in their abilities, proficiencies, training and in the successfulness of their actions. Information about practice profiles would allow patients to identify physicians whose proficiency is questionable (because they have been successfully sued for negligence, etc.) and those who have otherwise acted inappropriately as professionals and have been disciplined. Arguably, it is only when patients have this kind of information that they are adequately informed.[30] Some jurisdictions in the U.S. have accepted this reasoning and have put physicians' profiles on the Web for patients to consider.[31]

Likewise, there are data which show that the more a medical team works together or a physician performs a particular intervention, the better the outcome.[32] Therefore, arguably, part of the informed consent process should involve information about how often the physician or the medical team have performed the relevant intervention, and how successful they have been.

STANDARDS OF COMPREHENSION

However, information that is not understood is not information—at least, not as far as the recipient of that information is concerned. For instance, lectures on the eigenvalues of skew-Hermitian matrices or on enzyme-catalyzed chemical reactions given to junior high-school students who have no training in advanced algebra or in organic chemistry would contain information, but the information would be incomprehensible to the students; and a lecture on the Inuit sea god Aipalovik delivered in Inuktitut to cultural anthropology majors who spoke only English and French might be highly informative to someone who spoke the language, but would be just so much noise to the students who didn't speak Inuktitut.

The point is that there is a difference between information as an objective phenomenon and information as a subjective phenomenon. Standards of disclosure deal with information as an objective phenomenon—what is disclosed; standards of comprehension deal with information as a subjective phenomenon—what is understood. Unless the two coincide—unless what is disclosed is actually understood—there can be no informed consent. One might well make a decision, but the decision would be like an agreement to go gworking with a half-strung shrudlu at xingukraik. In other words, it would merely be opting uncomprehendingly for an alternative that one does not understand.

The relevance of these considerations to informed consent lies in the fact that consent is something given by a particular person relative to a set of specific facts that this particular person actually understands. Therefore, a modified objective reasonable person standard of disclosure is not enough for informed consent. All persons differ in their understanding, and one cannot simply assume that, just because an ordinary reasonable person in the patient's position would understand the information, *this* patient understands.

Moreover, the ordinary reasonable person in the patient's position is a statistical notion. However, the individual who is supposed to give consent is not a statistical entity. It is *this* particular person. This means that the level at which the information is disclosed—which is to say, the standard of comprehension—must be geared to the level of understanding of the individual who is supposed to give consent. In other words, it must be subjective.

This ethical fact is well understood by UNESCO when, in its statement on informed consent, it stipulates that[33]

> information must be communicated to the patient in a manner that is consistent with
> the patient's capacity to understand and in a form that maximizes such understanding.

and by the Canadian Medical Association when, in its Code of Ethics, it states that an ethical physician should "make every reasonable effort to communicate with . . . patients in such a way that information exchanged is understood."[34]

This fact is also what underlay the Supreme Court's decision in *Reibl v. Hughes*, when it said that a physician has a strict duty to explain to a patient, *in language that the patient can understand*, the essential nature and quality of the options that are open to the patient;[35] and that the physician must make sure that the patient *has in fact understood* the nature, gravity and extent of risks specifically attendant on the various options.[36] That is why physicians must gear the comprehension standard to the level of their particular patients.[37]

Therefore, both ethics and law agree that the standard of disclosure must be objective and adjusted to the particular position of the specific patient in question, whereas the standard of comprehension or understanding must be subjective. Unquestionably, this makes the physician's job more difficult, because the physician cannot pitch disclosure at a standard level of sophistication. Instead, the level must be adjusted anew to each situation and to the intellectual capacity and the education level of each patient.

However, that is neither unduly burdensome—after all, what lies at the very basis of the medical profession is the treatment of the patient as person—nor is it impossible. One patient's difficulty in understanding what another patient understands may simply be a function of lack of schooling, not intellectual capacity. It would be no more insurmountable than a dermatologist's difficulty in understanding the jargon of a nuclear physicist who designs single photon emission computed tomography devices for imaging, of an accountant who plans and runs the finances of a hospital or medical institution or of any other professional with whom the physician interacts. It is all a matter of adjusting the language and level of discussion to the sophistication and level of training of the individual in question.

This last point is important. It is tempting to assume that a patient's failure to comprehend what has been expressed in clear and objective language indicates a lack of competence on part of the patient, and that therefore the physician should look for a substitute decision-maker. (See Chapter 5 for an extended discussion of substitute decision-making.) However, that may not be the case. For instance, a twelve-year-old may not understand the options for treating her leukemia when this is explained to her at the level of a sixteen-year-old or even at the level of an adult, but she may understand it perfectly well when it is explained to her at her particular level of sophistication. The physician who wishes to treat her leukemia therefore has a duty to adjust the level of explanation to her ability to understand. This is not merely an ethical point. It is reflected in the legal case of *re K. (L.D.)*,[38] in which the court found that a twelve-year-old could understand the treatment options that were available for dealing with her leukemia when they were presented at her level, and therefore accepted that she had the capacity to make the treatment decision on her own behalf. (For further discussion of consent by children, see Chapter 5.)

The issue of children and consent will be discussed more fully in a moment and will also figure in the next chapter, which deals with substitute decision-making. For now, the important point to remember is that failure to understand is not necessarily a sign of lack of capacity. It may simply be a sign that the information has not been disclosed at the subjective level of the particular patient. In other words, it may be indicative of a failure in communication. Such a failure tends to be obvious when there is a language barrier—for example, when physician and patient speak different languages or when a patient is only partly fluent, as may happen with immigrants or with members of First Nations who have little opportunity to use either of the official languages. Here the physician's fiduciary duty to ensure that the modified objective reasonable person standard of disclosure and the subjective level of comprehension are met entails that the physician has to involve the services of someone who can function as an interpreter. This extends even so far as obtaining the services of someone who can convey the information in sign language if that should prove necessary.[39]

AGE AND CONSENT

As was mentioned a moment ago, Canadian courts have held that twelve-year-old children have the right to make their own health care decisions if they have capacity. It may be appropriate to discuss the matter at this point without, however, going into the issue of capacity itself, which is discussed in the next chapter. The matter is important because it goes to the very heart of the ethics of informed consent.

As was said in the beginning, the right to informed consent is nothing more nor less than an application of the Principle of Autonomy to the health care setting. Autonomy, however, is not a function of age. It is a function of capacity; and while age tends to be a good indicator of capacity, it is not necessarily a conclusive one. For example, a person may be twenty-five years old and lack capacity because of severe mental disability, whereas someone who is twelve or thirteen may be perfectly capable of making health care decisions. Likewise, someone may be forty-five years old but lack capacity because of severely impaired brain function due to a stroke, whereas another person may be one hundred and two and still be fully competent, loss of brain mass due to age-related neural degeneration[40] notwithstanding. Moreover, the Principle of Equality and Justice entails that one should not discriminate on the basis of ethically irrelevant differences. What is ethically central to consent is capacity. Therefore, if someone has capacity, then ethically, that is all that counts.

Canadian law captures these considerations very well. Thus, section 15 of the Charter of Rights and Freedoms stipulates that Canadian public policy may not discriminate on the basis of religion, ethnic extraction, disability or age, and section 1 of the Charter states that this may be overruled only if it is demonstrably necessary to do so for a free and democratic society. Therefore, the right to self-determination may be overruled on a given occasion but—and the case of *R. v. Oakes* spells this out very clearly—certain conditions must be met for this to be the case: There must be no other way of dealing with the situation, the limitation that is imposed on the rights of the individual must be directly connected with the aim to be achieved, and this limitation must follow the Principle of the Least Intrusive Alternative—which is to say, it must interfere with the rights of the individual only to the least degree necessary to achieve the otherwise legitimate end.

The Supreme Court specifically applied these considerations to the issue of consent by minors in the case of *A.C. v. Manitoba (Director of Child and Family Services)*.[41] A.C., who suffered from Crohn's disease, was almost fifteen years old when she was admitted to hospital with acute gastrointestinal bleeding. Her condition, although initially treatable without a blood transfusion, deteriorated over the next few days, and in the opinion of the attending physician it became necessary to give her a transfusion to stave off serious medical consequences and possibly death. A.C. was a Jehovah's Witness and therefore believed that, in accordance with God's commands, she should abstain from all blood and blood products. Shortly before her admission to hospital she had executed an advance directive (for more on advance directives, see Chapter 5), in which she clearly stated her refusal of blood and blood products under any circumstances, and she repeated this refusal explicitly when the issue came up during her treatment.

Her attending physician sought a court order to allow a blood transfusion under sections 25(8) and 25(9) of the Manitoba *Child and Family Services Act*. The relevant provisions of the Act state that[42]

> **25(8)** Subject to subsection (9), upon completion of a hearing, the court may authorize a medical examination or any medical or dental treatment that the court considers to be in the best interests of the child.
>
> **25(9)** The court shall not make an order under subsection (8) with respect to a child who is 16 years of age or older without the child's consent unless the court is satisfied that the child is unable
>
> > (a) to understand the information that is relevant to making a decision to consent or not consent to the medical examination or the medical or dental treatment; or
> >
> > (b) to appreciate the reasonably foreseeable consequences of making a decision to consent or not consent to the medical examination or the medical or dental treatment.

The order was granted. On appeal, A.C. argued that the relevant sections of the *Manitoba Act* violated her Charter rights. The appeal was denied, but the Supreme Court agreed to hear the matter and gave its decision on June 26, 2009. It upheld the Court of Appeal's decision in a majority decision of 6 to 1. However, it upheld the lower court's decision only because it accepted the lower court's finding that A.C. lacked capacity. Moreover, it stated that[43]

> a rigid statutory distinction that completely ignored the actual decision-making capabilities of children under a certain age would fail to reflect the realities of childhood and child development

and went on to say that[44]

> a young person is entitled to a degree of decisional autonomy commensurate with his or her maturity . . . with the child's views becoming increasingly determinative as his or her maturity increases.

In other words, Canadian law follows the ethics by decoupling consent from age and by rejecting an absolute or "rigid statutory distinction" that is based solely on age. Capacity is the key. Since all Canadian provinces and territories have child and family legislation similar to Manitoba's, the Supreme Court's decision means that all such legislation must be applied in accordance with the guidelines given in A.C. In particular, it means that physicians have to involve children in health care decision-making and must follow the child's wishes if there are clear indications that the child has capacity.[45]

PATIENT DELEGATION OF CONSENT

Given, then, that—subject to capacity—all patients have the right to informed consent, does this mean that the patient *must* make the decision, no matter what? The question is important because it sometimes happens that patients say to their physicians something like "You're the doctor, you decide!" or "I come to you as your patient. I don't want to make those decisions. That's your job."

By way of answer, it is important to remember that a right is not a duty. The difference between the two is not merely one of vocabulary but goes to the very heart of the issue. A right differs fundamentally from a duty in that it is a (justified) claim that a person has towards another. The person may take up that claim or not, as she wishes. A duty, on the other hand, is a justified claim that others have towards us. Therefore it is something that we must do when the relevant claim is exercised by the right-holder. We then have no choice. Since informed consent is a right and not a duty, it follows that patients may refuse to make a decision and simply allow others to decide for them. As the Royal College of Physicians and Surgeons put it, "Competent patients may waive this right to informed consent in full or in part,"[46] and as Chief Justice Bora Laskin expressed it in *Reibl v. Hughes*:[47]

> It is, of course, possible that a particular patient may waive aside any question of risks and be quite prepared to submit to surgery or treatment, whatever they be. If the physician is prepared to accept the decision-making burden such a situation presents no difficulty.

However, giving up the right to informed consent has consequences. For example, if a patient voluntarily and competently gives up that right, then the patient cannot legitimately complain if the decisions that are made by the health care professional are not the ones that he or she likes—or if they result in a negative outcome.

Moreover, a physician—or, for that matter, anyone else who is delegated such decision-making authority—does not have to accept what amounts to a delegation of decision-making authority. (For more on this, see Chapter 5.) It is not normally part of physicians' professional obligation to make decisions for their patients.[48] Things may have been different under the old paternalistic model of the physician–patient relationship, but it certainly does not hold in the fiduciary model. Of course, if a physician does agree, then the decision must be made in the patient's best interests; but, as was pointed out before, that may be problematic if the physician does not know the patient very well or does not know the patient's values. Therefore, if a patient really does not want to make a decision, the appropriate thing for a physician to do is to have the patient appoint a substitute decision-maker. Failing that, and if the physician is agreeable, the patient should be very clear about what values the physician should follow when making a decision on the patient's behalf.

INFORMED CONSENT: SOME CONSIDERATIONS OF PRACTICE

Obtaining Consent

At this juncture, two questions arise: Who should obtain informed consent? and What form should the consent take?

As to who should obtain the consent, the ethics of the matter is relatively simple—even though it is sometimes ignored in practice. Consent should be obtained by the person who is responsible for performing the procedure in question.

The reason for this lies in the nature of informed consent itself. Informed consent is agreeing to a procedure or an undertaking on the basis of information that has been disclosed according to the appropriate standard and that has been understood. It therefore requires that an appropriate exchange of information take place. (We here ignore the factor of voluntariness, which is dealt with separately later.) It follows that consent for a medical or surgical procedure cannot be obtained by anyone other than the physician who is performing or is responsible for the intervention. This is not to say that nurses may not enter the picture. After all, they do provide patient care, and usually on a more continuous basis even than attending physicians. Therefore, the information they can provide is relevant and may be an integral part of the information the patient should receive before deciding whether to give or withhold consent. But the significance of this information depends on the larger medical/surgical picture that only the physician who will perform or supervise the treatment can provide. The only exception is when the physician actually performing the procedure is not qualified to explain the risk—for instance, a resident who is working under the preceptorship of another physician.[49] Therefore, when nurses—or, for that matter, anyone other than the attending physician—are asked to obtain patient consent to a medical or surgical procedure, that consent is neither ethically nor legally valid. This can also be tied to the discussion of the physician–patient relationship in the preceding chapter (Chapter 3, "The Health Care Professional–Patient Relationship"). Under the fiduciary model, the patient's trust for medical care centres in the physician. That is why it is the attending physician—and no one else—who has the obligation to provide appropriate information and to obtain consent.[50]

Forms and Other Matters

Which brings into focus the second question: What form should consent take? The answer, again, is not very difficult. As long as the consent is competently given, voluntary and informed, it does not matter ethically or legally how it is expressed. For example, consent given in sign language is just as valid as consent given in written form, and verbal consent is equally legitimate. If it were otherwise, quadriplegic but competent patients could not give consent, and consent would not be possible if there were no writing tools or forms to sign.[51]

Consent also does not have to be on a special form or be accompanied by a signature either. In fact, as should be clear from what has already been said, a signature on a form will constitute consent if, and only if, the whole consent process that has been outlined in the preceding discussion has preceded the signing of the form.

The other thing to consider in this connection is that forms are geared to typical circumstances and to the average person. Consent, however, is specific to the individual who gives that consent and to the particular circumstances that obtain. A consent that does not take these particulars into account is neither ethically nor legally valid—which also means that a general consent is not valid either.[52]

This also means that a consent is valid only as long as the situation remains as was outlined in the consent process. As soon as the circumstances change in any way that an objective reasonable person in the patient's position would want to know, a new consent must be sought. The original consent will no longer be valid.[53]

Finally, consent is not a once-and-forever thing. Patients may change their minds. When patients change their minds and withdraw consent, the relevant procedures must be stopped precisely because consent has been withdrawn. Performing a procedure without consent is a violation of a patient's person and hence amounts to battery. The only exception is if stopping the procedure would present serious risk to the patient's health and welfare.[54]

TYPES OF CONSENT

Consent may either be assumed, entailed, implied or explicit. *Assumed consent* occurs when the health care professional assumes that because the patient has come to a health care facility, physician's office or a lab, the patient has in fact given consent to whatever medical intervention is usually provided in that setting. For instance, physicians and nurses tend to assume that if a patient has come to the emergency department of a hospital, the patient has given consent to the kind of care that is standardly provided in emergency departments, including intubation, blood transfusion and resuscitation if that should prove necessary to stabilize the patient. Similarly, health care professionals tend to assume that in the absence of any indication to the contrary, patients would want the kinds of treatment that Canadians generally agree to, and therefore they often do not seek an explicit consent from the patient.

This assumption, however, may not be justified. For instance, a patient may have gone to an emergency department simply to receive medication for the excruciating pain that he is experiencing but would have rejected any other intervention if he had been asked. Alternatively, suppose a patient is brought to the emergency department of a hospital with heavy blood loss as the result of an accident. The staff would be justified in assuming that she would want her injuries attended to; however, the staff would be unjustified in assuming that she agreed to (or would have agreed to) a blood transfusion even though most Canadians would normally agree to it. This particular patient might be different.[55] The general rule of thumb, therefore, is that unless the Doctrine of Emergency applies—which will be discussed in a moment—if consent can be had, it *must* be had. If the patient is unable to give consent (and the Doctrine of Emergency does not apply), the consent should be sought from a duly empowered substitute decision-maker.

Entailed consent is consent that is not explicitly sought but that follows from the consent given for another intervention. For instance, if a patient has given consent to major surgery that involves pain, such as a bowel resection or an appendectomy, consent to the surgery entails consent to anesthesia, since the surgery cannot realistically be performed without it (because of the patient's motion in response to the pain of cutting, shock, etc.). At the same time, there are limits even here. Specifically, if consent to a given procedure entails consent to another procedure but there are various options for performing that other procedure, then the patient must be asked which one of the options is acceptable. An example would here be the case of a woman who has consented to a C-section—which, of course, requires anesthesia. However, that anesthesia may be provided either as a general anesthesia, which renders her unconscious, or as a spinal anesthesia, which will merely deaden her to the pain but leave her conscious and aware.

Implied consent differs from entailed consent in that there is no need to obtain consent for a procedure or intervention that flows from a previous consent or an overt and unmistakable action. For instance, when someone goes to a lab to get a blood test and holds out his or her arm so that the phlebotomist can insert a needle to take the blood sample, nothing need be said or otherwise communicated. The act of holding out the arm in itself implies consent to the procedure. A possible exception to this, of course, would be if the patient felt coerced or if the patient's action did not have the same meaning in his or her particular socio-cultural subgroup that it has in Canadian society in general. Determining the latter, however, falls within the fiduciary duty to become familiar with relevant data about the patient.

Explicit—or, as it is sometimes also called, *express*—consent is the gold standard of consent in health care. Under explicit consent, the patient agrees to a particular intervention and indicates this verbally, in writing or by some other unequivocally clear method of communication. One should be careful, however, not to assume that because explicit consent has been given, it is therefore valid. Nothing can make a general consent valid, no matter how explicitly given, and a consent given under duress or influenced by power relationship, etc., will not be valid either.

FACTORS AFFECTING FREEDOM OF CONSENT

Cultural Parameters and Freedom to Decide

A final, albeit pivotal, assumption in informed consent is freedom: the ability of the decision-maker to make effective choices in an unconstrained fashion. We generally assume that we are free in the choices and decisions that we make and that we are unconstrained by influences not within our own control. That assumption, however, is unrealistic— even outside of the health care context. All of us, through the process of growing up in a particular culture and learning its language, acquire a conceptual framework that limits the range of what is meaningful to us. Each one of us is therefore constrained by the conceptual and valuational limits of the cultural and subcultural framework in which we are raised and in which we are embedded. It may influence the validity of our consent.

The point is graphically illustrated by the notion of illness itself. All of us assume that we know what the term means, and in our own contexts we surely do. Closer examination, however, reveals that its significance is culture dependent. So, for instance, it is entirely different in Hopi culture from what it is in English,[56] and it is different again in a Sikh[57] or Japanese-Canadian[58] setting.

In and of itself, this would not be particularly startling or important. However, it becomes important when we realize that the notion of illness defines a framework of appropriate behaviour—of sickness behaviour, or of what sometimes has been called the patient role—and this framework differs from cultural context to cultural context.[59] This difference holds not merely with respect to the notion of illness in general, but to particular illnesses and how they relate to the roles of the individual patients as actors in their social milieu. Because of that difference, options that are apparent from an Anglo-Canadian interpretation of illness may not even be relevant to someone not from that background; and the physician who simply assumes a common shared framework, and who bases his or her approach to informed consent on it, may commit a serious error.

Of course, the matter is obvious when it is stated so baldly. Things are not quite so clear, however, in the context of actual health care delivery. We tend to assume that because we speak the same language and because we function in the same national setting, we share the same general framework of concepts and values.[60] But this is not necessarily the case. Health care professionals are caught in this as much as patients are. Sometimes a commonality of language and vocabulary hides a dissimilarity of perspectives and values. And it is this absence of valuational and cultural congruity that may impair the freedom of the patient's decision-making.

More specifically, it may affect the range of options open to the patient because the patient may not understand and gauge the significance of the relevant terms in the same way as the physician, and *vice versa*. What are presented as reasonable alternatives by the physician, because within his or her framework they lack negative valuational associations, may in fact be quite unreasonable and not even exist as options within the patient's framework. For example, to a young Canadian woman of Anglo-Saxon background, the suggestion that she undergo a radical hysterectomy will be tinged with personal tragedy, all other things being equal, but it will lack the serious social and cultural overtones that such a suggestion would hold for a young woman of East-Indian or Asian extraction, for whom having children sometimes plays a crucial role in the spiritual life of the person and the family.[61] Therefore, even though a physician may outline the nature of the options open to the patient with what to the physician may seem to be exemplary clarity, and even though the patient may understand these options in a purely conceptual sense, their meanings as possible choices of actions may escape the patient because their significance as choices may not be part of the patient's valuational framework—or may have a significance that is not apparent to the physician.

A physician who proceeds in the consultative and consent process in ignorance of this sort of difficulty will run the danger of obtaining a consent that, because of the cultural variables, is not really free. This is part of the reason why the Supreme Court was quite correct when it insisted that to set the stage for truly free and informed consent, physicians must apprise themselves of whatever the subculturally unique aspects of their patients' value systems may be. Ethically, this is not only appropriate but necessary.[62] The cultural milieus of patients may impose freedom-limiting barriers that must be transcended if patients are to make choices that are truly voluntary and free—because in order for those choices to be truly voluntary and free, the situations must be presented to the patients in terms that are meaningful in their cultural and valuational contexts without allowing that context to rob them of the ability to transcend it, i.e., to make truly free choices. This, of course, is a tall order. However, the fact that Canada is a multicultural society, established by the Charter and recognized in case law, suggests that the attempt to transcend it should be made.

Non-Cultural Parameters

Other factors may also affect the freedom and hence the genuineness of consent: factors that reside not in a patient's embedding in a particular cultural or subcultural context but in the specific material facts of the case. Such material facts may be classified as being epistemic, external and internal in nature. The epistemic factors have already been dealt with in our discussion on the nature, amount and subjective availability of the information given to the patient. As was said then, insufficient or incomprehensible information limits the range of choices open to the decision-maker as much as the valuational and cultural framework in which the individual is embedded. It therefore acts as a constraint on liberty.

Freedom-Limiting Parameters—External External freedom-limiting parameters are different. They reside in certain aspects of the settings in which patients find themselves. They may be material or contextual. Material external freedom-limiting parameters include such things as forcible confinement and physical restraints. They require little comment. Any patient consent (or refusal) that is obtained under such conditions is not free and therefore cannot be considered binding.

Contextual freedom-limiting external parameters may be more subtle. They include such things as the very fact that the patient is in an institutionalized setting such as a hospital, clinic or even a nursing home. The reason for their potentially freedom-impairing effect is that institutionalization itself may interfere with the volitional capacity of a patient who is not used to such a setting.

That is to say, human beings are social animals. As such, at least part of the meaning in their lives comes from their familiar, everyday social relations. Not only do these provide comfort in a time of crisis (as well as pleasure in times of joy), they also help to define the identity of the individual as a member of the group. When these lines of connection are severed or when their normal functioning is interfered with, the identity of the individual is threatened. The individual therefore instinctively tries to compensate for this loss by attempting to strike new relations that will define his or her role, and thereby provide security and identity.[63]

In the institutionalized context, this usually expresses itself in the patient's heightened compliance with what is perceived as the accepted norm or with the wishes of the person perceived to be in authority. Thus, a patient in a hospital or a long-term care facility may well make choices that he or she would repudiate in a familiar domestic context. The following case illustrates this sort of situation:

> Mr. K. was an independent sixty-eight-year-old who had lived all alone after his wife had died. He had managed his own affairs without any help, and the very idea of being dependent on anyone evoked an extremely negative response from him. He fell and broke his hip, and as a result of this and complications that had occurred, he was now a resident in an extended care facility. It was standard custom in that facility that all residents who had trouble sleeping were issued sleeping medication as a matter of course and were expected to take it. It was simply part of the culture of the place. Mr. K. had always rejected the idea of sleep medication, and had always said that anyone who took it was simply asking for trouble. At entry into the extended care facility he had made his view known to the staff—who in turn let him know in no uncertain terms that this was the policy, everyone did it, and that he had better conform. Their behaviour and attitude—as well as their remarks—seemed to have the desired effect on him. After several days in the facility he started to take the medication even though he felt that he did not need it—and soon the whole thing became a matter of routine with him as well.

This case of Mr. K is not a high-profile one, and it certainly does not reflect standard procedure in extended care facilities. However, it does illustrate the point that institutionalization may affect the volitional stance of individuals to such a degree that they may succumb to what is presented as standard policy simply to establish and retain their place within the environment—i.e., to establish and maintain lines of connection.

Freedom-Limiting Parameters—Internal As to internal freedom-limiting factors that may undermine the validity of consent, they include such things as addiction, emotions, psychoses, neuroses and conditioning. For example, a patient may agree with his physician to quit smoking for medical reasons but be unable to carry out the decision because his addiction is too strong. Emotions may have a similar effect. A patient may be so emotionally overwrought by a diagnosis of breast cancer that she is simply unable to decide on which method of treatment to accept. Psychoses and neuroses can also interfere with the ability to choose and carry out a particular decision—not because the patient does not understand but because the patient simply cannot implement the decision.[64] Conditioning may have a similar effect—something that is especially worrisome for physicians when dealing with patients who have been raised in a particular religious setting that rejects certain types of therapy even though they may be life-saving. These and similar factors may interfere with a patient's ability to either make a free and uncoerced decision or carry out what they have freely decided.

There is one further parameter that is worth mentioning in this connection. It sometimes happens that a patient rejects a treatment where at first glance this refusal seems quite uncoerced. In actuality, however—and the physician may even suspect this—what is going on is something quite different. Either because of a cultural background or a psychological idiosyncrasy, the patient actually wants to agree but feels unable to do so unless repeatedly urged to do so by someone in authority, such as a physician.[65] In other words, whether for cultural or psychological reasons, a patient may feel that unless the treatment is pressed on her, she is not really considered a worthwhile human being. Therefore she may not agree, whereas in reality she really would like to. In this sort of situation the patient's refusal will not really be free and voluntary.

Factors like these are easily overlooked by health care professionals who are not sufficiently alive to the multicultural nature of the Canadian society. Their identification calls for special efforts and sensitivity, and may require special training in communication skills. That being said, however, this does not invalidate the previous considerations concerning the ethics of informed consent. The ethical parameters remain the same. The patient still has the right to self-determination and therefore the right to make the ultimate decision. In these cases, the parameters of the context have to be adjusted, so that the patient can effectively exercise that right. Again, the burden this places on physicians as communicators and facilitators of the decision-making process is great, but it is part and parcel of what it means to be a physician in Canada.

Power Relationships   A final but important freedom-limiting parameter is captured by the phrase "power relationship." The notion came to legal prominence in the case of *Norberg v. Wynrib*.[66] Ms. Norberg was addicted to Fiorinal, and in order to obtain a sufficient supply of the drug she acquiesced to the sexual demands of Dr. Wynrib. The case ultimately came to trial, and in his defence Dr. Wynrib noted that Ms. Norberg had understood the nature of their interaction and had consented to it. He argued that therefore he should not be found guilty of assault. The court rejected his argument:[67]

> The concept of consent . . . is based on a presumption of individual autonomy and
> free will. It is presumed that the individual has freedom to consent or not to consent.
> This presumption, however, is untenable in certain circumstances. A position of

relative weakness can, in some circumstances, interfere with the freedom of a person's will. [The] notion of consent must, therefore, be modified to appreciate the power relationship between the parties . . . In particular, in certain circumstances, consent will be considered legally ineffective if it can be shown that there was such a disparity in the relative positions of the parties that the weaker party was not in a position to choose freely.

In other words, a patient may be cognitively, emotionally and valuationally perfectly competent, but his or her autonomy may be compromised by the fact that the professional has greater authority and is in a position of control. While this is always the case in the sense that it is the professional—in this case the physician—who ultimately functions as gatekeeper to any care and any intervention, that control is misused and amounts to a sheer exercise of power if what the patient is required to do (or to agree to) has nothing to do with a therapeutic relationship and, moreover, the patient would not normally agree to it but for the power differential.

EXCEPTIONS TO INFORMED CONSENT

There are two assumptions that underlie the preceding discussion: One is that there is sufficient time to go through the informed consent process with the patient; the other is that disclosure of the relevant information will not interfere with the patient's ability to make a decision or jeopardize the physician's ability to act in a truly fiduciary manner. Neither of these conditions may, in fact, be met.

The Doctrine of Emergency

The first assumption may not be met when time is of the essence. In that case, the Doctrine of Emergency applies. According to the Doctrine of Emergency, if time is of the essence—in other words, if the physician must act immediately because otherwise the patient would suffer serious and irremediable harm—then the physician must do what is medically indicated without patient consent if the patient lacks capacity to give consent, if there is no reasonably available advance directive that is specific to the case, and if no substitute decision-maker is reasonably available to make the relevant decision.

The Doctrine of Emergency is rooted in the physician's fiduciary obligation to do the best for the patient. When a patient lacks competence but a treatment decision has to be made and acted upon without delay, and when no duly empowered substitute decision-maker is reasonably available—which is to say, is unavailable within the time frame necessary for making the decision—then for the physician not to act would be for the physician to become responsible for a preventable harm. That would violate both the Principle of non-Malfeasance and the Principle of Beneficence and thereby be in contravention of the physician's fiduciary duty to do the best for the patient. With due alteration of detail, it applies to all other health care professionals.

However, it bears repeating that this doctrine is very narrowly circumscribed. It does not apply if a clear, specific and relevant advance directive is reasonably available—for example, if the patient has a card in her purse that says that under no circumstances does she want any blood or blood products, as was the case with Mrs. Malette in the case already mentioned above. It also does not apply if a duly empowered substitute decision-maker is reasonably available, whether in person, by telephone or however. It also does not mean that the health care professional is entitled to make the decision on the basis of her or his own values. The decision must be the sort of decision that the objective reasonable person would be expected to make.[68]

The Doctrine of Therapeutic Privilege

Sometimes it happens that a patient is in such a condition that, in the opinion of the physician, if he or she were given the relevant information, the patient would suffer harm. That is to say, sometimes there are situations in which, in the opinion of the physician, the disclosure of the information that would normally be considered necessary for informed consent would be harmful to the patient: either directly, by hurting the patient; or indirectly, by resulting in a medically inadvisable choice on part of the patient; or, finally, by interfering with the effectiveness of the proposed treatment modality itself. In these sorts of cases it is tempting to argue that the patient should not be told the truth even though otherwise (as a competent person) he or she would be entitled to it. In other words, it is tempting to appeal to what has been called the Doctrine of Therapeutic Privilege.

The following case illustrates the sort of situation in which therapeutic privilege is sometimes claimed:

> A sixty-year old foundry-worker, married with three grown children, began to experience headaches and general malaise. After a thorough check-up he is found to suffer from essential hypertension. The patient is a rather assertive man with traditionally oriented masculine values that make him see illness as a shortcoming of the individual. He had previously indicated to his physician that he did not look positively on any prolonged treatment process for any disease, and that he certainly would never want to be on long-term medication that interfered with his ability to "act like a man." Furthermore there is some suspicion in the mind of the physician that disclosure of the results of the workup to the patient would only increase his anxiety level and elevate his blood pressure. The physician therefore decides not to tell the patient of his diagnosis nor that the medication he is prescribing is hypertension medication. Instead, he represents the symptoms as indicative of a passing condition which he wants to monitor and that could easily be controlled within a short time period with the medication prescribed—in reality an anti-hypertensive medication. He says that he would like to see the patient again within a few weeks just to follow up.

There is no denying the good will—the beneficence—of the physician. Rightly or wrongly, he genuinely believes that what he is doing is for the good of the patient, and that his duty as a physician forces him to withhold the true diagnosis. Otherwise, so he believes, the patient's health may be adversely affected by the disclosure itself; and there is the further danger that the patient might not do what is medically indicated. But is his action ethically appropriate?

To answer that question, we should really look at the relevance of the various considerations that could lead a physician to withhold information from a patient for so-called therapeutic reasons.

Reasons for Withholding Information

Harm Caused The first of these we identified as the possibility that disclosure of the information would actually and directly cause harm to the patient.

Let us begin our analysis by noting that there are cases in which this may actually occur, for example, situations where a borderline psychotic patient would actually acquire or evidence a full-blown psychosis, or an emotionally labile patient became fully compromised and unable to choose competently. Perhaps more extreme still would be the sort of situation indicated in the case above, in which a cardiac patient would be so deeply affected by the disclosure of the diagnosis and by the prognosis of the various treatment options that his health would be endangered, because the agitation produced by the disclosure would actually compound the potential for harm that existed prior to the disclosure.[69] In cases like these, so the reasoning would have it, the fundamental professional obligation not to produce harm requires that the patient not be told and that the relevant information be managed.

We believe that, in general, there is no quarreling with this line of reasoning so long as its limits are clearly adhered to. A health care professional cannot be obligated to become an agent of harm to his or her patient except in an accidental fashion, e.g., when the harm produced is instrumental for obtaining an otherwise ethically acceptable goal set by the patient in a competent fashion and exercising his or her right to self-determination. This includes such things as the harm of surgical incisions or the biochemical affront to the body by medications, all of which are normal and expected accompaniments of the relevant procedures themselves. These are acceptable so long as they are an inevitable and ineluctable concomitant of appropriate and consented-to medical treatment that is acceptable in itself.

But this is different from what is here at issue. In the sort of case under discussion, the potential harm is not an inevitable and ineluctable accompaniment of the *treatment*. It is a product of the *disclosure*. Therefore, if there is a reasonable expectation that the disclosure itself, no matter how it is handled, will produce harm or otherwise negatively affect the therapeutic conduct of the physician–patient relationship, then it is the physician's duty to refrain from disclosure.[70]

Still, it may be asked whether this reasoning really holds—and in a way, of course, it does. To start at a general level, the physician–patient relationship within which the duty of disclosure to the patient (i.e., the duty of honesty) is embedded is therapeutic in intent and design. Therefore, while the values of the patient have some bearing as to what precisely will be considered therapeutic insofar as valuational aspects of that concept are concerned, they are not completely determinative with respect to the notion of medical harm. This notion may be defined as encompassing the type of harm which in itself would be a reason why such a patient would want to consult a physician in the first place. We may therefore take it as a given that the conduct of the physician–patient relationship may not lead to harm that is not covered by exceptive clauses of the sort noted above. The logic of therapeutic privilege, therefore, is that there are some actions (or, of course, inactions—see our discussion of the active-passive distinction in Chapter 7) that will violate the injunction against harm in this sense.[71] This would also find support in the traditional injunction "Above all, do no harm!"

The claim that lies at the centre of the doctrine of therapeutic privilege is therefore the claim that the disclosure of some aspects of the condition of the patient, or of features of the treatment being advocated by the physician, will itself harm the patient in an identifiable fashion, mentally or physically. Therefore, if the reasoning that we have just sketched were to be followed consistently, it would mean that since such harm would be inconsistent with the very logic of the physician–patient relationship, as well as with the orientation or wishes of the patient or both, the physician does have an obligation not to reveal the relevant information to the patient. Instead, he has to manage it.

This sort of reasoning is surely defensible. If there is a real threat that harm in the sense that we have identified will indeed be produced by the disclosure, then such disclosure must not occur. However, at this juncture we must return to a point that we made in our discussion of standards of disclosure. Sometimes what the professional perceives to be a result of the nature of the information disclosed is not in fact a result of the nature of the information itself: It is a result of the way in which the information is presented. There is a place for empathy and compassion, for diplomacy and a "light touch" in the health care context, so long as these are not euphemisms for a paternalistic departure from truth.[72] Psychological preparation may well be a precursor for receiving information. Disciples of the Attila the Hun School of Tact have no place in a person-oriented profession.

Inadvisable Choice   Therapeutic privilege may therefore be claimed when there is reasonable certitude that physical or mental harm for this patient will result from the disclosure of this piece of information on this occasion.[73] But what about the sort of case in which disclosure of the information will not result in harm in any direct fashion but rather in an ill-advised or even completely mistaken choice by the patient?

The reasoning that may be advanced in favour of withholding information in such cases centres not in the probability of producing harm by the disclosure itself, but in the ethics of shared responsibility. If the professional discloses the information and, but for that information being known, the patient would probably have made the medically appropriate choice, then disclosure of the information must be considered a causal factor leading to the wrong choice, and therefore, to the harm that will eventuate from this wrong choice. Surely, so it may be argued, a claim of therapeutic privilege is appropriate in this type of case!

This line of reasoning has something very attractive about it. Its primary thrust is that a patient must not come to harm through the actions of the professional him- or herself. Nevertheless, its attractiveness notwithstanding, the reasoning itself is ultimately unacceptable. It contradicts the whole concept of informed consent. In the words of Chief Justice Laskin, what it really does is to "hand over to the medical profession the entire question of the scope of the duty of disclosure"[74]; and what is more, it does so on the basis of a paternalism that is only too apparent.

The ethical fact remains that competent patients (and here we are dealing only with competent patients or their proxy decision-makers) have the right to decide, even if the exercise of their decision-making power should not be medically optimal or even advantageous. If, as a result of appropriate disclosure along the lines that we have indicated, patients opt for what may only be described as medically less than optimal choices, physicians or other health care professionals who cannot live with this have no right to overrule patients, either directly or indirectly. Physicians do have the right to advise patients of the fact that their choice is less than optimal and to suggest that second options be sought and the decisions be reconsidered. If all else fails, and physicians cannot live with the decisions that the patients have made, they have the right to excuse themselves from such cases, on the condition that some other professional is available who would take their patients under these circumstances. But that is another matter.

Reduced Effectiveness It is sometimes argued that to reveal all relevant information to the patient in keeping with the legally and ethically mandated standards of informed consent is to make the very practice of medicine impossible.

That is to say, there is a certain element of placebo in the health care professional–patient relationship itself. Patients may get better simply because they have seen a physician or have been attended by a nurse. This aspect of the placebo effect is generally not deliberate. However, there are situations in which it may be, and sometimes is, used deliberately. For instance, pain can sometimes be controlled without drugs, simply by using a placebo. It is usually thought that if patients were to be told that they are receiving a placebo, they would not benefit from what in the end is harmless but effective therapy. The case of drug-dependent persons is an even better example. Sometimes the very possibility of curing drug addiction depends on fooling the patient, of weaning him or her away from the drug by the gradual substitution of an inert substance and then taking care of the psychological element of addiction that remains. The claim, then, is that to require fully informed consent in all such cases would be to do away with these and similar sorts of approaches, much to the detriment of the patient and to the possibility of health care delivery *per se*.

Again, as is so often the case in medicine, this sort of reasoning has much to recommend it, not the least point in its favour being that such an approach frequently works.

But once more, one has to ask whether it is ethically defensible. To answer this question, we have to take a brief look at the ethics of placebo use.

Placebos

Much has been written about placebos and their role in medicine, most of it from a psychological and psychiatric perspective. With but a few exceptions, the ethics of placebo use has remained relatively unexplored. Let us therefore begin by defining "placebo."

A placebo may be defined as "any therapy or component of therapy that is deliberately used for its non-specific, psychological or psycho-physiological effect, or that is used for its presumed specific effect but is without specific activity for the condition being treated."[75] We can distinguish further between *pure placebos*, which are pharmacologically inert substances prescribed by the physician, and *impure placebos*, which are pharmacologically active substances but which are not known to be specific or even appropriate for the condition in question.

If some commentators are to be believed, placebos are an integral, and one might even say unavoidable, aspect of medical practice. They are encountered in dentistry, podiatry surgery, electroconvulsive therapy "and in every medical specialty and for every treatment."[76] They have even been encountered in use for conditions[77] as diverse as angina, hypertension, diabetes, rheumatoid arthritis, peptic ulcers and above all pain.[78] So, for instance, a 1983 randomized trial of coronary bypass surgery showed that[79]

> bypass operations relieved pain in a substantially larger group of patients than did medical treatment, but in other respects the results of medical treatment were as good as those of surgery. People who had only medical therapy lived just as long as those who had undergone operation and were just as likely to return to work.

To take another example: In what by now has surely become a classic study, Beecher found that only 33 percent of soldiers found wounded on the battlefield required morphine, whereas 80 percent of patients with a similar degree of injury did.[80] The increased effectiveness was attributable to the relief felt by the soldiers at being injured, rather than killed, and the expectation of being taken away from the place of action to relative safety. In general terms, it is estimated that about 30 percent of people overall feel relief through the placebo effect,[81] and according to one researcher, 35 to 40 percent of treatments rely for their effectiveness on the placebo effect.

What we have just said may be taken to support the ubiquity of the placebo effect and the degree of its effectiveness. But what about the claim of inevitability? Here we can do no better than to quote from Spiro, one of the premier researchers in the area:[82]

> The therapists' faith, belief, enthusiasm, conviction, commitment, optimism, interest, positive and negative expectation, scepticism, disbelief, and pessimism about treatment has been established by research as a non-specific factor in most therapies.

In fact, more specifically still:[83]

In seven of our studies, there was a specific correlation between the physician's attitude to the patient . . . and improvement, accounting for about 25% of the improvement variance across studies . . . The results suggest that provider attitudes to the patient are important not only for placebo effects but also for active or specific treatment.

In other words, even when the placebo effect is not intended, it appears to be an inherent and irremovable component of the physician–patient relationship itself. If this is true, then surely it may be argued that the fact of placebo involvement in therapy presents no ethical problem. Surely it is an uncontrollable variable that insinuates itself into every therapeutic relationship. Therefore, it does not call for ethical objection but clinical investigation. And in a way, this response is appropriate—at least with respect to the placebo effect as it occurs as a matter of course in the health care setting—and one could well agree with Jospe's remark that[84]

really understanding the placebo effect will allow us not to eliminate it from the realm of therapy but rather to use it so that all aspects of the therapeutic endeavour may benefit.

But the placebo effect is sometimes used deliberately. For instance, it is sometimes deliberately used in the context of pain management and drug addiction; and sometimes it is used by physicians when they have no idea of the cause of a particular complaint and prescribe a placebo in the expectation that the statistical likelihood of relief will hold true in the particular case, and that therefore the complaint or symptoms will be dealt with without their having to resort to active but unknown therapy. A physician may even prescribe what in the end is a placebo, in the hope that the patient will simply be satisfied by the fact that something was being done.

It is against this sort of placebo use, and especially the second, that most critics have directed their fire. To quote a rather well-known statement on the subject, when placebos are prescribed in this fashion, the "physician does not seem to consider the sheer humiliation of being deceived."[85] Or again,[86]

To administer a placebo for any complaint is to perpetuate two widespread myths: that medicine can solve, and that medicine ought to be used to solve any problem a patient may bring to a physician.

To put it in terms that were used above, this use of the placebo effect—its deliberate employment—is characterized as paternalistic, deceptive, and as doing a disservice to medicine itself.

But an argument can be made for saying that the utter rejection of placebos may be pragmatically premature and ethically wrong.[87] To be sure, so the argument might go, the fact of deception as such is reprehensible. However, there are two kinds of deception: there is deception without patient involvement, and then there is deception in which the patient agrees to being deceived. This latter type of agreement lies at the basis of double-blind experimental studies. Here, the fact that the patient agrees to being deceived (without, of course, knowing the details of that deception) can be fully defended by an appeal to the Principle of Autonomy. Therefore, so the argument goes, could one not set up the placebo situation like this: The physician says to the patient something along the lines of: "This has helped others, although we don't know why. It's better that I don't tell you what it is; the likelihood of success lies between 30 and 60 percent.[88] Do you want to try it?" That would meet the critique that the ultimate effect of the public (or the individual) becoming aware of the deception are outweighed by its beneficial effects.[89] That would also satisfy the requirement of informed consent despite the fact of uncertain success rates. The patient would knowingly accept these parameters. And as to the claim that such usage would falsify the nature of medicine, this would simply be incorrect, because such placebo use would in fact be treatment—and possibly even curative. As such, it would be on a par with what is appropriately done in some other areas of health care, such as psychiatry.

Arguably, therefore, such placebo use may be defensible. However, while it may be defensible, it is unclear whether this type of use would really answer the objections that have been raised. In the *first* instance, it would be unrealistic and unworkable in practice. Everyone knows that successful placebo use depends on deception: on the patient not knowing that what is being given is in fact a placebo. *Second*, even if it turned out that there are cases in which this is not true, this would still not deal with the really hard cases: the cases in which deception is necessary for the placebo to work.

However, things are not quite that simple. Several studies suggest that the patient's knowing that something is a placebo has relatively little to do with the success of the placebo itself. What is of central importance is the attitude of the physician and the personality of the patient.[90] If that is true, then it may well be argued that the ethically correct procedure would be to present the patient with the option of not being informed about whether the treatment, therapy or procedure is genuine or placebo. Given the effectiveness rate even of informed placebo use, this option would allow the patient full exercise of autonomy without loss of the placebo effect as a genuine medical tool.

To sum up, what has just been outlined may be seen as a qualification of the usual understanding of the requirements of informed consent. It is based on the thesis that a patient can choose to be uninformed about certain aspects of the therapy that is being offered, because the patient understands that being uninformed may be an integral part of the therapy. The patient may even agree to be misinformed. As long as that fact and its consequences are explained clearly, the patient will still be giving consent, and that consent will still be informed. It is just that this informed consent is informed consent to being uninformed or misinformed within certain agreed-to limits.

However, to be acceptable, such lack of information (and such misinformation) would have to be carefully circumscribed. It would have to include a clear understanding that the placebo effect is inherently uncontrollable; that, at best, success may hold only for groups of individuals; and that it is quite unpredictable in particular cases.

As to cases in which deception is necessary for the placebo to be effective, here we have to go back to the fundamental nature of the physician–patient relationship itself.

When the physician enters into a fiduciary relationship with a patient, the physician acquires an obligation to determine what the relevant values of the patient are. That is to say, the physician acquires an obligation to determine those values that have a bearing on the patient's decision-making in the realm of health care.[91]

As far as deceptive placebo use is concerned, this means that the physician must find out where the autonomy, health and truthfulness stand in relation to each other in the patient's scheme of basic values. *If* the patient values health and autonomy over truthfulness, and *if* the patient comes to the physician of his or her own volition seeking help for a particular condition that makes deceptive placebo use medically appropriate, and *if* the use of a placebo stands a statistically better chance of being successful than anything else that is reasonably available, *then* the physician may consider using the placebo deceptively. Its use will here be sanctioned by the fact that the patient entered the therapeutic relationship not simply in pursuit of health, but more specifically to deal with a condition that includes a competence-impairing condition—namely, the fact that knowledge of the placebo as placebo would interfere with the medical effectiveness of the treatment sought by the patient. The fact that the patient sought the physician for treatment under such circumstances may therefore be seen as entailing consent.[92]

On the other hand, if the patient values truthfulness over health and autonomy, then a deceptive use of placebos is ruled out, nor would the fact that such use has a statistically significant success rate be relevant. The physician could not plead entailed consent because the value on which such an assumption was based would be missing.[93]

CONCLUSION

The competent patient has a right to informed consent as well as refusal. We have now explored some of the positive ramifications of this principle, as well as some of its limitations. On the side of the professional, it requires that the climate of decision-making be such as to optimize patient autonomy; on the side of the patient, it requires an attempt—a genuine and honest attempt—to grasp the relevant information and to use it appropriately, and to apprise the professional of any relevant aspects of the situation that might interfere with appropriate decision-making on the patient's part, insofar as they are known to the patient him- or herself and can be communicated. It must always be kept in mind that the parameters, conditions and guidelines that we have indicated above are but lifeless and formal expressions of a functional interrelationship between persons, and that health care decision-making is a living sort of affair that demands a give and take that can be determined only within the context of the actual situation itself. This is not to say that what we have said so far really doesn't hold after all, but that all of it must be applied by all parties to the health care delivery process in the spirit of a cooperative enterprise and of what we have called a fiduciary professional–patient relationship.

Further Readings

Brassington, I. "Is There a Duty to Remain in Ignorance?" *Theoretical Medicine and Bioethics* 32 (2011): 101–115.

Ciarlariello v. Schacter, [1993] 2 S.C.R. 119.

Freedman, B. "A Moral Theory of Informed Consent." *Hastings Center Report* 5.4 (1975): 32–39.

Hyun, I., "Waiver of Informed Consent, Cultural Sensitivity, and the Problem of Unjust Families and Traditions," *Hastings Center Report* 32.5 (2002): 14–22.

Kaufert, J.M., and R.W. Putsch. "Communication through Interpreters in Healthcare: Ethical Dilemmas Arising from Differences in Class, Culture, Language, and Power." *Journal of Clinical Ethics* 8.1 (Spring 1997): 71–87.

Malette v. Shulman et al. 72 O.R. (2d) 417. Ontario Court of Appeal.

McInerney v. MacDonald [1992] 2 S.C.R. 138.

Reibl v. Hughes [1980] 2 S.C.R. 880.

Sherwin, S., and M. Winsby. "A Relational Perspective on Autonomy for Older Adults Residing in Nursing Homes." *Health Expectations* 14.1 (Jun 2011): 182–189.

Endnotes

1. See J.G. Fleming, *The Law of Torts*, 9th ed. (Sidney: Law Books, 1998), Chapter 2; B.S. Markesinis and S.F. Deakin, *Tort Law* (Oxford: Clarendon Press, 1999), Chapter 4.

2. Reibl v. Hughes, (1980) 2 S.C.R. 880, 114 D.L.R. (3d) 1, 33 N.R. 361, 14 C.C.L.T. 1.

3. A.C. v. Manitoba (Director of Child and Family Services), 2009 SCC 30.

4. Malette v. Shulman (1990), 67 D.L.R. (4th) 321 (Ont. C.A.).

5. Compare R. Dworkin, *Life's Dominion: An Argument about Abortion and Euthanasia* (London: Harper Collins, 1993), at 224: "The . . . value of autonomy . . . derives from the capacity it protects: the capacity to express one's own character—values, commitments, convictions, and critical as well as experiential interests—in the life one leads . . . It allows each of us to be responsible for shaping our lives according to our own coherent or incoherent—but, in any case, distinctive—personality. It allows us to lead our lives rather than be led along them, so that each of us can be, to the extent a scheme of rights can make this possible, what we have made of ourselves."

6. Mulloy v. Hop Sang [1935] 1 W.W.R. 714 (Alta. C.A.).

7. Nancy B. v. Hôtel-Dieu de Québec (1992), 86 D.L.R. (4th) 385 (Que. S.C.).

8. Loc. cit.

9. Starson v. Swayze (2003), 225 D.L.R. (4th) 385 (S.C.C.), at 412.

10. World Medical Association, International Code of Medical Ethics (2006), accessed 31 Mar 2011 at www.wma.net/en/30publications/10policies/c8/index.html

11. Canadian Medical Association, Code of Ethics (Update 2004), clause 24; accessed 31 Mar 2011 at http://policybase.cma.ca/PolicyPDF/PD04-06.pdf

12. CMA Code of Ethics, clause 21.

13. S.E. Ross and C.T. Lin, "The Effects of Promoting Patient Access to Medical Records: A Review," *J Am Med Inform Assoc.* 10.2 (Mar–Apr 2003): 129–138; B. Fisher, V. Bhavnani and M. Winfield, "How Patients Use Access to Their Full Health Records: A Qualitative Study of Patients in General Practice," *J R Soc Med.* 102.12 (Dec 2009): 539–544; J.J. Cimino, V.K. Patel and A.W. Kushniruk, "What Do Patients Do with Access to Their Medical Records?" *Stud Health Technol Inform* 84(Pt 2) (2001): 1440–1444.

14. It does not matter whether patients pay directly or indirectly through third parties such as provincial or private health care insurers. Health care insurers act as agents for the insured persons, who pay for what is produced through their premiums.

15. Strictly speaking, the situation is a bit more complicated. Focusing only on the contractual nature of the relationship, *prima facie* it is the party who contracts the physician's services who pays. This would seem to suggest that unless the patient contracts the services, it is the direct-paying party—usually the insurer or some such agency—that owns the record. However, the insurer (whether a state agency—in which case the payment is ultimately from the insured through the taxation structure—or the private insurer) has a contractual arrangement with the patient to fund the services of the physician, where this arrangement is the result of some benefit that is due to the patient because of employment, fees paid, etc. Unless it is contractually agreed to the contrary between the insurer and the patient, the record belongs to the patient because it is paid for by the patient through the financial arrangement underlying the relationship. With due alteration of detail, similar considerations apply to any third-party arrangement for providing health services, inclusive of government agencies in countries that have socialized health care.

16. For a recent Canadian case in agreement with this, see McInerney v. MacDonald 93 D.L.R. (4th) 415. Of course, one can distinguish between the material medium or instrument of the record and the material of the record itself. The preceding refers to the latter, not the former. Ownership of the material medium is a matter of the fiscal arrangement and the terms of service between physician and patient in the physician–patient interaction. This is also recognized in McInerney.

17. McInerney v. MacDonald [1992] 2 S.C.R. 138.

18. For a legal reflection, see Picard and Robertson, op. cit., Chapter 3, "Informed Consent: The Doctor's Duty of Disclosure," and A. Kent, op. cit., *Law*, Chapter 5, "Consent." See also Moskop (1981), Veatch (1972) and the special issue of *Theoretical Medicine* 5.1 (1984), "Autonomy and the Doctor Patient Relationship."

19. Kelly v. Hazlett, (1976), 15 O.R. (2d) 290, 1 C.C.L.T.1, 75 D.L.R. (3d) 536 (H.C.).

20. Kelly v. Hazlett.

21. Sometimes also called the fallacy *ad verecundiam*. See D. Walton, "Reasoned Use of Expertise in Argumentation," *Argumentation* 3 (1989): 59–73.

22. Reibl v. Hughes (1980), 14 C.C.L.T. 1(S.C.C.).

23. P. Kortum, C. Edwards and R. Richards-Kortum, "The Impact of Inaccurate Internet Health Information in a Secondary School Learning Environment," *Journal of Medical Internet Research* 10.2 (30 Jun 2008); R. Kiley, "Quality of Medical Information on the Internet," *Journal of the Royal Society of Medicine* 91 (1998): 369–370; J. Silberg, "Assessing, Controlling and Assuring the Quality of Medical Information on the Internet: *Caveat Lector*—Let the Reader and Viewer Beware," *JAMA* 277 (1997): 1244–1245.

24. Canterbury v. Spence (1972), 464 F. 2d, 790–791.

25. Reibl v. Hughes, 21, emphasis added.

26. Reibl, at 894.

27. See Chester v. Afshar [2004] 4 All E.R.

28. Cf. Thibault v. Fewer (2001), [2001] M.J. No. 382, 2001 CarswellMan 418 (Q.B.)

29. The World Medical Association, *Declaration of Lisbon on the Rights of the Patient*, editorially revised at the 171st Council Session, Santiago, Chile, October 2005; accessed 6 Apr 2011 at http://dl.med.or.jp/dl-med/wma/lisbon2005e.pdf

30. E.-H.W. Kluge, "Physicians' Practice Profiles and the Patient's Right to Know," *J Eval Clin Pract* 6.3 (Aug 2000): 235–239.

31. See Association of State Medical Board Executive Directors, DocFinder, accessed 6 Apr 2011 at www.docboard.org/docfinder.html, which lists specializations of physicians and whether disciplinary actions have been taken against them.

32. H.K. Westli, B.H. Johnsen, J. Eid, et al., "Teamwork Skills, Shared Mental Models, and Performance in Simulated Trauma Teams: An Independent Group Design," *Scandinavian Journal of Trauma, Resuscitation and Emergency Medicine* 18.47 (2010).

33. UNESCO, *Informed Consent*, accessed 3 Apr 2011 at http://unesdoc.unesco.org/images/0014/001487/148713e.pdf

34. CMA Code of Ethics, clause 22.

35. Reibl v. Hughes 14 C.C.L.T. [1980]1, 14–22.

36. Reibl v. Hughes, 16–17, and 59, which specifically mentions the physician's duty to make "certain that he was understood." See also Starson v. Swayze.

37. Reibl v. Hughes, 16.

38. Re K. (L.D.) (1985), 48 R. F. L. (2d) 164 (Ont. Prov. Ct.).

39. Eldridge v. British Columbia (Attorney General) [1997] 3 S.C.R. 624.

40. D.E. Bredesen, R.V. Rao and P. Mehlen, "Cell Death in the Nervous System," *Nature* 443.7113 (Oct 2006): 796–802.

41. A.C. v. Manitoba (Director of Child and Family Services*)*, 2009 SCC 30.

42. *Child and Family Services Act*, available at http://web2.gov.mb.ca/laws/statutes/ccsm/c080ei.php

43. A.C. v. Manitoba (Director of Child and Family Services*)*, 2009 SCC 30, at 116.

44. Ibid., at 114.

45. For further discussion of the ethics involving children, see C. Harrison, N.P. Kenny, M. Sidarous and M. Rowell, "Involving Children in Medical Decisions," *CMAJ* 156.6 (Mar 1997): 825–828.

46. *Code of Ethics of the Royal College of Physicians and Surgeons of Canada.*

47. Reibl v. Hughes, (1980) 2 S.C.R. 880, 114 D.L.R. (3d) 1, 33 N.R. 361, 14 C.C.L.T. 1.

48. The reason for the qualifier will be discussed when dealing with the Doctrine of Emergency, *infra*.

49. Cf. Ferguson v. Hamilton Civic Hospital (1983), 144 D.L.R. (3d) (Ont. H. C.) affirmed (1985) 33 C.C.L.T. 56 (C.A.).

50. Cf. Picard and Robertson, op. cit., at 169–171. An exception to providing the information may be when the patient already knows on other grounds and from a creditable source—e.g., the patient has been told by an allergist that she is allergic to a particular type of medication.

51. Cf. Picard and Robertson, op. cit.

52. Cf. Picard and Robertson, op. cit., at 49 ff.

53. Cf. Ciarlariello v. Schacter, [1993] 2 S.C.R. 119. "[T]he patient must be advised of any material change in the risks which has arisen and would be involved in continuing the process. In addition, the patient must be informed of any material change in the circumstances which could alter his or her assessment of the costs or benefits of continuing the procedure."

54. Op. cit., at 30. "When a patient withdraws consent during a procedure to its continuation the procedure must be stopped unless to do so would seriously endanger the patient."

55. Cf. Malette v. Shulman, *supra*.

56. See R.B. Brandt, *Hopi Ethics: A Theoretical Analysis* (Chicago: University of Chicago Press, 1954). See also R.B. Brandt, *Ethical Theory* (Englewood Cliffs, NJ: Prentice Hall, 1959), 97–99, for analogous remarks.

57. J. Ramakrishna, "Health, Illness, and Immigration. East Indians in the United States,"*Soc Sci Med* 27.5 (1988): 471–477.

58. See E. Ohnuki-Tierney, *Illness and Culture in Contemporary Japan: An Anthropological View* (Cambridge: Cambridge University Press, 1984).

59. M.Z. Varul, "Talcott Parsons, the Sick Role and Chronic Illness," *Body & Society* 16.1 (June 2010): 72–94.

60. Compare Brandt and D. Lee, "Individual Autonomy and Social Structure," in D. Lee, *Freedom and Culture* (Englewood Cliffs, NJ: Prentice Hall, 1959), 5–14.

61. See S. Firth, *Dying, Death and Bereavement in a Biritch Hindu Community* (Leuven: Peeters, 1997), Chapter 5; E.L. Dvis (ed.), *Encyclopedia of Contemporary Chinese Culture* (Oxford: Routledge, 2005).

62. Reibl v. Hughes, at 16.

63. In the criminal context, this is known as the Stockholm Syndrome. See N. de Fabrique, S.J. Romano, G.M. Vecchi and V.B. van Hasselt, "Understanding Stockholm Syndrome," *FBI Law Enforcement Bulletin (Law Enforcement Communication Unit)* 76.7 (July 2007): 10–15, retrieved 8 Apr 2011 at www.fbi.gov/stats-services/publications/law-enforcement-bulletin/2007-pdfs/july07leb.pdf/ at_download/file. For the non-criminal context, see the classic discussion by A. Freud, *The Ego and the Mechanisms of Defence* (London: Hogarth Press, 1937).

64. J.L. Cummings, "Frontal-Subcortical Circuits and Human Behavior," *Arch Neurol* 50 (1993): 873–880; A.A. Grunsfeld and I.S. Login, "Abulia Following Penetrating Brain Injury during Endoscopic Sinus Surgery with Disruption of the Anterior Cingulate Circuit: Case Report," *BMC Neurol* 6.4 (23 Jan 2006).

65. S.M. Alaoui, "Politeness Principle: A Comparative Study of English and Moroccan Arabic Requests, Offers and Thanks," *European Journal of Social Sciences* 20.1 (2011): 7–15, at 5.2: "Traditionally in Moroccan offer has to be repeated and declined a number of times before it is accepted. Accepting from the first offer is regarded as bad form, so S/H go through this ritualized behaviour where each one has a defined role." See also C. Taleghani-Nikazm, "Politeness in Persian Interaction: The Preference Format of Offers in Persian," *Crossroads of Language, Interaction, and Culture* 1 (1998): 3–11.

66. Norberg v. Wynrib, [1992] 2 S.C.R. 226.

67. Op. cit., at 27.

68. The reason for not requiring that it be the sort of decision that an objective reasonable person in the patient's position would make is that under these circumstances it may be impossible to determine whether the patient's values depart from standard values or what the patient's particular circumstances are.

69. Compare E. Picard, *Legal Liability of Doctors and Hospitals in Canada* (Toronto: Carswell, 1984), 99.

70. See M. Somerville, *Consent to Medical Care*, Study Paper for the Law Reform Commission of Canada (Ottawa, 1980), 16 f, for an analogous statement, although she does not go as far in her position as we do.

71. "In this sense," because the notion of harm must always be patient relative in that the values of the patient may have bearing on the matter. If the physician cannot accept the value system of the patient as determining in these matters, the physician has the option (all other things being equal) of asking to be excused from the case.

72. Compare Reibl v. Hughes, 17, and 21–22.

73. Compare H.T. Engelhardt, Jr., *Foundations of Bioethics* (New York and Oxford: Oxford University Press, 1986) 276 f, and T.L. Beauchamp and J.F. Childress, *Principles of Biomedical Ethics* (New York and Oxford: Oxford University Press, 1979), 74, who see it as involving an "impracticality of communicating," and who construe the notion loosely. For a better expression, see M. Somerville, "Structuring the Issues in Informed Consent," *McGill Law Journal* 26 (1981): 767: ". . . the physician may rely on therapeutic privilege to justify non-disclosure of risks where the reasonable physician in the same circumstances would have believed that the disclosure *in itself would physically or mentally harm the patient to some significant degree*" [Emphasis added].

74. Reibl v. Hughes, at 882.

75. H.K. Spiro and E. Spiro, "Patient-Provider Relationship and the Placebo Effect," in J.D. Malarazzo, S.M. Weiss, J.A. Hurd, N.E. Miller and S.M. Weiss, *Behavioral Health: A Handbook of Health Enhancement and Disease Prevention* (New York: John Wiley and Sons, 1984), 372.

See also H.K. Spiro, "Definitions" in *Doctors, Patients and Placebos* (New Haven: Yale University Press, 1986), 10–22.

76. Spiro, op. cit., 33. See also M. Lipkin, "Suggestion and Healing," *Perspectives in Biology and Medicine* 20 (1984): 121–126.

77. Spiro and Spiro, op. cit., 377. See also T. Killip, E. Passamani and K. Davis, "Coronary Artery Surgery Study (CASS): A Randomized Trial of Coronary Artery Bypass Surgery," *Circulation* 68.5 (1983): 939–950; B.R. Cassileth, E.J. Lusk, D.S. Miller et al., "Psychological Correlates of Survival in Advanced Malignant Disease," *New England Journal of Medicine* 312 (1985): 1551–1555; B. Klopfer, "Psychosocial Variables in Human Cancer," *J Prog Tech* 21 (1957): 331–340; C.W. Gowdy, "A Guide to the Pharmacology of Placebos," *Canadian Medical Association Journal* 128 (1983): 921–925; M.M. Katz and G. Benil, "Blood Sugar Lowering Effects of Chlorpropamide and Tolbutamide: a Double Blind Study," *Diabetes* 14 (1965): 650–657.

78. See L.D. Egbert, E. Battit, C.E. Welch, and M.K. Bartlett, "Reduction of Postoperative Pain by Encouragement and Instruction of Patients: A Study of Doctor-Patient Rapport," *New England Journal of Medicine*, 270 (1964): 825–827; see CASS (ref. note 77); R. Melzack, *The Puzzle of Pain* (New York: Basic Books, 1973); H.K. Beecher, "The Powerful Placebo," *JAMA* 159 (1955): 1602–1606.

79. CASS, quoted in Spiro, 42.

80. See Beecher (ref. note 78).

81. M. Jospe, *The Placebo Effect in Healing* (Lexington, MA: Heath, 1978), 31. See also Park et al., "Effects of Informed Consent in Research Patients and Study Results," *Journal of Nervous and Mental Diseases* 195 (1976): 349–357.

82. H.K. Spiro, "The Placebo Response," in *Modern Perspectives in World Psychiatry*, 2nd ed., ed. J.G. Howells (Edinburgh: Oliver and Boyd, 1971), 606.

83. Spiro and Spiro (ref. note 76), 378; Compare Jospe (ref. note 80), 142; Egbert et al. (ref. note 77), 824–827.

84. Jospe, 148.

85. B. Simmons, "Problems in Deceptive Medical Procedures: An Ethical and Legal Analysis of the Administration of Placebos," *Journal of Medical Ethics* 4 (1978): 172–181.

86. Simmons, 176.

87. For an analogous discussion, see E.-H.W. Kluge, "Placebos: Some Ethical Considerations," *CMAJ* 142.4 (15 Feb 1990): 293–295.

88. Compare H.K. Spiro, "The Placebo Response" in *Modern Perspectives in World Psychiatry*, ed. J.G. Howells (Edinburgh: Oliver and Boyd, 1971).

89. See also Simmons, 172–181, and S. Bok, *Lying: Word Choice in Public and Private Life* (New York: Pantheon Books, 1978).

90. M.S. Templin et al., "Placebos: How Much Do You Know about Them?" *Nursing Life* 4 (Nov–Dec 1984): 52–53; H. Brody, "The Lie That Heals: The Ethics of Giving Placebos," *Annals of Internal Medicine* 97.1 (1982): 112–118; C.W. Gowdy, "A Guide to the Pharmacology of Placebos," *CMHA* 128 (1983): 921–925; and L.C. Parks and L. Covi, "Non-Blind Placebo Trials," *Archives of General Psychiatry* 124 (1965): 334–345.

91. See Reibl v. Hughes, 16.

92. Since the patient is otherwise competent, no proxy decision-maker needs to be involved here.

93. Part of this discussion is based on E.-H. W. Kluge, "Placebos: Some Ethical Considerations," *CMAJ* 142.4 (15 Feb 1990): 293–295.

Chapter 5
Substitute Decision-Making

This chapter considers the issues that arise when health care professionals are faced with patients who, for one reason or another, are considered incompetent and cannot make their own treatment decisions. In all such cases, it becomes important to identify who should act as substitute decision-maker, what criteria the substitute decision-maker should use and how previous, competently expressed wishes (if any) should factor into the decision-making process.

Questions to Keep in Mind While Reading this Chapter:

1. What is substitute decision-making? Is all substitute decision-making the same? What is the underlying ethical reason for substitute decision-making?

2. Who is an appropriate substitute decision-maker? Under what circumstances? Can substitute decision-makers be replaced?

3. What criteria should substitute decision-makers use? Should these criteria be the same for all types of substitute decision-making?

4. What is the role of health care professionals in substitute decision-making? What is the role of the courts? Of significant others or next-of-kin?

INTRODUCTION

People who are competent have the right to make health care decisions about what should happen to them not only here and now but also when they are no longer capable of making such decisions. As we saw in the preceding chapter, such decisions are called advance directives. But what about cases like the following?

1. A fifty-three-year-old man who had a stroke a year ago that left him physically somewhat disabled—slurred speech, some balancing problems and weakness on the left side of his body—suffers another stroke. This last stroke has left him hemiplegic with elevated blood pressure, completely aphasic with what appear to be intermittent periods of awareness and, according to a psychiatric assessment, overall cognitively severely impaired and incompetent. He is fed by a nasogastric tube, which he has

pulled out on occasion. On other occasions, he has apparently assisted the nursing staff in replacing the tube and at times even "assists" by holding it during his feeding. His overall behaviour is unpredictable. His wife tells the most responsible physician (MRP)[1] that he often told her after his first stroke that if he were ever left seriously compromised by another stroke, he would not want to live. His wife therefore wants the nasogastric tube removed and would like him to be allowed to die a quiet death, in accordance with his previous wishes.[2]

2. A six-year-old child, K.L.F., was admitted to the Hospital for Sick Children on February 26 to have a tonsillectomy and an adenoidectomy. The surgery was performed the same day. Immediately after surgery, in recovery, the child suffered from recurring bleeding, which continued off and on until March 3. He lost about 200–250 cc. of blood in that time. He is suspected of having thrombocytopenia, which affects the ability to clot. So far, he has been stabilized without blood or blood-products—which is important to his parents, who are Jehovah's Witnesses and who refuse to consent to medical treatment that involves blood or blood products. It is eight days after the surgery, and a critical time when secondary bleeding may occur. Shortly after midnight (March 6) K.L.F. suffers a rapid bleed and loses 80 cc. His total blood loss before this bleed had been 40 percent of his blood volume. The MRP wants permission to transfuse if more blood is lost. The parents refuse because the use of blood is against their religion. The Children's Aid Society is called in to seek a court order for custody, so that it can order a transfusion.[3]

3. A mentally profoundly disabled twelve-year-old girl requires twenty-four–hour care from her mother. The girl tends to "smear" her stool, and has what has been diagnosed as an incurable phobia of blood. Among other things, she becomes self-abusive when bleeding from even small injuries or scratches that show blood on her body. She is also taking anticonvulsant medication. She is at Tanner stage 4 and about to experience menarche. In theory, it would be possible to stop her from menstruating with otherwise appropriate medication. However, all such medications are counter-indicated because they would interact with her anticonvulsant medication and present a serious risk of stroke. Her mother requests that the girl have a radical hysterectomy. After due consultation with a psychiatrist and a gynecologist, the physician agrees and schedules her for surgery. A nurse on the ward notifies a pro-life group, which pickets the hospital. The physician quickly cancels the surgery and discharges the girl. The mother is frustrated and angry.[4]

4. A.C., who suffers from Crohn's disease, was almost eighteen years old when she was admitted to W.H.S. Hospital suffering from acute gastrointestinal bleeding. Her condition, although initially treatable without the administration of a blood transfusion, deteriorated over the next few days. In the opinion of the MRP, a transfusion was necessary to stave off serious medical consequences and possibly death. A.C. is a Jehovah's Witness, and it is part of her belief system that, in accordance with God's commands, she should abstain from the use of all blood and blood products. She had

executed an advance directive a short while before her admission to hospital, clearly stating her refusal of blood and blood products under any circumstances, and she explicitly refused consent to a blood transfusion on this occasion. The Ministry of Child and Family Services alleged that she was incompetent and needed a substitute decision-maker, and further alleged that for obvious reasons her parents were not an appropriate choice.[5]

In all of these cases, substitute decision-making is a central issue. Other instances in which substitute decision-making becomes important include cases such as those of comatose or unconscious accident victims who are brought into the emergency departments of hospitals; situations in which persons suffering from Alzheimer's disease require medical treatment, but there is no advance directive; or situations involving severely disabled newborns who can be saved but will live a life of pain and suffering. Still other examples include patients who have been given pre-op medication and are asked to agree to a change in medical procedure, or elderly persons who live on their own but suffer from Diogenes syndrome[6]—the list is almost endless. Dealing with these sorts of situations is made immeasurably easier if one can identify some general principles that should be followed.

The operant assumption underlying all of this, of course, is that someone should function as substitute decision-maker for incompetent patients in the first place. Why is this assumption correct? In brief, the need for substitute decision-makers follows from the Principle of Autonomy and Respect for Persons and the Principle of Equality and Justice, which were subjects of discussion in Chapter 1. The need for substitute decision-making is also reflected in the various declarations of medical, ethical and legal authorities, which stipulate that (mental) handicap is not a reason for discrimination; and substitute decision-making is legally mandated by section 15 of the Canadian Charter of Rights and Freedoms, which outlaws policies, rules and regulations that discriminate on the basis of disability.

That is to say, as we saw in Chapter 1, a right is a justified claim that someone may exercise if he or she so chooses. Now, one of the most fundamental rights in health care is the right to decide what shall happen to one's body. (There are, of course, limits to this right. For example, it does not extend to refusing appropriate treatment for highly infectious diseases such as cholera or open tuberculosis because this would violate other people's right not to be infected and would pose a danger to everyone else. See Chapter 4, "Informed Consent.") The crucial point here is that deciding what shall happen to one's body involves decision-making. However, deliberately deciding or choosing to do something is different from merely doing something—from merely acting. Thus, cutting someone because of an involuntary spasm of the hand that holds the scalpel is different from deliberately using the scalpel to cut during an operation. The former does not involve choosing or decision-making, whereas the latter does. It involves understanding *that* a choice is possible, *that* various options are open from among which one can be chosen and *that* these options have different consequences. In other words, decision-making involves understanding.

But more is involved. Decision-making also involves values. Merely being aware of options and understanding their implications is not the same as actually making a choice. Making a choice requires something that motivates the individual to actually select among these options, and it is here that values enter. As one commentator so aptly put it, values are "concepts of the desirable with motivating force."[7] In other words, values function as action potentials. Absent values, choices cannot and will not be made.

Incompetent patients may be compromised in terms of both understanding and values. That is to say, they may lack any awareness, as in case (1); they may lack values altogether, as in case (2); they may lack an understanding of the choices that are open to them, as in case (3); or, as in case (4), although they may be cognitively competent, it is unclear that their values have been adopted freely and without coercion.

In cases (1) to (3), the inability to exercise the right of choice clearly is the result of circumstances beyond the patients' control. Therefore, if someone does not step in and exercise the right for them, they would actually be punished for being the victims of bad luck. Ethically, that is unacceptable. As to case (4), if we assume for the moment that A.C. has not adopted her values freely and without coercion, then to allow her to decide what should happen to her would be to honour her decision-making authority, but in a perverse way. That is to say, A.C. understands—she is cognitively competent—but to honour her wishes would be to punish her for an accident of fate that saw her acquire values that are out of keeping with the standard values of society without having had the opportunity to make them authentically her own.[8]

In these and similar cases one must consider the patient's level of cognitive capacity and, when that level is insufficient for competent decision-making, one must make arrangements for an appropriate substitute decision-maker. Similar remarks apply in the case of questionable values and other aspects of competence. Not to arrange for substitute decision-making would be to punish the individuals for their lack of competence.[9] What follows examines substitute decision-making under three headings:

1.   What constitutes competence?
2.   Who should function as substitute decision-maker?
3.   What values should a substitute decision-maker use?

WHAT CONSTITUTES COMPETENCE?[10]

There are different ways of approaching the notion of competence. For instance, it can be approached from a psychiatric, a psychological, a legal, or even a sociological perspective. From an ethical perspective, however, one can distinguish four parameters. These are conceptual, emotional, valuational and volitional in nature.

Conceptual Competence

One of the most important aspects of competence—and indeed the parameter that historically has tended to predominate in legal considerations involving health care—is conceptual competence.[11] So, for instance, the Alberta *Personal Directives Act*, which identifies decision-making competence in terms of capacity, defines capacity as "the ability to understand the information that is relevant to the making of a personal decision and the ability to appreciate the reasonably foreseeable consequences of the decision";[12] the Ontario *Mental Health Act* defines an incompetent person as someone who lacks "the ability to understand the subject matter in respect of which consent is requested and able to appreciate the consequences of giving or withholding consent."[13] The Nova Scotia *Hospitals Act* is even more explicit, stating that "in determining whether or not a person is capable of consenting to treatment the examining psychiatrist shall consider whether or not the person being examined (a) understands the condition for which the treatment is proposed; (b) understands the nature and purpose of the treatment; (c) understands the risks involved in undergoing the treatment; (d) understands the risks involved in not undergoing the treatment; and (e) whether or not his ability to consent is affected by his condition."[14] Legislation in the other Canadian provinces is essentially similar.

Conceptual competence centres in what has sometimes been called the reasoning or intellective ability of a person.[15] However, that is not a simple notion. It covers several distinct parameters. First, there is the *cognitive* aspect: It consists in the ability to understand or grasp the relevant information. This component of conceptual competence is clearly illustrated by the Ontario *Mental Health Act*, referenced above, which states that it is "the ability to understand the subject matter in respect of which the consent is requested."[16] It is very important, however, to avoid equating cognitive competence with educational sophistication. As we saw in Chapter 4, and as the leading case of *Reibl v. Hughes* makes very clear, cognitive competence centres in the individual's ability to understand the information that is presented at an appropriate level. (For a full discussion, see Chapter 4, "Informed Consent.") By contrast, educational sophistication has nothing inherently to do with an individual's ability to understand in that sense. It goes to the training that the individual has received.[17] Medical information that is presented in language that is suited to communication only among highly trained health care professionals will not be understood by the ordinary person—not, however, because the ordinary person lacks the capacity to understand but because the information is presented at an inappropriate educational level. (See Chapter 4 for a discussion of the subjective standard of comprehension, as outlined in *Reibl v. Hughes*.)

Conceptual competence also has an *inferential* aspect. This consists in the individual's ability to see connections among the information that is presented, and in the ability to draw appropriate conclusions.[18] This is what underlies the question, "Do you understand the consequences of your decision to accept or forego the proposed treatment?" It also plays an important role in legal competence assessments, and is reflected in the Ontario *Mental Health Act*'s requirement that a competent person must be "able to appreciate the consequences of giving or withholding consent."

In other words, inferential competence refers to the ability to discern the implications of the information that is presented. Here again, it is important to distinguish between competence and sophistication. Almost invariably, a highly trained health care professional will be able to identify more—and possibly different—consequences than the ordinary reasonable person who lacks such education. Therefore, someone will be inferentially incompetent only if that person cannot discern the consequences and implications that a comparatively placed reasonable person would normally be able to identify.

Finally, *mnemonic* component refers to the ability to remember, i.e., to function intellectually in more than the immediate present. That is to say, decision-making is more than a momentary affair. It extends into the past because it draws on memories that lend conceptual significance to the data that are being presented, and it extends into the future because it requires the individual to project into an expected future that will be shaped by whatever decision is made.[19] People whose mnemonic capacity is so impaired that they live only in the specious present—that is to say, people who live only in a narrowly extended time frame in which significant past decisions and experiences are not remembered—such individuals cannot adopt such a stance. Being mnemonically impaired, they cannot make decisions that have more than merely momentary significance. Alzheimer's patients whose temporal awareness is confined to the specious present lack cognitive competence in precisely this sense, even if their conceptual and inferential competence is unimpaired.

Clearly, given its various components, conceptual competence is not an all-or-nothing affair. Not only does it involve variations as to the presence or absence of the various components, their degree of presence (or absence) may also vary, as may the depth of inferential structure, the extent of the time-consciousness involved and so on.

Evaluations of conceptual competence are therefore never easy. Of course, there are clear-cut—or at any rate relatively clear-cut—and obvious cases. For instance, someone suffering from Down's syndrome and having the functional intelligence of a one-and-a-half-year-old clearly will be cognitively incompetent. Such a person will be unable to grasp the concepts necessary for orienting in the world, to understand the nature of a particular medical condition or to comprehend the various treatment choices. Such a person will also be inferentially incompetent, because he or she will be unable to engage in reasoning of sufficient depth to be able to make a decision among the various options that are available, to grasp their implications and so forth.[20] More than likely, the person will also be mnemonically incompetent with respect to the various data, their significance, previous decisions reached and so on.

On the other hand, someone suffering from Alzheimer's disease and living wholly in the present, as sometimes happens in such cases, may well be conceptually and inferentially quite competent within that temporal framework, despite overall mnemonic incompetence; or a child of nine may be inferentially and mnemonically quite competent and yet fail to be completely competent on the cognitive level. Consequently, the child's overall competence may be impaired.

There are also situations in which someone's conceptual competence is only temporarily impaired, as for instance when someone is recovering from anesthesia, is severely sleep-deprived or suffers from other transient causes. The claim that someone is conceptually incompetent, therefore, always has to be carefully circumscribed and treated with extreme care. Perhaps a useful rule of thumb is this: One should always assume conceptual competence unless there are reasonable and convincing grounds to the contrary, rooted in the nature or condition of the individual and his or her situation. In fact, that is the legal default position.[21]

Emotional Competence

The notion of emotional competence acknowledges the fact that human beings are not automata but living beings who are embedded in psychosocial contexts and interact with other persons on more than merely cognitive terms. It also acknowledges that the choices we make, or indeed how we make them, may be influenced by the emotions that we experience on a particular occasion.

Emotional competence has two parameters: appropriateness and strength. Appropriateness, as the term indicates, refers to the appropriateness of the emotions to the circumstances. For example, all other things being equal, someone who laughs uproariously on being told the news of her child's diagnosis of colon cancer is expressing an inappropriate emotion. The individual is probably in what could reasonably be called emotional shock. Such a person is hardly in a position to make a competent choice at that point in time. On the other hand, an emotion may be appropriate but may be experienced so strongly that it interferes with the ability to reason, to appreciate the implications of the various options, or to make a choice at all. Expressions such as "being overcome with emotion" and "being stunned" capture this sort of situation fairly well. Usually, such emotional incapacity is of short duration. Emotional incompetence, therefore, is the inability to reach a reasoned (and reasonable) decision either because of emotional aberrations or because of the intense emotional feelings or pressures that are experienced at that time.

It is usually negative emotions that are implicated in this context: emotions such as grief, sorrow or despair. This is what underlies the standard rule that people whose loved one has died in hospital should be approached for possible organ donation only by professionals who are specially trained to deal with such emotional turmoil and who can assist the bereaved individuals in making a rational decision. Positive emotions such as joy, delight or pleasure are rarely if ever considered when assessing whether someone is emotionally too compromised to make a competent decision. Why exactly that should be the case is not clear. Clearly, positive but extremely violent emotions ought to be considered just as incapacitating as negative ones. That aside, however, the standard rule is this: If the emotions differ significantly from what is the social norm in that particular context, or if they are so extreme that they interfere with rational decision-making, then the individual's competence is put in question.

Valuational Competence

While conceptual and emotional competence are necessary conditions for decision-making competence, they are not sufficient. As we saw before, there must be something that actually motivates the individual to choose among the available options and to act on that decision. This additional element is contributed by the individual's values. Valuational competence is one of the most difficult aspects of competence to assess and is one of the most easily mishandled. In what follows, we examine the notion with special attention to two central questions: What makes certain values ethically unacceptable? and What values should a substitute decision-maker use?

What makes certain values ethically unacceptable?   There are several reasons why certain values are ethically unacceptable for decision-making. One lies in the very nature and role of values in decision-making as such. If, as has been suggested, values are action potentials, then mutually inconsistent values will in fact be contradictory action potentials.[22] Therefore, as a general principle, having mutually inconsistent values may make it impossible for a decision-maker to make consistent and reasoned choices. The decision—if a decision could be made at all—would be, so to speak, not reasoned but random.

At the same time, it would be foolish to ignore the fact that most people hold inconsistent values without being valuationally incompetent. Arguably, therefore, valuational incompetence obtains only when someone holds contradictory values and continues to hold them even after their mutually conflicting character has been demonstrated.

But even this would be too stringent. People may reasonably continue to hold conflicting values because these values strike them as justified in their own right—for example, the value of sustaining human life and the value of ending suffering. Suppose a particular patient is suffering from an incurable and irremediable condition that makes life a living hell—Sue Rodriguez claimed that her particular version of amyotrophic lateral sclerosis fell into that category[23]—then that person may well continue to believe that there is an obligation to sustain life but at the same time maintain that it is also ethically acceptable to end that life in order to end the suffering. Such a person would not necessarily be incompetent. For a comparison, one might consider the statement by Pope Pius XII that even though there is a duty to preserve life, it is ethically acceptable under certain circumstances to end that suffering life by allowing the individual to die.[24] (For a more detailed discussion of the ethical issues surrounding the ending of life, actively or passively, see Chapter 7, "The Ethics of Deliberate Death.")

In other words, in apparent contradiction to what has been said above, inconsistent values may motivate a person without the individual thereby becoming valuationally incompetent. The solution to this conundrum lies in the fact that values may be ranked. In other words, a value system will be inconsistent and unusable for rational decision-making only if the values cannot be ranked or balanced relative to each other. (This is similar to W.D. Ross's claim that rights and duties as such hold only *prima facie*, subject to the conditions that prevail. See Chapter 1, "Ethics as a Discipline.") Only then will it become impossible for the individual to reach a (reasoned) decision. Consequently, the logical condition for valuational incompetence must be amended like this: Persons are valuationally incompetent if they hold contradictory values, refuse to change these values after due reflection and cannot balance the conflicting values in a reasoned fashion in order to reach a decision.

At the same time, valuational competence requires more than merely valuational consistency or the ability to rank conflicting values. Values that change from moment to moment are not a secure basis for making decisions that have implications beyond the immediate moment. That is to say, while competent persons may change their values, their value framework must be more or less stable over a given period of time, since otherwise no consistent plans can be developed and the resultant actions may well be in conflict with each other. The Supreme Court recognized this in its decision in *A.C. v. Manitoba (Director of Child and Family Services)*, which formed the basis of case (4) above, when it said that one of the criteria for evaluating the competence of a mature minor is whether "there [is] reason to believe that the adolescent's views are *stable* and a true reflection of his or her core values and beliefs."[25]

The last clause in the Court's decision introduces another aspect of valuational competence. Competently held values must be *authentic* values.[26] That is to say, a decision-maker may give every appearance of making a valuationally competent decision by using consistent and stable values, yet the values may have been acquired as a result of the social embedding of the individual—as it were, through a process of social conditioning. Case (4) above raises just that possibility. While A.C.'s values would be acceptable if she had come to believe them on her own and without undue pressure, it was not at all clear to the Court that she had done so, given that she had grown up in a Jehovah's Witness household where she was probably conditioned from early childhood to consider the value of not accepting blood or blood products as cardinal features of a morally responsible life. In other words, as one commentator put it, valuational competence must satisfy the "authenticity condition—the qualification . . . that those values which guide the actions and decisions of autonomous persons must be authentically 'their own' and not the products of wholesale indoctrination or manipulation."[27]

This does not mean that patients who have acquired their values in a particular social context or as a result of having been raised in a family with particular values are therefore valuationally incompetent. If that were the case, then almost everyone would be valuationally incompetent. It merely means that if the values that a particular patient has and that form the basis of the patient's decision-making differ importantly from the social norm, it is appropriate to consider the *possibility* that they may not be authentic values but a result of conditioning. This is especially important in cases like that of A.C. above. Children tend to stand in a dependence relationship to their family unit, and that dependence may interfere with their ability to form authentic values. In fact, the same issue arises in any situation in which the patient is in a dependence relationship, whatever the age of the patient in question. It involves the issue of volitional competence, or capacity, which will be discussed in a moment. Another aspect of valuational competence centres in the question of whether the values properly recognize people—whether that be the individuals themselves or others—as persons. For example, values that treat individuals only (or primarily) as production units—that is to say, as entities whose value resides solely in what they can contribute either to society or to the social unit in which they are embedded—are values that are ethically unacceptable because they deny the individual's status as a person. (They violate the Principle of Autonomy and Respect for Persons. See Chapter 1.)

Such values are sometimes encountered in the geriatric setting when elderly persons decide that they do not deserve health care because they have "outlived their usefulness" and are "mere mouths to feed." Their decision-making may be cognitively and emotionally competent, but it will be valuationally flawed. (This issue will be addressed further in Chapter 10, "Resource Allocation.")

Another example along these lines involves values that deny equal status to persons who are cognitively impaired or who belong to different ethnic or religious groups. An example of the former would be the values that would underlie a parental decision not to treat an infant suffering from Down's syndrome simply because that infant will never be cognitively competent; an example of the latter would be the values that would allow a particular ethnic or religious group to use members of another ethnic or religious group for medical experiments—as happened in Nazi Germany[28] and in Manchuria under Japanese occupation.[29]

Finally, not all values are what, for want of a better term, one might call appropriate. For instance, there are values that are simply too radical or bizarre. An example here would be the case of the medical student from Chicago who reportedly castrated himself surgically for no discernible reason (and who did so in a surgically exemplary fashion) except that he felt that such a state was better than one of sexual normalcy.[30]

However, it would also be incorrect to say that simply deviating valuationally from social norms makes someone valuationally incompetent.[31] Nor would the reverse automatically be true. The ethical acceptability of values is not simply a function of their social acceptance. One need only look at the values that licensed the non-consensual sterilization of mentally disabled people in Canada (see Chapter 11, "Reproductive Ethics and the Right to Have Children") or the ethnic cleansing of Armenians in Turkey[32] to appreciate this point; or consider the fact that conscientious objectors did not share general social values in the 1940s, and that people who were opposed to slavery in the 18th century—or those who favoured women's suffrage in the 19th century—were out of step with social values.

The main aspects of valuational competence could therefore be summed up like this:

1. The values must be in keeping with the facts of reality. They must not set up action potentials that can never be satisfied even in principle, for example, the value of eternal biological life, of unlimited physical prowess and so on. (For further and more detailed discussion of this, see Chapter 7 "The Ethics of Deliberate Death.")

2. The values must reflect the nature of the individual as a person. That is to say, if a person is someone who has the present capacity for cognitive self-awareness (and this will be spelt out in greater detail in Chapter 8, in our discussion of personhood and abortion), then the values of the individual must be consistent with the nature of the individual as a person. This entails that values which deny the status of the individual as a person must be rejected.[33]

3. The values of a competent person must be part of a more or less stable framework. This does not mean that the values cannot change, but it does mean that they cannot change from moment to moment.

4. The values must be authentic values.

5. A valuationally competent individual must be willing to examine (and if necessary change) her or his values when presented with evidence of their inconsistency or their unreasonableness.

Finally, the following point bears emphasizing: Valuational incompetence is not the same as being unethical or morally evil. It is unacceptable to violate the legitimate and effective (moral) rights of others. However, such a violation will be unethical only if whoever acts in this fashion does so freely and knowingly, or if he or she should have known that such a violation would be the reasonable predictable outcome of that particular act.

Moreover, there is no logical (or, for that matter, psychological) reason to suppose that incompetence in one area automatically carries over into another.[34] In health care, this finds legal reflection in the case of *Starson v. Swayze*, in which the Supreme Court ruled that even though someone may suffer from a mental illness such as schizophrenia, this does not automatically mean that the person is incompetent to make health care decisions—even about whether or not the person should be treated for that very mental illness.[35] Analogously, elderly persons may have lost the right to make financial decisions on their own behalves and have someone assigned to exercise power of attorney regarding financial matters, but this does not automatically mean that they cannot still make health care decisions for themselves. Further, if someone who is incompetent while unmedicated is competent while on medication and makes a health care decision, that decision is binding, even if the decision is against treatment and, as a result, the person will be confined to a mental institution for the rest of his or her life. How competence comes about—i.e., the *cause* of competence—is not what is important; what is important is whether the person is in fact competent at the time of decision-making.

The three-axis notion of competence that has just been sketched can be represented graphically, as in Figure 5.1:

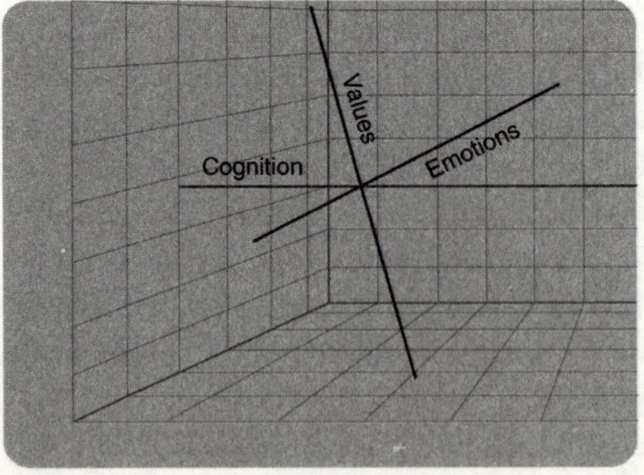

Figure 5.1 Competence

Volitional Competence

However, competent decision-making involves more than being cognitively capable, emotionally uncompromised and having appropriate values. It also involves the ability to actually make an authentic choice and to translate that choice into action.

This ability may be impaired in two ways. For want of better terms, these may be referred to as *internal* and *external freedom-impairing parameters* respectively. Addiction is an example of an internal freedom-impairing parameter. Some addicts clearly understand the implications of their substance abuse, are unhindered by inappropriate emotions and use appropriate and authentic values in deciding to break their addiction and yet are unable to act on this decision precisely because they are addicted.[36] Conditioning provides another example. Some persons may be unable to choose authentically because they have been conditioned to accept certain sets of values. Even though such persons may be presented with a range of options, and even though they may fully understand and appreciate the implications of the various choices, these individuals will inevitably select only particular options because the value sets into which they have been conditioned effectively constrains them in that direction.[37] People from abusive situations sometimes find themselves in this position. Likewise, some individuals may be unable to make "free" choices because of mental illness or be unable to act on choices that they have rationally made. Pedophilia provides a good example. Pedophiles are not necessarily conceptually compromised. They may even share standard social values, intellectually reject the sexual abuse of children and may be emotionally horrified by their own actions—and yet be unable to "help themselves." In these sorts of cases, internal conditions prevent the individuals from either making or acting on otherwise competent choices.

As to external freedom-impairing parameters, these are generally grounded in the situation in which the individual is embedded. An example here could be prisoners in jail or residents of a rigidly controlled long-term care facility. These individuals may be perfectly competent in all other respects and may even be free of internal freedom-impairing parameters. However, they may be volitionally compromised because the rules, regulations and even physical restraints that they encounter prevent them from translating their decisions into action.[38]

Similarly, dependence and power relationships may constrain the will of the individual and constitute a freedom-impairing parameter.[39] Something like this sometimes occurs in the geriatric setting when elderly persons feel dependent on other individuals—say, on their caregivers or on someone perceived to be in authority—and powerless, and do not want to make a choice that might give offence.

Undue enticement is still another example where the will of the individual is overborne by the particulars of the situation.[40] (For further detailed discussion of the Guidelines, see Chapter 6, "Research Using Human Subjects.") Thus, the young mother who is in prison for a criminal offence but agrees to participate in a particular piece of research because she is offered the prospect of early parole is volitionally impaired, because the very prospect of seeing her children constitutes undue enticement. The same holds true for the elderly person in a long-term care facility who agrees to conform to certain rules or to engage in certain activities (e.g., take her medication) because of the promised reward of seeing her grandchildren.

It is interesting to note that the common law has long recognized some of these factors—in particular the fact that someone's will may be overborne by undue pressure, or that the will of an otherwise competent individual may be overcome by undue enticement or be impaired by an unequal power relationship. The law even recognizes that although the will of the weaker party may not actually be dominated or overcome in any overt sense, the situation itself may be of such a nature that the consent is neither genuine nor authentic, because the various factors constitute *de facto* freedom-impairing parameters. This notion, which was initially developed in the context of contract law,[41] has increasingly found application in the context of health care and has received explicit expression in the case of *Norberg v. Wynrib*, when the Supreme Court said that[42]

> It is presumed that the individual has freedom to consent or not to consent. This presumption, however, is untenable in certain circumstances. A position of relative weakness can, in some circumstances, interfere with the freedom of a person's will. Our notion of consent must, therefore, be modified to appreciate the power relationship between the parties . . . In particular, in certain circumstances, consent will be considered legally ineffective if it can be shown that there was such a disparity in the relative positions of the parties that the weaker party was not in a position to choose freely.

It bears emphasizing that the previous considerations regarding competence and capacity have focused specifically on health care decision-making. They cannot automatically be applied to situations in which the individual in question is the agent. Thus, it is not at all clear that the courts would accept a plea of incompetence from a pedophile, even though the International Classification of Diseases includes pedophilia as a distinct

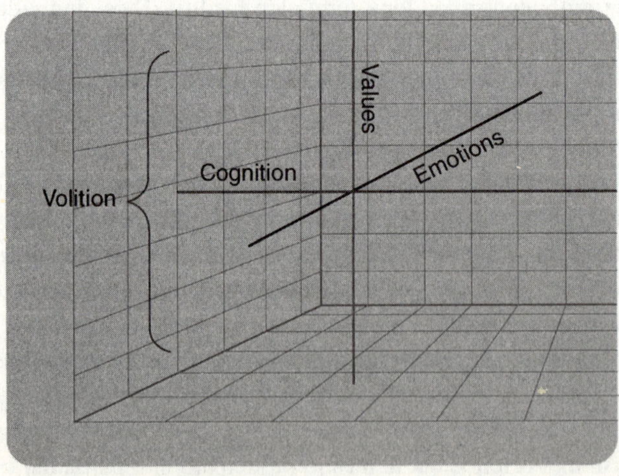

Figure 5.2 Competence and Capacity

classification (F65.4). At the same time, it is interesting to note that drug addiction—albeit not an actual state of intoxication—has sometimes been recognized in common law countries as excusing the addicted person if the individual satisfies what is called the "settled insanity" or "M'Naghten rule." However, in the latter case, the individual must have been unable, by virtue of mental disorder, to appreciate the nature and quality of the act or know that it was wrong. Arguably, this points to a discrepancy between the law and social policies. An exploration of this, however, transcends the scope of this discussion.

To sum up, then, competence in the extended sense of the term includes capacity, as indicated in Figure 5.2.

WHO SHOULD FUNCTION AS SUBSTITUTE DECISION-MAKER?

Having achieved some clarity on what constitutes competence, it is now time to consider the question of who should act as substitute decision-maker in health care matters for someone who is incompetent.

The Physician

It used to be said that when a patient was incompetent, it was the MRP who should make the health care decisions for the patient. Historically, we encounter this stance in Percival's *Medical Ethics*, where the physician is exhorted to make the decisions for the patient by "[uniting] tenderness with steadiness, and condescension with authority";[43] and it persisted well into the 20th century in what in Chapter 3 was described as a paternalistic or priestly model of the physician–patient relationship. The reason for giving physicians this decision-making authority—insofar as a reason was given at all—was that health care decisions dealt with medical facts, and that physicians had incomparably greater expertise and practice in these matters than next-of-kin or anyone else. Medical knowledge and medical decision-making was what their training was all about. Therefore, decision-making power should reside with physicians.[44]

However, this model of the physician–patient relationship has long been discarded. Even if one were to grant the point about training and practice, it is generally agreed that all other things being equal—certain types of emergencies being an exception—it is not physicians who ought to be the substitute decision-makers for incompetent patients. First of all (and we already saw this in Chapter 3), the assumption that because someone makes decisions frequently—and, clearly, physicians do make medical decisions incomparably more frequently than anyone else—does not mean that the decisions the person makes are therefore ethically appropriate. They may be medically appropriate, but that is another matter.

Secondly—and here again we are merely restating what was said before in the preceding chapters—one has to distinguish sharply between a decision that is made in a professional capacity on matters involving technical expertise, and a decision about whether that technical expertise ought to be exercised in the first place. As the Supreme Court put it in *Reibl v. Hughes,* to allow physicians to make (substitute) treatment decisions because of their technical expertise would be to "hand over to the medical profession" the whole extent of health care decision-making. It would undercut the Principle of Autonomy and would make a mockery of the very notion of informed consent.

As we saw in Chapter 4, every patient has the right to accept or reject any intervention, and the values of the patient play a crucial role in such decision-making.[45] The mere fact that a patient has become incompetent does not rob the patient of that right or of the right to have those values reflected in health care decision-making about that patient. It merely means that someone has to implement those values for the patient. While it is possible that a physician may be familiar with these values—especially if the patient has expressed them to the physician in an advance directive (which will be discussed in a moment)—this is generally not the case. Nor is a physician as well-placed as others—in particular not as well placed as significant others or persons who have been explicitly identified by the patient when competent—to interpret what those values would mean on a given occasion. Therefore, as a general rule, physicians must defer to duly empowered substitute decision-makers in health care decision-making for incompetent patients.

The Doctrine of Emergency

Of course—and herewith we return to the exception noted above—there are situations in which time is of the essence and a health care decision must be made without delay. Emergency rooms of hospitals provide the most graphic examples of these sorts of situations. But to say that in emergencies the primary decision-making power invariably belongs to the physician and that it is the physician who should function as substitute decision-maker is to ignore the fact that the incompetent patient may previously have given an applicable advance directive or may have identified someone as substitute decision-maker for just that sort of situation—or that some other substitute decision-maker is available who could make an appropriate decision.

To be sure, there are situations in which this is not possible: for instance, when there is no advance directive, an otherwise duly empowered substitute decision-maker is not reasonably available and the patient would suffer serious or irremediable harm if a decision were not made. In that case, the so-called *Doctrine of Emergency* empowers the physician to act as substitute decision-maker. However, such a decision will always be subject to later review to see whether it respected the values of the patient insofar as these were reasonably available at the time and, if these values were not reasonably available, whether the decision was made in keeping with established social values. The decision may never be based on purely medical values or on the physician's personal values.

Furthermore, even this conclusion is subject to certain conditions because there are different types of emergencies. Specifically, it is ethically relevant to distinguish between unforeseeable and foreseeable emergencies. Unforeseeable emergencies are situations that could not reasonably have been foreseen; foreseeable emergencies are situations in which the chance that an emergency may arise is reasonably foreseeable. An example of the first kind of emergency would be an unexpected stroke or a berry aneurysm; an example of the second kind of emergency would be cardiac arrest in a patient who was known to have a cardiac problem and to be at risk.

Only in unforeseeable emergencies will there be no time to consult beforehand in order to establish the direction or even precise nature of the patient's values and wishes. Here indeed, all other things being equal,[46] the physician must have, and does have, both ethically and legally, primary decision-making power. In fact, all other things being equal, the physician has not only the right but the duty to act in the appropriate fashion without obtaining informed consent. This follows from the fiduciary nature of the physician–patient relationship. However, it does not hold in the second sort of case. Here the physician's obligation is to establish beforehand what the patient would want, should the emergency occur. For the physician not to do so—not to establish this valuational direction beforehand—is for the physician to abandon the fiduciary role.

A second limitation on emergency decision-making powers comes into play when an appropriate substitute decision-maker for the patient is available and can be consulted. Next-of-kin usually fall into this category, as do legally appointed substitute decision-makers.[47] They may not be ignored as decision-makers unless the time is so precious that consultation is impossible, the fact of their present availability notwithstanding. In that case, the Doctrine of Emergency once more applies.

Physicians and Advance Directives

Finally—and this clarifies the notion of an advance directive—a patient may, when competent, have made a clear and autonomous decision about what direction treatment should take if the patient were ever unable to indicate his or her wishes. Jehovah's Witnesses usually act in this way, but so do many other patients—including elderly patients who do not wish to be resuscitated if they should arrest. If such an advance directive is reasonably accessible to the physician—for example, on a signed (and possibly even witnessed) card of the sort frequently kept by Jehovah's Witnesses—and if the situation is covered by that statement, then the physician must abide by it.[48] The Supreme Court of Newfoundland already recognized this as a legal duty in 1987, in the case of *Little*,[49] and it was reaffirmed in the classic Ontario case of *Malette v. Shulman et al.*[50] Likewise, all Canadian provinces have enacted legislation giving legal recognition to advance directives, and these need not necessarily be registered or have a physician's signature to be valid.

Both ethically and legally, therefore, if there is a competently executed advance directive that is reasonably available in emergency contexts, the physician must follow that advance directive even if it is against the physician's better medical judgment and even if it means that the patient might die. The physician cannot simply step in as substitute decision-maker and do what is medically appropriate. That is why it is generally recommended by the various medical licensing bodies that ethical physicians should explore the concept of an advance directive with their patients as part of their fiduciary duty, so as to have clarity in emergency situations.

Duly Empowered Substitute Decision-Makers

All other things being equal, therefore, physicians are not the duly empowered substitute decision-makers. But if not physicians, who then should act in that capacity? In case (1) above, the wife functions as substitute decision-maker; in case (2), the parents and the Children's Aid Society compete for that role; in case (3), the mother wants to act in that capacity; and in case (4), the Ministry claims to be the appropriate substitute decision-maker, the fact that parents are available notwithstanding. Another sort of case would be one in which the incompetent patient lives in a "stable relationship" with a partner, the two are not married, but the partner claims to be the appropriate substitute decision-maker even though consanguineous next-of-kin are available.[51]

Significant Others   This last sort of case really brings us to the very core of substitute decision-making. As was pointed out above, the ultimate reason for substitute decision-making is that incompetent patients should not lose their right to be treated according to their own values. Therefore, one of the more important questions in substitute decision-making is that of who is best placed to know those values and to act on them.

In our society, it is usually significant others. The interpersonal relationships that exist between significant others and the patient usually mean that the significant others tend to know the incompetent person better than anyone else. It is therefore both reasonable and appropriate to assume that significant others are better placed than anyone else to use the patient's values when acting as decision-makers on behalf of the incompetent. It is simply unrealistic to think that a physician who has a practice of 2,000 patients can know these patients as well as the members of the patients' families.

Another consideration, purely ethical in nature, contributes to this conclusion. The assumption of substitute decision-making power does not involve the *transfer of a right*: It is the *assumption of a responsibility*. That is why the substitute decision-maker has an obligation to exercise the right of the incompetent person in as close a manner as possible to the way in which the individual him- or herself would have done so, had he or she been able. Next-of-kin usually have the patient's welfare more strongly at heart than does the physician—who is a professional and a stranger, and who has thousands of other patients to worry about—and they usually have more time to devote to appropriate value-based decision-making.

Of course, if the matter were left there, it could create more problems than it solved. Often there are several people who can legitimately claim to be next-of-kin. Parents, siblings, spouse (however the notion of spouse may be defined) and other relatives all fall into this category. Therefore, unless there is a way of ranking them in terms of priority, it may well happen that all of them would become involved and make conflicting decisions.

Health care professionals would then have no way of deciding whose decision should be followed. In the recent past, this has sometimes happened over such issues as to whether to continue life-saving or -sustaining treatment, whether to remove organs for donation, and the like.

To avoid this problem, most jurisdictions have statutes that detail the ranking order of the various next-of-kin with respect to substitute decision-makers. The order usually goes something like this:[52]

1. the spouse (which includes a common-law spouse), who may be of any age or gender provided that she or he is competent;
2. if there is no spouse, or if the spouse is incapacitated or not reasonably available, any of the children, provided they are of age and are themselves competent;
3. if there are no children, or if they are not of the age of majority or are incompetent, either of the parents who is mentally competent;
4. if there are no parents reasonable available, or if they are incompetent, any of the siblings who have attained the age of majority and are competent; and
5. if none of the above is reasonably available or competent, any other next-of-kin who has attained the age of majority and is mentally competent.

While this goes some way towards solving the problem, it does not go far enough. For instance, suppose that there are several children, and they do not agree: Who, then, has priority? For that matter, what if the parents are the appropriate substitute decision-makers, but they don't agree?

Another problem arises if the next-of-kin do not discharge their role as one would normally expect in our society. This would be true, for example, if the wife in case (1) really wanted to be free of the burden of an invalid husband in hospital, wanted to pursue her own life plans, and therefore misrepresented what her husband had told her. It would also be true if parents wanted to have a certain operation for their child—for instance, sterilization—not because it was in the best interests of the child but because it would serve their own convenience. This might well be a version of case (3) above.

In short, to think that the next-of-kin will function consistently and make decisions that are in the best interests of the incompetent person may sometimes be a questionable assumption. Inheritance conflicts, personal animosities and convenience may play a role even in families. Prudence and justice therefore demand that there be some way to guard against this sort of eventuality.

Here the physician has to step in—not as an adjudicator, because that role belongs to the courts, but as someone who identifies the problem and who initiates appropriate steps to solve it. This duty is rooted in the fiduciary nature of the physician–patient relationship that was discussed in Chapter 3. After all, the incompetent individual is the physician's patient, and the fact that a third party enters into the decision-making process does not mean that the elements of trust and care that are characteristic of the physician–patient relationship disappear. Physicians must exercise just as much care when considering the decisions of substitute decision-makers as they would when considering the choices of patients themselves. In fact, physicians must examine these choices even more closely, specifically with an eye to whether they follow the rules that bind acceptable substitute decision-making.

To some degree, of course, whether the substitute decision-making process has gone awry is a matter of subjective assessment. But not entirely. In cases in which the patient was once competent, the physician, before initiating review procedures, will have to balance the quality of life that may be expected from the relevant treatment options against the wishes and expectations that were expressed by the patient when the patient was competent. The physician must then compare this with the choice made by the substitute decision-maker. The less contact the physician has had with the patient prior to the onset of incompetence, the more difficult this will be. In general, the physician in these cases should be guided by the choices that, in his or her estimation, the objective reasonable patient would make.

In this context, it is worth noting that the physician's task is helped tremendously by consultation with other health care professionals, and in particular with the nurses. In most cases, it is the nurses who provide ongoing care for the patient. Therefore, they are much more likely to be attuned to the nuances of the patient's expressions, the values that the patient might hold or might have held, the relationship that the patient has or has had with next-of-kin and so on.

The *Parens Patriae* Powers of the Court

A final note on who may act as substitute decision-maker. As a matter of law, the courts have the power to appoint a substitute decision-maker, and such a substitute decision-maker will take precedence over any other substitute decision-maker—even over one who has previously been appointed by the now incompetent patient. This is called the *parens patriae* powers of the court.[53]

The historical origin of the courts' *parens patriae* powers is unclear. It probably goes back to old English law, when Edward I took over the right of feudal lords to administer the property of persons of "unsound mind" who could no longer fulfill their feudal duties. Beginning around 1660, this power was gradually combined with the Court of Chancery's power to assume the wardship over persons of "unsound mind," and it ultimately evolved into the *parens patriae* powers as these are understood today.[54]

However, the notion of *parens patriae* powers also has an ethical basis. In a just and equitable society there should be some way to ensure that the rights of those who cannot exercise these rights for themselves are in fact exercised, and that they are exercised in an appropriate fashion. Ideally, the duly empowered substitute decision-makers that were identified above would function in this role. However, as we have seen, it is possible that, for some reason or other, duly empowered substitute decision-makers may fail to carry out their mandate appropriately. If there were no independent authority that could look into such matters and, if necessary, provide someone who would carry out that task in an ethically appropriate fashion, the incompetent's rights might well be subverted. Equality and Justice, therefore, entail that there should be such an independent body, and that this body have the necessary power to enforce its decisions. The courts are such a body, and the *parens patriae* powers of the courts are a reflection of this fundamental ethical consideration.

In this connection, it may be worth mentioning that it would be illogical for the courts, when they invoke their *parens patriae* powers, to appeal to considerations of best interest in order to overrule a decision that was competently made by a patient. As Mr. Justice Binnie pointed out in his minority judgment in A.C., considerations of best interest become relevant only once there has been a finding of incompetence. If individuals are competent, it is up to them to decide what is in their best interests, and while their choices may be tragic in the eyes of the court, that opinion would not allow the court to overrule the autonomy or section 7 Charter rights of individuals.

WHAT VALUES SHOULD A SUBSTITUTE DECISION-MAKER USE?

Having identified who the substitute decision-maker should be, we turn to the next question: "What values should a substitute decision-maker use?"

Previously Competent Patients

The guiding rule when trying to answer this question is that the choice made by the substitute decision-maker should come as close as possible to the choice that the incompetent person would make if that person were competent. This follows from the Principle of Autonomy (because every patient has the right to accept or reject any intervention) and the Principle of Equality and Justice (because this right to self-determination should not be removed from the patient simply because of disability).

This rule really presents few difficulties if the patient has previously, while competent, given a clear indication of exactly what should be done. The only question that then arises is whether the situation that was outlined by the patient's directive fits the situation at hand. That may present difficulties in certain cases—for instance, if the patient's advance directive stipulates non-resuscitation in case of a cardiac arrest, but the cardiac arrest was precipitated by the inadvertent administration of antagonistic drugs as a result of medical error, and was not a consequence of the cardiac problems that were considered by the patient when executing the advance directive. However, it is usually quite clear from the wording of the advance directive—or at least it should be clear if the directive is properly executed.

It is also possible that an advance directive does not identify specific interventions to be followed or omitted but simply indicates the core values that should be followed in substitute decision-making. In this event, the work of the substitute decision-maker becomes more difficult, because outcome considerations enter the picture, and these outcomes have to be interpreted in light of the valuational framework specified in the directive. In these cases, the decision cannot be made by the substitute decision-maker independently of medical advice, because the identification of possible outcomes is a professional medical matter. Therefore, if only values are identified in the directive, substitute decision-making will consist in cooperative interaction between the substitute decision-maker and the MRP (or the health team, as applicable), whereby the latter supplies the information that is interpreted by the substitute decision-maker in light of the patient's values.

Things become more difficult when the patient has left no indication of what specific interventions should or should not be followed or of what values the substitute decision-maker should follow in making a decision. In such instances, the substitute decision-maker is faced with two possibilities: He or she can identify relevant values on the basis of the actions, statements and general lifestyle of the patient before the onset of the incompetence; if that is not (reasonably) possible, the substitute decision-maker will have to use the values that an objective reasonable person in the patient's position would use to make a decision.

That is to say, there is no reason to assume that someone whose lifestyle has given no indication of being structured by unusual values or who has not, in any reasonably accessible way, indicated that he or she held unusual or non-standard values, would not in fact subscribe to the general values of the society in which he or she lives. Therefore, one may justifiably assume that such an individual would accept the values that guide other members of society. It follows, therefore, that not to use such values would in fact be to discriminate against the incompetent patient because of this incompetence—and that would be neither just nor fair. Consequently, Equality and Justice entails that when the incompetent patient's values cannot be identified with any degree of certainty, the substitute decision-maker should use the values of the objective reasonable person in that society, insofar as these values are ethically defensible.[55] And since a substitute decision-maker has a fiduciary duty to act in the best way possible and in the best interests of the incompetent person, Fidelity underwrites this conclusion as well.

All of which means that unless an advance directive explicitly stipulates the contrary, a substitute decision-maker may never use her or his own values when acting as substitute decision-maker. Not only is there no guarantee that the incompetent patient would share the values of the substitute, to use one's own values would also be to act as though the decision to be made had become the substitute's own decision, and this might possibly result in a decision that deviated seriously—and without discernible reasons that would be acceptable to the incompetent person—from societal norms.

Patients Who Have Never Been Competent

Children The discussion so far has dealt with substitute decision-making for patients who have previously been competent. That does not include young children and patients who have never been competent because they were born mentally disabled. While the underlying principles that govern substitute decision-making also apply in these cases, they are sufficiently different to deserve separate consideration. Let us begin with considering whether parental values should be guiding.

In the case of young children, what enters into the equation is the fact that as children mature, they tend to acquire the values of the immediate social unit in which they grow up. Case (4) is a good example of this. A.C. may well have acquired her values because of being raised in a Jehovah's Witness family; and if statistics are anything to go by, it is highly likely that when she reaches the age of nineteen, she will still have the same values.[56] Since she would then no longer fall under the relevant legislation that allowed the Manitoba Director of Child and Family Services to intervene in her case, it is also highly likely that her decision against blood transfusions would be binding. Therefore, if the duty of the substitute decision-maker is to make the decision in a way that most closely approximates the kind of decision the incompetent person could make if he or she was in a position to make a decision, it seems *prima facie* reasonable that the parents of children who have never been competent should be permitted to use their own values. After all, it is likely that those would be the values that the children, if competent, would use.

However, the fact—if it is a fact—that people are likely to acquire the values of the family unit in which they grow up does not mean that they will invariably do so. These are merely statistical data. The individual person is not a statistic, especially when it comes to making personal decisions. What is true of a group of people cannot automatically be applied to a particular member of that group. To argue otherwise is to commit the fallacy of division. This person might be different. There is no way of knowing, therefore, whether this particular child would in fact grow up to share the values of its immediate social setting and accordingly reject the relevant treatment.

Moreover, the statistics which supposedly show that children who are born into a particular family unit will come to share in the beliefs and values of the group have not gone unchallenged. Some studies that have looked at value transmission within the family suggest that the relationship is much more complicated. They suggest that there is a "zeitgeist effect," according to which the overall social embedding of the individual, rather than merely the embedding of the individual in the family unit, plays an important formative role. Moreover they suggest that the alleged similarity between parents' and children's values may be more an artifact of cultural stereotyping than of robust reality.[57]

As well, the Principle of Autonomy and Respect for Persons says that everyone has the right to self-determination, subject only to the equal and competing rights of others. That right to self-determination includes the right to develop one's own values. An incompetent child, as in case (2) above, has not yet had that opportunity. It can develop these values only if it grows older. However, it has to be alive in order to grow older. Therefore, its right to self-determination, as guaranteed by the Principle of Autonomy and Respect for Persons, entails that it should be given that opportunity.

Finally, substitute decision-makers have a fiduciary obligation to treat the incompetent person as justly and fairly as possible. This does not simply mean that the incompetent child should be treated like any other child *within that particular family setting*. That would be to draw the boundaries for decision-making too narrowly. Instead, it means that the child should receive the treatment that any other child *within society* is likely to receive. In other words, since in Canada health care is a matter of social right, the standard of what constitutes a level playing field with respect to health care decisions is not what is equitable within the particular family unit but within society as a whole. Therefore, while a competent person may decide to depart from the social norm in matters of values, a substitute decision-maker cannot, in equity, assume that someone who has never been competent has departed from that norm or would in fact do so.

Of course this does not mean that all life-saving or -sustaining treatment modalities are therefore obligatory. The very same reasoning that argues in favour of providing the child with the relevant treatment even against the wishes of the substitute decision-makers—in this case, the parents—also places a limit on the nature and extent of the treatment in question. The treatment must have a reasonable chance of success, whereby the degree of reasonableness is not defined by the health care professionals or the substitute decision-makers. These are interested parties who have a position to defend. It must be defined in terms of what members of society would normally accept.

An ancillary question is whether to treat incompetent persons—say, children who have been found to lack decision-making capacity—against their will if they actively resist. Arguably, the answer must be in the affirmative if certain conditions are met. Specifically, a treatment must have a greater than fifty-fifty chance of success, it must be the sort of treatment that the objective reasonable person would accept and it must be in keeping with the bests interests of that person—whereby the notion of best interests must pay due attention to any psychological harm that would result from being forcibly treated.

Assent and Involving Children in Decision-Making

As has been pointed out above, decision-making capacity is not an all-or-nothing affair. This is especially true in the case of children as they mature. To entirely cut them off from input into the decision-making process would be to ignore the fact that their understanding and their values may have some degree of competence. Not to allow children to have input into the decision-making, and not to pay due regard to their interests and values, would not only denigrate them as persons but could also undermine their cooperation—which in turn could mean that treatment might not be as successful as it would otherwise be. Finally, to ignore children's views entirely might well have tragic consequences for the subjective experiences of the children as persons.

The realization of these factors has evolved over the years and has found expression in two respects. *First*, it is generally agreed that in the context of therapeutic treatment decisions, children should be involved in the decision-making process as much as possible, with the nature and degree of their involvement geared to their level of capacity and understanding.[58] This does not mean that children's decisions should automatically be accepted as binding. That would be to ignore the possibility of their decisional incompetence. Rather, it means that it should not automatically be assumed that the children's position is entirely unreasonable and need not be heard. Due weight should be given to their considerations, values and concerns. In current terminology, this is expressed by saying that whenever possible, substitute decision-makers should seek a child's *assent*. While not binding, either in favour of or against treatment, it should be a relevant consideration commensurate with their maturity and understanding. The age of seven is usually considered an appropriate age at which to involve a child in this fashion. However, here as in all other cases involving consent, what is ultimately telling is not some abstract number but the actual ability of this child under these circumstances to participate in these deliberations. *Second*, when treatment is experimental—this usually refers to Phase III Trials,[59] which will discussed more fully in Chapter 6, "Research Using Human Subjects"—children should in fact have the final say unless there is no other treatment available, the failure to treat at all would have serious or even life-threatening consequences, and the experimental treatment holds out a reasonable expectation of success.[60] In all other cases, the assent should not only be sought but, as was said a moment ago, should be considered binding.[61] This is reflected clearly in the Consent Guidelines that have been promulgated by the medical research centres in Canadian universities, such as the one at the University of Manitoba, which states that[62]

> [t]he child's objection to participating in research should be binding unless the intervention holds out a prospect of direct benefit that is important to the health or well-being of that child and is available only in the context of research.

Substituted Judgment: Permanently Incompetent Patients

The difficulties that substitute decision-makers face in the case of children are magnified in the case of permanently incompetent patients—more specifically, in the case of patients who, unlike normal children, will never attain to competence. The difficulties are magnified because the quality-of-life criteria that would otherwise be appropriate in normal substitute decision-making may well be inappropriate for such patients.

That is to say, one of the considerations that enter into substitute decision-making is the expected quality of life of the patient. This is not a terribly difficult consideration for children who will develop normally because, all other things being equal, their quality of life can be projected on the basis of standard experiences and can be measured with quality-of-life measures. Over the years, a consensus has emerged that, minimally, these quality-of-life measures should have an objective physical and a subjective psychological component.[63] The objective physical component should include measures that assess the patient's physical health and well-being, the ability to function and interact physically with other persons, the absence of pain or discomfort, and in general the ability to take advantage of the opportunities that society offers its members. The psychological component should include measures that assess the patient's cognitive and emotional status, self-perception, stress and in general the degree to which the person can achieve life satisfaction. Some quality-of-life measures also add a spiritual element as a separate component.[64] Moreover, many contemporary measures recognize that quality of life differs from age group to age group. Accordingly, they differ in the number and nature of the variables they measure and emphasize different considerations for people at different stages of their lives.[65]

However, the subjective quality of life of permanently incompetent persons in the sense identified above may differ so fundamentally from that of other persons that neither the objective reasonable person standard nor that standard as adjusted to the level of a child—nor, finally, the patient's own subjective expression (insofar as such an expression is available at all)—can be used as a guide.

The objective reasonable person standard assumes a subjective life experience that simply does not exist in these cases. To use that standard as a guide would therefore be to use something that by its very nature would be inappropriate. The same thing is true of the standard of the reasonable person as adjusted to the level of a child. Even here, one can assume a fundamental commonality of quality perception that is absent in the case of congenitally incompetent patients who will never mature.

The individuals' subjective expressions do not provide much of a guide either. These expressions have to be interpreted. By definition, however, any interpretation will be an interpretation by people who themselves experience the world through an objective reasonable person perspective. That means that the significance of these subjective expressions may be radically misconstrued, because such an interpretation would be based on a world experience that in no way parallels that of incompetents themselves.

The matter was considered by the B.C. Supreme Court in 1983 in *In the Matter of Stephen Dawson.*[66] The Court stated that

> [i]t is not appropriate for an external decision-maker to apply his standards of what constitutes a liveable life . . . The decision can only be made in the context of the disabled person viewing the worthwhileness or otherwise of his life in its own context as a disabled person—and in that context he would not compare his life with that of a person enjoying normal advantages. He would never know of a normal person's life having never experienced it.

In enunciating this position, Mr. Justice L. Mackenzie, who decided the case, was adopting what had become known as a substituted judgment approach[67] for congenitally incompetent persons. It asked the substitute decision-makers to place themselves into the position of the congenitally incompetent person and make the decision from that perspective.

However, closer examination soon showed that this approach presented substitute decision-makers with an insuperable problem. The demand that they put themselves into the position of the incompetent person and judge from that perspective was logically incoherent. If the incompetent person lacks sapient cognitive awareness, then the demand that the substitute decision-makers make a decision from the perspective of the incompetent person is the demand that the substitute decision-makers decide without assuming any vestige of sapient cognitive awareness themselves. Either that, or they would have to project some criteria or some awareness into the situation. In either case, however, it would be to treat the congenitally incompetent person as though that person were not in fact congenitally incompetent. That, however, would be contradictory. The notion of substituted judgment therefore amounted to pure fiction.

The problem was pointed out in the literature. It found judicial recognition in the case of *re Eve*,[68] which formed the basis of case (3) above. Mr. Justice LaForest, in stating the majority judgment, rejected the very concept of substituted judgment roundly as follows:[69]

> [C]hoice presupposes that a person has the mental competence to make it. It may be a matter of debate whether a court should have the power to make the decision if that person lacks the mental capacity to do so. But it is obviously a fiction to suggest that a decision so made is that of the mental incompetent, however much the court may try to put itself in [the incompetent's] place. What the incompetent would choose if she or he could make a choice is simply a matter of speculation.

Mr. Justice LaForest went on to speak of "the sophistry embodied in the argument favouring substituted judgment" and quoted with approval from *Matter of Eberhardy*— a U.S. case, in which the court had stated:[70]

> We conclude that the question is not of choice because it is sophistry to refer to it as such, but rather the question is whether there is a method by which others, acting on behalf of the person's best interests and in the interests, such as they may be, of the state, can exercise the decision.

This, of course, left the substitute decision-maker with the original problem. How should substitute decision-making in such cases proceed? What criteria should be used?

To date, the issue remains unresolved from a legal perspective.[71] A viable solution would need to be based on the fact that if substitute decision-making is appropriate at all, the individual for whom such decisions must be made will still be a person. This means that no matter how different the quality of life of that individual may be it still must be assumed to have a person-oriented nature. That in turn entails that when deciding on treatment or non-treatment, or when deciding the direction that a particular treatment ought to take, the substitute decision-maker need not attempt the impossible task of trying to put her- or himself into the position of the incompetent and decide on the basis of the quality of life that she or he would then (expect to) experience. Nor should the substitute decision-maker simply project what the ordinary person would choose under such circumstances. That would be to ignore the very real difference between the congenitally radically incompetent and the ordinary person. Ethically, therefore, one can offer the following suggestion: The substitute decision-maker should focus on the type of decision that would be appropriate in the case of a normal individual with a similar medical problem and the effect on the quality of life for the affected person relative to treatment and non-treatment.[72]

That is to say, using the medical problem as a basis, the substitute decision-maker could consider the relative changes that would result in the quality of life of the incompetent patient if the treatment options in question were to be employed. Here, any subjective expression of satisfaction with life, psychological affect and other evaluative parameters would have to be taken into consideration and be balanced against the likelihood of improvement (or retention) of sapient cognitive awareness, the possibility of meaningful social interaction, and the general cost of the treatment to the patient in purely human terms irrespective of the individual's values (if any). These changes would have to be expressed in numerical terms. They could be called a comparative quality-of-life coefficient.

The substitute decision-maker should then perform a similar evaluation for an otherwise normal person with a similar medical problem or constellation of problems—if such a case were available and independent of the mental disability of the patient in question—and derive a similar comparative quality-of-life coefficient. The substitute decision-maker could then compare the two coefficients and consider the range of comparative quality-of-life coefficients under which the normal person would opt for treatment. If it turns out that on balance the comparative quality-of-life coefficient of the congenitally incompetent person under treatment would fall below the range considered acceptable for the normal person, the decision would reasonably be against treatment; in all other cases it would be in favour. This would not provide a perfect tool, but it would give substitute decision-makers who find themselves in this situation an objective way of making a decision rather than relying on their own subjective feelings.

CONCLUSION

Incompetent patients are persons. That is a truism—but it is a truism that has serious ethical implications for health care decision-making. It means that the ethical rights that belong to all other patients also belong to incompetent patients, despite their incompetence. This is clearly reflected in the various declarations of medical, ethical and legal authorities, which state that mental handicap is not a reason for discrimination. It is also legally mandated by section 15 of the Canadian Charter of Rights and Freedoms, which outlaws policies, rules and regulations that discriminate on the basis of disability.

Since medical treatment may be administered only on the basis of informed consent, this means that the right to informed consent also belongs to the incompetent patient. The complicating factor, of course, is that the incompetent patient cannot exercise that right because of the fact of incompetence. That is why an incompetent patient has to have a substitute decision-maker whose role is to exercise that right for the incompetent individual. For this notion to be operationalized, however, not only must there be some way of identifying who should function as substitute decision-maker, but there must also be some way of identifying what values such a decision-maker should use.

The discussion in this chapter has tried to shed some light on these issues, with special emphasis being placed on why substitute decision-making is ethically mandated in the first instance, who should function as substitute decision-maker and what should be involved in such decision-making. The discussion has not dealt with the particular ethical issues that arise in the context of specific types of medical and health care situations. The chapters that follow deal with just such issues: issues such as abortion, experimentation, euthanasia and reproductive health care. With due alteration of detail, the concepts that have been developed in this chapter apply there as well.

Further Readings

A.C. v. Manitoba (Director of Child and Family Services), 2009 SCC 30.

Boyle, E.H. *Female Genital Cutting: Cultural Conflict in the Global Community* (Baltimore: Johns Hopkins University Press, 2002), 2, 31.

Buchanan, A., and D. Brock. *Deciding for Others: The Ethics of Surrogate Decision Making* (Cambridge, U.K.: Cambridge University Press, 1989).

Gabor, J.Y. "The Role of Children in Decision-Making and Consent to Cancer Treatment." *University of Toronto Medical Journal* 10.3 (2003): 203–207.

Gaylin, W., and R. Macklin (eds.). *Who Speaks for the Child? The Problems of Proxy Consent* (New York: Plenum Press, 1982).

Heylan, D.K., et al. "Decision-Making in the ICU: Perspectives of the Substitute Decision-Maker." *Intensive Care Medicine* 29.1 (2003): 75–82.

Kluge, E.-H. "Quality-of-Life Considerations in Substitute Decision-Making for Severely Disabled Neonates: The Problem of Developing Awareness." *Theoretical Medicine and Bioethics* 30.5 (2009): 351–366.

Lazar, N.M., et al. "Substitute Decision-Making." *Canadian Medical Association Journal* 155.10 (1996): 135–137.

Peisah, C., O. Forlenza and E. Chiu. "Ethics, Capacity, and Decision-Making in the Practice of Old Age Psychiatry: An Emerging Dialogue." *Current Opinion in Psychiatry* 22.6 (2009): 519–521.

Endnotes

1. The term *most responsible physician*—which is usually abbreviated as MRP—refers to the physician who is in charge of the care of a patient when the patient is in a multi-physician clinical setting.

2. Adapted from a case encountered by the author as an ethics consultant.

3. Adapted from "In the Matter of Kristie Lee F." P.C.C. (F.D.) Ontario (1072/88).

4. Adapted from Re Infant K, Supreme Court of B.C. Jan. 30, 1985, Vancouver Registry A 842 616.

5. Based on A.C. v. Manitoba (Director of Child and Family Services) (2009) SCC 30.

6. C.A. Reyes-Ortiz, "Diogenes Syndrome: The Self-Neglect Elderly," *Comprehensive Therapy* 27.2 (Summer 2001): 117–121.

7. C. Hodgkinson, *The Philosophy of Leadership* (Oxford: B. Blackwell, 1983), 36. See also O. O'Neill, "Practical Principles and Practical Judgment," *Hastings Center Report* 31.3 (2001): 1–23.

8. I. Hyun. "Waiver of Informed Consent, Cultural Sensitivity, and the Problem of Unjust Families and Traditions," *Hastings Center Report* 32.5 (Sep–Oct 2002): 14–22, reprinted in E.-H.W. Kluge, ed., *Readings in Biomedical Ethics: A Canadian Focus*.

9. For a slightly different analysis from a legal perspective, see H. Savage and C. McKague, *Mental Health Law in Canada* (Toronto and Vancouver: Butterworths, 1987), 121–124. See also E.I. Picard

and G.B. Roberts, *Legal Liability of Doctors and Hospitals in Canada*, 4th ed. (Toronto: Thomson-Carswell, 2007), 67–92.

10. For an interesting discussion and analysis of competence, see A.E. Buchanan and D.W. Brock, *Deciding for Others: The Ethics of Surrogate Decision Making* (Cambridge and New York: Cambridge University Press, 1989). For a Canadian legal perspective, see Picard and Roberston, op. cit., Chapter 2.

11. See Picard and Robertson, op. cit.; C.A. Kent, *Medical Ethics: The State of the Law* (Butterworth: Toronto, 2005), Chapter 5, "Consent."

12. *Personal Directives Act* R.S.A. 2000, c. P.

13. *Mental Health Act* R.S.O. 1990, c. M; see also the *Substitute Decisions Act*, 1992 S.O. 1992, c. 30.

14. *Hospitals Act* 1989, Revised Statutes of Nova Scotia, Chapter 208, amended 1994–95, c. 7, ss.29–37, 150; 2000, c. 6, s. 102; 2000, c. 29, ss. 15, 16; 2001, c. 5, s. 4.

15. Johnston v. Wellesley Hospital (1971) 2 O.R. See also Booth v. Toronto General Hospital (1910), 170. W.R. 118. For a more recent case, see Steinback v. Jaffe [1988] O.J. No. 1081. For legal commentary, see A. Kent, Picard and Roberts, loc. cit..; C.A. Kent, loc. cit., A. Linden, *Canadian Tort Law*, 3rd ed. (Toronto: Butterworths, 1982), 60; M. Stauch, K. Wheat and J. Tingle, *Sourcebook on Medical Law* (London: Cavendish Publishing Limited, 1998), 119–126. See also Beauchamp and McCullough, op. cit., 123; Beauchamp and Childress, op. cit., 69.

16. *Mental Health Act* R.S.O. 1990, c. M; see also the *Substitute Decisions Act*, 1992 S.O. 1992, c. 30.

17. This statement assumes a normal or average level of cognitive ability. Clearly, there is a relationship between conceptual ability and education. Someone who is conceptually disabled cannot benefit from higher levels of education.

18. See H. Morreim, "The Concepts of Patient Competence," *Theoretical Medicine* 4.3 (October 1983): 231–251, especially 234–236.

19. A.E. Buchanan and D.W. Brock, *Deciding for Others: The Ethics of Surrogate Decision Making* (New York and Melbourne: Cambridge University Press, 1989).

20. This is similar to the evaluative component that Morreim, *supra*, calls "performance competence" (237 f), although Morreim's notion also includes a volitional parameter.

21. Picard and Robertson, loc cit.; Kent, loc. cit. For the position on children, see below.

22. See O'Neill, op. cit.

23. Personal communication of Sue Rodriguez to the author, who acted as ethics consultant in the case. For formal expression, see Rodriguez v. British Columbia (Attorney General), [1993] 3 S.C.R. 519.

24. Pope Pius XII, "Prolongation of Life: Allocution to an International Congress of Anesthesiologists," *Osservatore Romano* (24 Nov 1957).

25. A.C. v. Manitoba (Director of Child and Family Services), (2009) SCC 30, emphasis added. See also C. Elliott, "Patients doubtfully capable or incapable of consent," in *A Companion to Bioethics*, ed. H. Kuhse and P. Singer (Oxford: Blackwell, 1998), 452–462.

26. I. Hyun, "Authentic Values and Individual Autonomy," *The Journal of Value Inquiry* 35.2 (2001): 195–208, and "Waiver of Informed Consent, Cultural Sensitivity, and the Problem of Unjust Families and Traditions," *Hastings Center Report* 32.5 (2002): 14–22. See also O. Gostin, "Informed Consent, Cultural Sensitivity, and Respect for Persons," *JAMA* 247 (1995): 844–845; S. Benhabib, "Cultural Complexity, Moral Interdependence, and the Global Dialogical Community," in *Women, Culture, and Development: A Study of Human Capabilities*, ed. M.C. Nussbaum and J. Glover (Oxford: Clarendon Press, 1995), 235–255.

27. Hyun, "Waiver of Informed Consent," op. cit., at 16.

28. G. Annas and M. Grodin (eds.), *The Nazi Doctors and the Nuremberg Code: Human Rights in Human Experimentation* (New York: Oxford University Press, 1992).

29. D. Barenblatt, *A Plague upon Humanity* (New York: HarperCollins, 2004); S.H. Harris, *Factories of Death: Japanese Biological Warfare 1932–45 and the American Cover-Up* (London: Routledge, 1994).

30. N.H. Kalin, "Genital and Abdominal Self-Surgery. A Case Report," *Journal of the American Medical Association* 241.20 (May 1979): 2188–2189.

31. See T.S. Szaz, *Ideology and Insanity* (New York: Doubleday, 1970) and *The Myth of Mental Illness: Foundations of a Theory of Personal Conduct* (New York: Hoeber-Harper, 1961).

32. V.N. Dadrian, *The History of the Armenian Genocide: Ethnic Conflict from the Balkans to Anatolia to the Caucasus* (Oxford: Berghahn Books, 1995).

33. This holds even under a utilitarian approach. "Good" would here be defined in terms of good for persons. Therefore, if an act resulted in or aimed at a reduction of personhood, it would be in conflict with the basic principle of utility. This raises the question of how far a hedonistic utilitarian approach can consistently be purely materialistic in orientation. Presumably, that is why Mill ranked pleasures and advocated those that retain awareness and higher human capacities. See J.S. Mill, *Utilitarianism*, Chapter 2.

34. For a legal perspective on a clinical tool in this regard, see *Starson v. Swayze,* [2003] 1 S.C.R. 722, 2003 SCC 32. See also P.S. Appelbaum and T. Grisso, "The MacArthur Treatment Competence Study: I. Mental Illness and Competence to Consent to Treatment," *Law and Human Behavior* 19 (1995): 105–126; T. Grisso et al., "The MacArthur Treatment Competence Study: II. Measures of Abilities Related to Competence to Consent to Treatment," *Law and Human Behavior* 19 (1995): 127–148; and T. Grisso and P.S. Appelbaum, "The MacArthur Treatment Competence Study: III. Abilities of Patients to Consent to Psychiatric and Medical Treatment," *Law and Human Behavior* 19 (1995): 149–174.

35. Starson v. Swayze, [2003] 1 S.C.R. 722, 2003 SCC 32. For an interesting discussion of this case, see J.E. Gray and R.L. O'Reilly, "Supreme Court of Canada's 'Beautiful Mind' case," *Int J Law Psychiatry* 32.5 (2009): 315–322.

36. Tobacco addicts who try to quit smoking but find themselves unable do so fall into this category.

37. Clearly, there is an overlap between authenticity in values and volitional compromise.

38. M. Somerville, *Consent to Medical Care*, Study Paper for the Law Reform Commission of Canada (Ottawa: 1979), 95–103. See also D.C. Martin et al., "Human Subjects in Clinical Research—A Report of Three Studies," *New England Journal of Medicine* 279 (1968): 1426; and A. Jameton, *Nursing Practice: The Ethical Issues* (New York and Toronto: Prentice Hall, 1984), at 128. On the compromising effects of illness and institutional and legal arrangements, see S. Ketchum and C. Pierce, "Rights and Responsibilities," *Journal of Medicine and Philosophy* 6 (1981): 271–279, and G. Annas, "The Emerging Stowaway: Patients' Rights in the 1980s," *Law, Medicine and Health Care* (1982): 32–35, 46. This lack of personal confidence may even affect nurses in the institution; see C.K. Hofling et al., "An Experimental Study in Nurse–Physician Relationships," *Journal of Nervous and Mental Disease* 143 (August 1966): 171–180.

39. For examples of how this may affect the physician–patient relationship regarding sexual contact, etc., see *The Final Report of the Task Force on Sexual Abuse of Patients*: An Independent Task Force Commissioned by The College of Physicians and Surgeons of Ontario (25 Nov 1991).

40. Tri-Council. *Ethical Conduct for Research Involving Humans* (Ottawa: 1998), article 2.2. The whole set of guidelines is available at www.umanitoba.ca/research/media/TCPS_gov_canada_statement.pdf

41. Lloyds Bank Ltd. v. Bundy, (1975) Q.B. 326, at 339. As Lord Denning put it, "a person's capacity may be impaired . . . when his bargaining power is grievously impaired by reason of his own needs or desires, or by his own ignorance or infirmity, coupled with undue influences or pressures brought to bear on him by or for the benefit of the other."

42. Norberg v. Wynrib, (1992) 2 S.C.R. 226, 12 C.C.L.T. (2d) 1, at 257. See also Picard and Robertson, at 44.

43. Percival, *Medical Ethics*, Chapter 1.

44. See R. Veatch, "Models for Ethical Medicine in a Revolutionary Age," *Hastings Center Report* 2 (June 1972): 5–7, for a classic discussion of the so-called "priestly model." For a classic discussion of a middle-of-the-road perspective, see B. Freedman, "A Moral Theory of Informed Consent," *Hastings Center Report* (Aug 1975): 149–157.

45. See *supra* concerning exceptions that centre in the health and welfare of others.

46. That is to say, there having been no previous competently executed indication by the patient of his or her wishes about what direction health care should take should he or she be incompetent and unable to decide for him- or herself. See *Malette vs. Shulman*. On emergency powers from a legal perspective, see Picard and Robertson, op. cit., 56–61.

47. Picard and Robertson, op. cit., 67 ff; Kent, op. cit., Chapter 5. Various provinces specify the identity and ranking of substitute authority. Specific identification of a substitute by the patient aside, the ranking usually follows degree of familial propinquity.

48. Linden, op cit., 63; Picard and Robertson, loc. cit.; Kent, op. cit. For the classic legal case on this, see *Malette v. Shulman*.

49. Matter of C.P. Little, Supreme Court of Newfoundland (1987) No. F87111, at 57.

50. Malette v. Shulman et al. [1990] 67 D.L.R. (4th) 32. For a good discussion of relevant legal cases, see Health Law Institute, Dalhousie University, *Case Summaries: Advance Directives, Do-Not-Resuscitate Orders and Withholding and Withdrawal of Potentially Life-Sustaining Treatment Cases* (April 2004) accessed 8 June 2010 at http://as01.ucis.dal.ca/dhli/cmp_documents/documents/case_studies_2.pdf

51. Mawdsley v. Austin [1985] 1 W.W.R. 369 (B.C.S.C.), 14 DLR 4th 315.

52. Cf. Picard and Robertson, 72–79.

53. Kent, 147 ff; Picard and Robertson, Chapter 2, *passim*. For a discussion of these powers from the court's own perspective, see *Eve*.

54. See *Eve*, which cites *Cary v. Bertie* (1696), 2 Vern. 333, at p. 342, 23 E.R. 814, at 818; Morgan v. Dillon (Ire.) (1724), 9 Mod. R. 135, at p. 139, 88 E.R. 361, at p. 364, as authorities. See also L.B. Costin, "The Historical Context of Child Welfare," in J. Laird, *Handbook of Child Welfare* (New York: Free Press, 1985), 34–60. See also Kent, op. cit., 146 ff.

55. The reason for the phrase *in that society* is that what counts as reasonable will be partly a function of the social context.

56. P. Vedder et al., "The Intergenerational Transmission of Values in National and Immigrant Families: The Role of Zeitgeist," *Journal of Youth and Adolescence* 38.5 (May 2009): 642–653; K. Boehnke, A. Hadjar and D. Baier, "Parent–Child Value Similarity: The Role of Zeitgeist," *Journal of Marriage and Family* 69.3 (2007): 778–792.

57. A.M.C. Roest, J.S. Dubas and J.R.M. Gerris, "Value Similarities among Fathers, Mothers, and Adolescents and the Role of a Cultural Stereotype: Different Measurement Strategies Reconsidered," *Journal of Research and Adolescence* 19.4 (2009): 812–833; K. Boehnke, "Parent–Offspring Value Transmission in a Societal Context," *Journal of Cross-Cultural Psychology* 32.2 (2001): 241–255; K. Boehnke, A. Hadjar and D. Baier, "Parent–Child Value Similarity: The Role of Zeitgeist," *Journal of Marriage and Family* 69.3 (2007): 778–792.

58. C. Harrison et al., "Involving Children in Medical Decisions," *Canadian Medical Association Journal* 156.6 (1997): 825–882.

59. These are studies where the new treatment/drug has passed safety screening (Phase I Trials) and has shown some promise (Phase II Trials).

60. Health Canada Research Ethics Board, *Ethics Review of Research Involving Humans—Administrative Policy and Procedures Manual*, available at www.hc-sc.gc.ca/sr-sr/pubs/advice-avis/reb-cer/index-eng.php#t3_4, s. 3, esp. 3.2–3.5; D. Tomlinson and N.E. Kline, *Pediatric Oncology Nursing: Advanced Clinical Handbook* (Berlin: Springer, 2005), Chapter 16.

61. See Harrison et al. For a slightly different view, see S.L. Berg, "Ethical Challenges in Cancer Research in Children," *The Oncologist* 12.11 (2007): 1336–1343. It should be noted that Berg's position is formulated within the legal context of the U.S., which differs somewhat from Canada in this regard.

62. Informed Consent Guidelines, University of Manitoba, available at www.umanitoba.ca/faculties/medicine/research/ethics/consent_guidelines.htm

63. W. Spitzer, A. Dobson and J. Hall, "Measuring the Quality of Life of Cancer Patients: A Concise QL-Index for Use by Physicians," *Journal of Chronic Diseases* 34 (1981): 585–597; University of Toronto Quality of Life Project, accessed 24 Jul 2008 at www.utoronto.ca/qol/; S.A. Shumaker and M.J. Naughton, "The International Assessment of Health-Related Quality of Life: A Theoretical Approach," in *The International Assessment of Health-Related Quality of Life: Theory, Translation and Analysis*, ed. S.A. Shumaker and R. Berzon (Oxford: Rapid Communications, 1995), 3–10.

64. University of Toronto Quality of Life Project, available at www.utoronto.ca/qol/

65. University of Toronto Quality of Life Project, available at www.utoronto.ca/qol/; S.A. Shumaker and M.J. Naughton, "The International Assessment of Health-Related Quality of Life: A Theoretical Approach," in *The International Assessment of Health-Related Quality of Life: Theory, Translation and Analysis*, ed. S.A. Shumaker and R. Berzon (Oxford: Rapid Communications, 1995), 3–10.

66. In the Matter of Stephen Dawson (1983) 3 W.W.R. 618 (B.C.S.C.) reversing (1983) 3 W.W.R. 597 (B.C. Prov. Ct.).

67. The concept of substituted judgment was introduced in the U.S. case of Superintendent of Belchertown State School v. Saikewicz, 370 N.E. (2d) C 417 (Mass. S.C. 1977).

68. Re Eve, [1986] 2 S.R.C. 388 (S.C.C.).

69. Re Eve, 64.

70. Re Eve, 65.

71. For an interesting discussion of some of the variables involved from a judicial perspective, see Savage and McKague, 121–122. See also E.-H.W. Kluge, "After Eve: Whither Proxy Decision-Making?" *Canadian Medical Association Journal* 137 (1987): 715–720.

72. What follows is based in part on E.-H.W. Kluge, "Quality-of-Life Considerations in Substitute Decision-Making for Severely Disabled Neonates: The Problem of Developing Awareness," *Theoretical Medicine and Bioethics* 30.5 (2009): 351–366.

Chapter 6
Research Using Human Subjects

Experimentation has been an integral part of health care from the beginning. It could scarcely be otherwise. Even traditional medical knowledge is based on experiments. After all, one cannot tell ahead of time what will work, how it will work and what the side effects will be. One has to look and see. Therefore, the question is not *whether* one should experiment but *how*. Should it be haphazard and opportunistic, or should it be scientifically structured so that the results are usable in all analogous cases? Moreover, is good science automatically good ethics, or do other considerations enter?

This chapter attempts to clarify these and related topics. It begins with a brief historical introduction and then goes on to deal with more particular matters, such as the difference between therapeutic and non-therapeutic research, informed consent, the ethical design of research projects and the question of inclusiveness or subject selection. The role of pharmaceutical companies will also be explored as well as issues such as offering rewards for participating in research, the use of placebos and deception.

Questions to Keep in Mind While Reading this Chapter:

1. What is a medical experiment? How does it differ from ordinary health care procedures?

2. How does informed consent in medical research differ from informed consent in the therapeutic setting?

3. What are some of the conditions that an ethically acceptable medical experiment should satisfy?

4. Is there a difference between therapeutic and non-therapeutic experimentation? If so, what is it?

5. Is it acceptable to pay the subjects of medical experimentation?

6. What is meant by "inclusiveness" in subject selection, and why is it important?

7. What is the role of pharmaceutical companies and other funders in the conduct of medical experiments?

INTRODUCTION

Research using human subjects—or, to use more traditional terminology, human experimentation—is as old as medicine itself. In the beginning, it was rather unsophisticated and was conducted on an essentially hit-or-miss basis, using naturally occurring substances or traditional procedures in the hope they might be effective. What worked—or more correctly perhaps, what seemed to work—was retained and became part of traditional medicine; and as health care became the province of specially trained individuals such as shamans, surgeons, midwives and apothecaries, the various traditional practices were incorporated into their training. It was only in the Middle Ages, with Ibn Sina, that medical experimentation was put on a scientific footing and the groundwork was laid for scientifically valid research in medicine.[1]

Scientific validity was not the only thing that was slow in developing. Ethics was another. It was only when the world became aware of the atrocities committed by Nazi physicians—for various reasons, Japanese experimentation was not publicized by the Allies and was not common knowledge until the 1980s[2]—that global concern about the ethics of human experimentation emerged and a concerted effort was made to develop international guidelines.[3] This concern initially surfaced in the Nuremberg Trials of 1945–46,[4] when Nazi physicians and health care administrators were tried for "crimes against humanity." It led to the formulation of the *Nuremberg Code* in 1948.[5] This Code was refined and restated by the World Medical Association in the *Declaration of Helsinki*,[6] and has since found reflection in the *Operational Guidelines for Ethics Committees that Review Biomedical Research* of the World Health Organization,[7] the *International Ethical Guidelines for Biomedical Research Involving Human Subjects* of the Council for International Organizations of Medical Sciences[8] and the *Convention on Human Rights and Biomedicine* of the Council of Europe.[9] It was also foundational to the rules, guidelines and laws that regulate health-related research in countries as diverse as Australia,[10] Canada,[11] the U.K.,[12] the U.S.[13] and China.[14] While these differ in expression and in how they are enforced, the underlying principles are the same and have become integral to modern research ethics.

Focal to the ethics of research using human subjects are several interrelated sets of questions. One set centres in consent: Is informed consent always necessary? Who should give it? What criteria should be used to determine whether it is genuine? Another set of issues centres in the need for experimentation itself: Is it necessary to experiment with human beings at all, or will experimentation on non-human animals suffice?[15] Moreover, is anything "fair game" or are there limits? What is the relationship between scientific validity and ethical acceptability when experimenting with human beings?

There are still other questions. For instance, who should be enrolled in an experiment and under what circumstances? Should people who volunteer for medical experiments receive some kind of material recognition or gratuity? Would this constitute undue enticement? What about compromised populations, such as children, fetuses, people who suffer from dementia and so on? Moreover, what should one do when it becomes clear in the course of a study that the treatment being investigated is superior to the standard treatment but the strict scientific standards that have to be met before the treatment will be approved by licensing authorities have not yet been satisfied? Similarly, should patients who suffer from otherwise untreatable conditions be allowed access to experimental treatments even if they are not enrolled in the projects?

There are also issues that arise when it comes to the funding of research.[16] For instance, could the source of their funding unconsciously bias researchers? Do those who fund the research have the right to impose conditions on the publication of research results? On the analysis of the data that have been developed? These and similar questions are not merely the stuff of academic debates but the subject of bitter litigation.

EXPERIMENTATION: SOME PRELIMINARY ISSUES

Before we address these matters, some preliminary comments about the difference between medical experimentation and therapy, and about why medical experiments are ethically mandated.

What is Distinctive about Medical Experimentation?

All medical interventions have an element of uncertainty. The reason is simple: No two human beings are the same, not even identical twins.[17] Minute changes in DNA as well as differences in organ placement, exposure to diseases and everyday life experiences result in bodies (and minds) that differ from person to person. Therefore, every time a physician treats a patient, there is an element of uncertainty that surrounds the intervention. That is why the Canadian Medical Association (and other medical associations) treat medicine not as a purely scientific enterprise but talk about the "art and science of medicine."[18]

Keeping in mind, then, that all medical interventions involve uncertainty, perhaps the best way to capture what makes research using human subjects different from therapy is to highlight their difference in purpose and design. Two factors distinguish research from therapy: *First*, the main intent in research is not to provide therapy but to discover something new or to remove uncertainty regarding effectiveness, side effects and outcomes. While part of the intent may be therapeutic—for instance, in Phase II and III trials (which will be discussed later)—this is not at the forefront of a researcher's mind. *Second*, research is designed to maximize the possibility of developing scientifically valid and generalizable data applicable to groups of patients, whereas therapy is intended to maximize the chance of successful treatment of the individual patient, using established therapeutic means.

Why Experiment?

Which brings us to the next question: Why engage in medical research at all? This, in turn, can be broken down into two further questions: Why not simply continue with traditional and proven procedures and treatments, and expand on these as the occasion warrants and as one sees fit? and Why perform research on human subjects instead of non-human animals?

The answer to the first question is simple. Physicians have a fiduciary obligation towards their patients. Ethical physicians, therefore, cannot simply accept traditional drugs or procedures merely because they have been handed down for generations. They must be certain—or at least as certain as possible—that these will work appropriately and that there is no better way of providing the relevant care. The only way to ensure this is to subject traditional treatments to careful scrutiny, to examine and improve existing modalities, and to develop new treatments where none exist or are effective. And the only way to do this is to engage in scientifically controlled experimentation.

A great deal of research has been devoted to determining what this means in actual practice. The standard conclusion is that it all depends. The same scientific approach is not appropriate for all types of situations. For instance, a statistical retrospective study may be more appropriate in the case of traditional remedies than a controlled double-blind placebo study; whereas a controlled double-blind placebo study (with or without crossover) may be just the thing to determine the efficacy of a new drug or procedure.

But whatever method is appropriate, it is generally agreed that *experimentation itself* is both appropriate and necessary. Otherwise, unless the parameters of a particular treatment modality are appropriately determined, treatment itself becomes experimentation— but in an uncontrolled fashion.

However, this must be qualified. It does not mean that experimentation is appropriate in all situations. For instance, when the drug, treatment or procedure is well-known and has proven itself effective and appropriate for a particular condition, it would clearly be ethically inappropriate to embark on a new trial to test it. That might well deprive patient-participants of the drug or treatment they would normally receive. The Principle of Fidelity would therefore be violated, and the participating physicians would fail in their obligation to their patients. The potential benefit of trials must always outweigh the potential risks.[19] This has become known as the condition of *equipoise*: There must be genuine uncertainty as to the comparative benefit of the interventions in question.[20]

Another example of an instance in which trials would be inappropriate would be when initial analysis has shown that the drug or treatment being investigated is no better than what is already available, has greater potential side effects or will probably be more expensive, without compensating benefits. Likewise—for reasons that will be discussed more fully later on, when dealing with informed consent in research and experimentation—the continuation of a trial is inappropriate when it has become apparent during the course of the trial that the modality under investigation is more effective or otherwise preferable to the modality against which it is being measured as a control.

As to the second question—Why not confine biomedical research to using non-human animals?—the answer is also simple: While human beings are animals and share a lot of characteristics with other animals, they are not physiologically and biochemically the same. What may work in animal "models" may not work in human beings—or it may work differently and have different side effects. For instance, a study that looked at the predictability of drug toxicity for humans on the basis of animal studies found that transferability ranged from 43 to 71 percent—which meant that simply transferring animal results to human beings would run a 29 to 57 percent risk of failure.[21]

As to the question of why not to dispense with both human and non-human animal testing entirely and use computer models, *in vitro* models derived from human cells, etc., the answer is twofold: Not only would one have to do human testing to acquire the data necessary for constructing the computer models in the first place, but such models—and this includes *in vitro* cultures, etc.—do not mimic how medications or procedures work in human bodies as integrated organ systems.[22]

In the end, therefore, research using human subjects is inescapable in health care. The choice is not *whether* to experiment but *how*. Using anything but the best scientific standards and statistical means would be to violate the fiduciary obligation of physicians towards their patients and of the health care profession towards society.

THE DESIGN OF CLINICAL TRIALS

When looking at the scientific design of research with human beings, it is important to keep in mind that research using human subjects uses human beings. The statement is a tautology, and the point seems trivial—but it has far from trivial implications. The Principle of Autonomy and Respect for Persons stipulates that human beings should always be treated as ends in themselves, never merely as tools or as means to an end. Moreover, the subjects of such research are volunteers. Researchers therefore have an obligation not to abuse the good will of participants and to use their services in the best way possible. This means that research using human subjects should always be structured around the Principles of Autonomy and of Fidelity—which in turn means that it should be preceded by consent and be scientifically valid. It should therefore have a clearly formulated research question, the methodology used to answer that question should be appropriate, the analysis of the data that are developed using that methodology should be logically sound and the study should answer the question it claims to answer. This rules out poorly designed research projects as ethically unacceptable and imposes on administrative bodies such as Research Ethics Committees, whose function it is to supervise human research, the obligation to carefully scrutinize research projects not merely for ethical issues but also for scientific validity. The Tri-Council Guidelines stipulate at 6.4 that such a committee shall have at least two members who "have expertise in relevant research disciplines, fields and methodologies." Therefore, the requirement that Research Ethics Committees vet research proposals for scientific validity seems to be accepted by the Tri-Council, which sets the standards for all publicly funded research in Canada.

Scientific Validity

Scientifically valid medical research—particularly pharmacological research—involves four phases. Phase I studies are "first-in-human" baseline studies to determine the toxicity and safety levels of a drug when it is used on healthy human beings. They usually involve only a small number of people (twenty to one hundred), and participants are generally paid for their participation. Phase II trials are conducted with pharmaceuticals that have passed Phase I trials and usually involve larger numbers (fifty to three hundred). They involve both healthy volunteers as well as patients, and are designed to assess dosing requirements (how much of the drug should be given to show an effect) and to study efficacy (how well it works at the prescribed dosage levels). Phase III studies are randomized, controlled, multi-centred trials in different locations with different health care providers, and potentially involve thousands of patients, depending on the disease or condition being targeted. Their purpose is to provide a definitive assessment of how effective a drug is and what its side effects are. They are generally double-blind, placebo-controlled and randomized. Phase IV studies—sometimes called post-marketing surveillance studies—are designed to identify effectiveness, side effects and other issues once a drug has been licensed and is actually used in therapy, and they do not involve the controlled population groups of clinical trials. Since even the best designed research cannot control for all possible conditions that might affect how a particular drug functions, it is at this Phase IV stage that latent problems begin to emerge.

It is generally accepted that the gold standard for Phase III trials is a randomized, placebo-controlled, double-blind design. In such trials, participants are randomly selected from a stratified list of potential participants, i.e., from a list of individuals who are grouped according to the kinds of health conditions or genetic or physiological makeup that are reasonably expected to react differently to the proposed intervention. They are then divided equally into those that receive the intervention and those that receive a placebo, and neither research subjects nor researchers know who receives the intervention and who receives the placebo.

While the use of placebos is scientifically appropriate, it may on occasion be ethically problematic. Sometimes—and this is particularly true in pharmaceutical research—the object of the research is not to develop a therapy where none exists but to develop one that is more effective, less burdensome or less expensive. In these cases, using placebos instead of established therapy would deprive the participant patients of that therapy if they end up in the placebo group. This would violate the Principle of Fidelity.[23]

There are two ways of dealing with the problem. The standard way is to design such trials by using what are called *active placebos* rather than *pure placebos*, that is to say, using the existing therapy as a placebo rather than something that has no known (or expected) clinical effect on the condition of such participants. The other option is to use a pure placebo, but to inform potential participants that a pure placebo will be used and that the existing therapy will be unavailable if they agree to participate.

Numbers

Research that enrols a large number of participants (such as Phase III trials) may be scientifically valid—the more data points the better—but may go beyond what is strictly necessary to obtain statistically significant results. It is here, once more, that science and ethics intersect. Enrolling more participants than necessary for a statistically significant result is to ignore that human beings are persons and to treat them as mere counters. It would violate the Principles of Fidelity and non-Malfeasance, because it would expose more participants than necessary to the possibility of harm. Therefore, researchers whose research requires human subjects should always be sure that the number of human subjects they enroll is the minimum that is statistically necessary to produce significant results.

For analogous reasons, studies that simply replicate what has been studied before in scientifically valid protocols are inherently unethical, unless there are good grounds to suppose that the previous results were somehow inconclusive or that they did not apply to newly emerging illnesses.

Subject Selection

Another issue under the rubric of scientific validity is subject selection. The reason for conducting research using human subjects is not to develop data that apply only to the individuals enrolled in the study but to develop generalizable data that can be applied to all patients with similar conditions. To this end, not only must the number of subjects enrolled in a study be sufficiently large to yield statistically valid results but the subjects themselves must constitute a representative sample of the patient pool that is supposed to benefit from the research. Therefore, selection criteria must focus solely on relevant medical considerations and issues such as age, race, gender, etc., may not play a role in the selection process unless they are relevant to the scientific matter at issue.

This is not only good science, it is also good ethics, because it is mandated by the Principle of Fidelity (one should do the best one can for people in one's care) and by the Principle of Equality (one should not discriminate on the basis of ethically irrelevant differences). If subject selection were not truly representative of the potential patient pool, it would leave uncertain how the therapy would work with patients who are unrepresented in the study group and would turn the use of the new treatment into an uncontrolled experiment for those who were unrepresented. This happened when women were excluded from studies involving cardiac conditions and children from studies involving anesthesia and analgesics.[24] While this exclusion may not have been deliberate, it did occur. It is perhaps also worth noting that the deliberate exclusion of persons who lack decision-making capacity would fall under the same rubric. While in their case it may be difficult to structure an appropriate consent protocol, it is possible to do so by using the distinction between consent and assent—which will be explored a little later.

Minimal Risk

A somewhat more difficult matter is the concept of minimal risk. The Tri-Council Guidelines permit a researcher to conduct research that would be too risky in his or her own community in another location if the risk factor in the experiment would constitute no higher than "minimal risk" for persons in that other location—where minimal risk is defined as "the probability and magnitude of possible harms implied by participation in the research [being] no greater than those encountered by participants in those aspects of their everyday life that relate to the research."[25]

The Guidelines do go on to say that the inclusion of persons whose daily lives expose them to relatively high levels of risk should not "exacerbate their vulnerability,"[26] but this is still problematic, because it encourages "venue shopping." An example would be choosing Africa as a location to conduct research on the effectiveness of an antimicrobial gel to prevent the transmission of HIV/AIDS, because condom use there is low, infection rates are high, and the research protocol, following locally prevalent practice, does not require the use of condoms. This violates the Principle of Equality. The Principle demands that all persons be treated equally as persons. However, if a risk factor is too high for participation by someone in the researchers' own community, then to go to another community where the risk factors are higher is to treat the relevant parties differently as persons. Ethically, it is irrelevant that the potential participants encounter a high risk level "in those aspects of their everyday life that relate to the research." The fact that the research does not introduce a new risk level is logically independent of the fact that the researchers are taking advantage of the higher risk level. If the Principle were adhered to consistently, the ethically appropriate risk level would not be that of the milieu in which the potential participants are embedded but that of the researchers themselves. Moreover, the safety standards that would be applied in the researchers' own community should also be applied in the experimental setting—standards which would be violated in the example just cited because condom use is not part of the research protocol. Not applying these safety standards would be to take advantage of the misfortune of the potential participants—and that would constitute discrimination.

Balance of Risk and Benefit

Another issue is that of acceptable risk–benefit ratio: i.e., the balance between the risk of harm to the subject and the benefit to be gained. This has nothing to do with science and everything to do with ethics. The reason lies in the fact that harm as such is not a scientific concept. Thus, speaking purely scientifically, the amputation of an organism's limb is just that—the removal of a limb—and a research protocol that looked at whether an organism goes into shock or suffers other effects would look at how the organism's overall functioning is affected by this intervention. Speaking purely scientifically, this can be described in terms of cytokines, coagulation, inflammation, epithelialization, formation of granulation tissue, tissue remodelling, etc. Harm would not be a scientific category that one would include in the description. It becomes meaningful to speak of harm only when one attaches a value to the organism and to its functioning in a particular manner. Harm is therefore a value-based concept and belongs to ethics. With due alteration, similar remarks apply to the concept of benefit.

A research protocol may, therefore, be scientifically valid but involve a risk of harm to its participants that is out of all proportion to the importance of the information to be gained. For instance—to continue with the previous example—if one wanted to find out at what point human beings go into terminal shock from injuries, one could design a scientifically valid protocol that involved vivisection without analgesia or anesthetic. (This was in fact done to prisoners in World War II by Japanese surgeons.)[27] The information that would be gained by such research would be useful for developing ways of dealing with injured persons in real life; however, it would treat the human subjects as mere objects, and the harm that would be done to them would be out of all proportion to the information that was gained. Likewise, infecting mentally disabled children with hepatitis to obtain baseline data on the progression of the disease and to see whether gamma globulin would assist in controlling the infection—as was done in Willowbrook, NY, in the 1960s[28]—might yield useful and possibly important data for dealing with hepatitis, but the harm that such research would produce on its subjects would make it ethically indefensible. Or, finally, while LD50 research designs—designs that determine the dose required to kill half the subjects enrolled in a particular study after a specified test duration[29]—would yield valuable data, they are ethically unacceptable for research using human beings, because they treat the subjects as mere objects.

Health Researchers and Research Ethics Boards (REBs) or Committees

Finally, a few words about REBs and their relationship to the professionals who are involved in medical research. In a sense, it is the professionals who really are the primary players in research. To be sure, research cannot proceed without research subjects, but it is the professionals who initiate and conduct it, and who determine its direction.

Health researchers like to emphasize that their research is intended to benefit society. They rarely point out that they themselves benefit as well. That is to say, much of health research is conducted in hospitals that are associated with universities and medical schools, and most researchers hold academic appointments. At times, this has some potentially disquieting repercussions. Academic careers depend on publications or on the development of new techniques, methods, agents, devices and so on. Researchers, therefore, are motivated at least in part by professional self-interest. This may make researchers whose careers are closely associated with the success of their projects unconsciously somewhat lax in their observance of relevant ethical niceties.

It is here that REBs come in. REBs are part of the surveillance mechanism that society has developed to ensure that human research is conducted as ethically as possible and in accordance with the standards that have been developed since Nuremberg. In Canada, this means that the protocols for all publically funded research or for research that is carried out in public institutions have to be vetted by a duly constituted institutional REB on the basis of the Tri-Council Guidelines. If, in the REB's opinion, there is anything amiss in the protocol, or if it could be improved in some fashion, the REB either withholds approval or gives conditional approval, subject to appropriate changes being made. Moreover, approval usually comes with the condition that a report be made by the principal investigator(s) to the REB at the conclusion of the project.

In years gone by, REBs (or their equivalents) included a preponderance of health care professionals. While these were well trained in their areas of specialization, most had very little training in ethics. Moreover, health care professionals, and especially those who are also academics, tend to live and work in a subculture whose perspectives and values differ from the rest of society. Not surprisingly, therefore, their decisions were sometimes out of step with general social values. To avoid such problems, contemporary REBs include laypersons and individuals trained in ethics. In fact, this is a requirement that is codified in the Tri-Council Guidelines' stipulations on the constitution of REBs.[30]

Of course, the fact that a research protocol has been approved by an REB does not guarantee that it will actually be carried out in an ethically appropriate fashion. That is why the Guidelines also stipulate that REBs have an oversight function over approved projects for the lifetime of the research.[31]

However, no matter how diligent REBs may be in their operation, their effectiveness as monitoring agencies depends to a considerable degree on the willingness of researchers to report discrepancies in ethical practice. There are fairly recent cases other than from Nazi German and wartime Japan when such reporting did not take place. The Tuskegee study in the U.S. is a case in point.[32] Several generations of health care professionals and senior health care administrators knew that the study was unethical, and that reporting mechanisms were available that would have brought the study under scrutiny even in the absence of modern REBs. The Willowbrook experiment is another example. In neither case did anyone associated with the research "blow the whistle."

The U.S. has no monopoly on such cases. The research on "psychic driving" and "depatterning" performed by Ewen Cameron in the late 1950s and early 1960s at the Allen Memorial Institute of McGill University—the so-called MKULTRA experiment[33]— is merely one of a series of Canadian examples. Cameron carried out psychiatric research to develop brainwashing techniques for the Western intelligence community.[34] The research involved subjecting patients to rather unusual procedures that included the use of psychotropic drugs such as LSD, keeping the patients asleep for prolonged periods of time (sometimes for more than eighty-five days at a stretch), the use of chlorpromazine, barbiturates, sodium amytal, repeated electroconvulsive shock treatments and so on. Cameron's colleagues were apparently aware that these treatments contravened standard medical and research practice—in particular, that they contravened the *Nuremberg Code*—that they had dubious therapeutic value and were performed without informed consent from either the patients themselves or duly empowered substitute decision-makers.[35] The colleagues were also aware that the procedures violated the traditional medical-ethical tenet of *primum non nocere!* (Above all, do no harm!) and thus contravened not only the Principles of Autonomy and Fidelity but also the Principles of Beneficence and non-Malfeasance. Yet no colleague or co-worker informed the relevant authorities.[36]

The point of recounting these examples is not to suggest that all of this has changed with the advent of modern REBs and their oversight role. The point is that even when oversight mechanisms exist—and they existed at that time as well—they will work only if those who are in a position to engage them actually do so. In other words, it requires forthrightness on part of the research community itself. All researchers, whether junior or senior, have a duty to take appropriate steps when they have doubts about the ethical acceptability of a procedure or practice. This duty holds all the more strictly, the more innovative or the more experimental the procedure and the greater the potential harm. The prestige of a senior colleague—Cameron was President of the American Psychiatric Association and became President of the World Psychiatric Association—or even of a teacher, should not be allowed to obscure this fact.[37] Not to take the necessary steps when appropriate is to fail the research subjects. In the case of Cameron's research, several people suffered irreversible destruction of fundamental parts of their personalities. The fact that they did not die, as did many in the Tuskegee experiment, is of little ethical consolation.

Therapeutic and Non-Therapeutic Experimentation

Finally, a brief note about the distinction between therapeutic and non-therapeutic research.[38] Therapeutic research is research on medical conditions shared by the patient-subjects, conducted on the understanding that there is some possibility it will benefit them. In the words of the Tri-Council, it is research that is "conducted with populations whose therapeutic options have been exhausted" and whose purpose is to see whether the new treatment has any chance of success.[39] Phase II and III trials in pharmacological research are classic examples, because only patients who might benefit from the therapy would be enrolled in these trials.

By contrast, therapy is not an issue at all in non-therapeutic research. The sole intent here is to advance knowledge or perfect a technique. If there is any benefit for the subjects, this will be incidental. Phase I pharmaceutical trials fall into this category. They are "first-in-human" trials in which the subjects are healthy persons. They may sometimes include patients for whom conventional treatment has failed. However, even then the explicit purpose is to establish baseline data. There is little if any likelihood of clinical benefit for the participants.[40]

While the distinction between therapeutic and non-therapeutic research seems intuitively clear, not everyone agrees with it. Some have argued that the experimental component of so-called therapeutic research automatically disqualifies it as genuine therapy, and that the inclusion of patients in Phase II and III trials may well conflict with the fiduciary obligations of the attending physicians.[41] This opinion is not generally shared in the health care community, and it is argued that any concerns that might arise in this connection can be met by ensuring that participation in medical research is only on the basis of proper informed consent.

CONSENT IN EXPERIMENTATION

Which brings us to informed consent in the research setting. It is important to be clear what informed consent here amounts to because it is different from informed consent to therapy.

Consent in Research versus Consent in Therapy

To clarify the point, it may be useful to go back to beginnings. The difference between consent to being a research subject and consent to being treated as a patient is grounded in the difference between research and therapy, and the different roles of researchers and therapists.

More specifically, the therapeutic physician–patient relationship is a therapeutic relationship based in trust. Hence its name: *fiduciary*. Patients can trust that their physicians will do what is in their best interests and will not deceive them. It also is understood that unless it is clearly stated otherwise, the therapy is of a standard and validated nature. When that is not the case, the patient has the right to know this, and the physician has to inform the patient, unasked, of that fact.

By contrast, the subjects in human experiments are voluntarily exposing themselves to indeterminate risks, and are agreeing to interventions whose primary purpose is not to provide therapy for themselves but to benefit others. The consent process must therefore be still more scrupulous and encompassing than the consent process for therapy. The researcher must disclose, *unasked*, not simply what the objective reasonable person in a patient's position would want to know but *everything* that is known about the research protocol, including all anticipated and known risks and outcomes. In other words, while the standard for informed consent in the therapeutic setting is the (modified) objective reasonable person standard, the standard in the research setting is the complete disclosure standard.

This is not only a matter of ethics; it is also a matter of law. It is clearly expressed in the 1965 case of *Halushka v. University of Saskatchewan*.[42] The case involved a university student who had volunteered to participate in a non-therapeutic experiment involving a new anesthetic. He had not been told that the anesthetic was new, that a tube would be advanced through a vein and into his heart to monitor the effect of the anesthetic, or that the procedure involved a low but quantifiable degree of serious risk. The risk did materialize, and Mr. Halushka was left half paralyzed. He sued the University—and won. As the Court stated,[43]

> There can be no exceptions to the . . . requirements of disclosure in the case of
> research . . . The subject of medical experimentation is entitled to a full and frank
> disclosure of all the facts, probabilities and opinions which a reasonable man might
> be expected to consider before giving his consent.

It was not always this way. Aside from the examples of German and Japanese experiments already mentioned, one of the best-known examples of research conducted without appropriate informed consent involved the discovery of the vaccination against smallpox. Edward Jenner believed that fluid taken from blisters raised by cowpox would yield immunity to smallpox. To test this, he inoculated an eight-year-old boy without consent from the boy or his parents. The experiment was a success and resulted in treatment that led to the eradication of smallpox, thus saving hundreds of millions of human lives.[44] But that is hindsight. There was no way Jenner could have known this at the time. He had a well-founded suspicion, to be sure—milkmaids who came down with cowpox rarely if ever contracted smallpox—but it was merely a suspicion. What he was doing was uncontrolled research without consent.

Different Ethical Perspectives

The stunning success of Jenner's experiment raises the question of whether concern over study design and informed consent in research is really all that important, given the potential for tremendous gains.

The answer sketched so far has been framed from a deontological perspective. Specifically, it was grounded in the Principle of Autonomy and in the fiduciary nature of the physician–patient relationship, both of which have a deontological basis. However, a utilitarian might well see this differently. A utilitarian could argue that the Jenner case clearly demonstrates that there are occasions when the greatest good for the greatest number outweighs by far any injury that individual people (or even to a small minority of persons) might suffer. Of course, one should always have good reasons for embarking on research in the first place—utility itself demands that resources not be wasted—and research protocols should be scientifically designed to maximize the likelihood of meaningful (and hopefully successful) outcomes. But one should not rule out the very possibility of arriving at such answers by insisting on the niceties of informed consent. If one did, one would forever be barred from doing certain kinds of research and from developing treatments that might advance the welfare of all humanity.

Likewise, a communitarian could argue that societies are not simply aggregates of individual person-atoms, each distinct and separate in its own sphere of self-determination. Societies are made up of people who are interconnected. They can exist and function only if the individuals do not insist on their autonomy at the cost of social welfare—because if they do, their own welfare will be imperiled as well. Therefore, there are occasions when informed consent to research must be dispensed with, and health research is just such a case. Here, the very nature of society demands that common interests transcend self-interest.

Clearly, which conclusion is valid depends on the ethical system one adopts. If the analysis of the preceding chapters is correct, the appropriate approach is deontological. It is certainly the approach that underlies current guidelines both in Canada and in the global community as a whole.

The "Forbidden Fruit" Controversy: Using Unethically Derived Data

A related issue is whether medical results that have been obtained by unethical means may be used by health care professionals to help their patients. In the case of Jenner's experiment, it may be relatively easy to answer in the affirmative. At least, nothing in the literature has suggested that Jenner's results should not have been used to eradicate smallpox. However, the use of Nazi experimental results—but, interestingly enough, not of Japanese data—has stirred up considerable debate.

The argument against using these results centres in what has been called the "forbidden fruit doctrine." This is the doctrine that if one comes into possession of something by unethical means, then that thing is tainted by its origin and may not be used.[45] It maintains that the data from German and Japanese research are indelibly tainted by their origin, and that to use them is not only unethical in itself but also encourages the deliberate ignoring of ethical standards simply to obtain interesting and important results.

The argument for using the data has two strands. One strand is essentially pragmatic. It centres in the fact that this research provided data that could not be derived using modern ethical standards but that were—and continue to be—invaluable in developing modern therapies. For example, the Nazi data have been used to develop hyperbaric treatment for decompression sickness and for air embolisms as well as for dealing with hypothermia, and have proved invaluable in the development of sulfonylureas and thiazide diuretics. Similarly, Japanese experiments on frostbite and dehydration have laid the foundation for therapeutic measures to deal with these conditions, and their experiments of infecting prisoners with virulent infectious diseases have provided important data for developing protocols to deal with epidemics and pandemics.

The second strand for using the data is more ethical in orientation. It begins with the fiduciary obligation of physicians towards their patients and combines this with the thesis that the deliberate failure to intervene in a causal chain of events when one has a duty to do so constitutes a moral failure on part of the person who has that duty. (For more on this in the context of active/passive euthanasia, see Chapter 7.) On that basis it argues that the failure to use the relevant Japanese data is not only to become unethical through inaction but is also to become a passive agent of patient harm.

The positive strand—in particular the second version—has quite a bit of plausibility. By contrast, the negative stance is more difficult to defend, its gut-level appeal notwithstanding. Among other things, it has to assume that things—in this case data—can have ethical properties in and of themselves and independently of how they are used. Without this assumption, it makes no sense to say that unethically obtained data are tainted. It also requires the assumption that once something has acquired an ethical property, that property remains an integral aspect of its nature no matter how it is used. That would mean that most medical interventions and techniques could not be used either, because they were developed unethically. While this is not a logical reason for rejecting the negative stance, it should give anyone who advances it pause to consider what its acceptance would entail from a metaphysical perspective and, perhaps more importantly, whether it can be consistently maintained in practice.

But what is perhaps more important is that the negative stance must either deny that one can become an agent of harm by not doing something—in this case, by not using therapeutic means that are at one's disposal—or say that unethically derived means are not means that are at one's disposal. The first would contradict the concept of negligence. It would also invalidate the Principle of Beneficence and undermine the "Good Samaritan" legislation of Quebec (and most European countries). They stipulate that everyone has a duty to come to the assistance of a person in need if they can do so without undue danger to themselves. As to the second, it simply defines unethically derived means as non-available means. It therefore begs the question.

As was said, the positive stance is much more easily defended. It follows standard ethical and logical reasoning by distinguishing between a thing and its use. By the same token, however, it runs the danger of retroactively sanitizing unethical acts because of their positive effects. Anyone who adopts the positive stance, therefore, has to be careful to make it very clear that he or she is not condoning unethical acts, i.e., is basing his or her stance on the simple logical position that to use what is obtained unethically is not thereby to endorse the unethical act itself.

Innovative Procedures

Another controversial issue is the use of what are sometimes called innovative procedures. "Off-label" drug usage is a good example.[46] Innovative procedures are modalities that have been validated for conditions other than the one being treated. Because they are not validated for the new condition, their use involves an element of research. For instance, using propranolol (which was initially approved for tachyarrhythmias) as an antihypertensive and antianginal agent constitutes innovative use, as does the use of recombinant factor VIIa (an anticoagulant originally approved for the management of hemophilia patients who have developed inhibitors to factor VIII) for patients who have undergone cardiovascular surgery or suffer from trauma and intracerebral hemorrhage.[47] Their established track record in their validated contexts removes some uncertainty. Indeed, the uncertainty surrounding their use in the new context may be minimal. However, the degree of uncertainty that surrounds their use here is greater than the degree of uncertainty when they are used in their validated setting. Therefore, logically speaking, innovative use constitutes uncontrolled experimentation, and patients have a right to be aware of this. Ethically, they should be asked for an explicit informed consent that satisfies research standards.

THE TRI-COUNCIL GUIDELINES AND CONSENT IN THE RESEARCH SETTING

In Canada, research is subject to the Tri-Council Guidelines. Among other things, these stipulate that research must not proceed without consent, and that the consent process should make clear the reason for the study, the techniques that will be involved (such as randomization of treatment), the reason why the prospective subject(s) is (are) being invited to take part in the study, the reasonably anticipated benefits and consequences of the study in general and for the prospective subject(s) in particular. If benefits are not anticipated, this should be stated; and foreseeable risks, including discomforts and inconveniences to the prospective subject(s) or third parties should be made clear. The consent process should also indicate how the confidentiality of subjects will be protected, where and how long the data will be kept, their ultimate disposition, who will have access, and whether they will be published or used in any other way inclusive of secondary use in other projects. It should also clearly state the anticipated time commitments of the subject(s), the intent (if any) to conduct follow-up studies, the conditions under which the study will be stopped and the fact that participants may withdraw at any time for any reason unless withdrawal will jeopardize their well-being.[48] All of this must be disclosed at a level and in a manner that the research subjects can and do understand.

If the person who participates is also a patient who is currently undergoing treatment, the consent process must also disclose whether and how the research may interfere with his or her current therapy and what therapy will be unavailable as a result of participation. Moreover, it must be made clear which procedures will be part of the research protocol and which will be a part of usual patient care.[49]

Deception and the Possibility of Harm

At first glance, this raises a serious problem for the use of placebos in Phase II and III trials. Arguably, the use of placebos involves deception. *Prima facie*, this contradicts everything that has been said about consent.

However, the difficulty is more apparent than real. While researchers have a duty to be truthful, research subjects can competently agree to waive the right to be told the truth about what they are being given or whether the intervention they receive is genuine or a sham. The only condition is that their waiver must be based on a full understanding that the latter may in fact be the case. Therefore, if a project involves the use of placebos, that fact must be disclosed at the outset and as part of the information that is given to potential research subjects before they make a decision about participation.

A more difficult situation arises when deception is necessary because of the very nature of the research itself. Some psychiatric research falls under this rubric. The Tri-Council Policy stipulates that deception should be used only when the research deals with an important issue, could not practically be carried out without deception and involves no more than minimal risk to the subjects, and when the subjects can be debriefed about the fact of deception without harm or detriment to their welfare at the conclusion of the project.[50]

However, this assumes that it is possible to tell beforehand whether someone can be debriefed without harm. This may be problematic. For instance, it is impossible to tell beforehand whether or not someone, who as a result of participating in an experiment becomes aware of unpleasant character traits of which he or she was previously unaware, will sustain damage to his or her self-image and self-esteem. Nor can one guarantee that "debriefing" will deal with the problem. Likewise, it may happen that a participant develops psychological traits or tendencies which, but for the experiment itself, would never have developed.

Of course, *any* medical intervention may introduce a new element or activate a latent condition that, but for that intervention, would not have arisen. In the case of physiological experiments, however, this possibility of iatrogenic harm can usually be guarded against by proper controls on the parameters of the experiment, either in terms of cut-off points, quality control or simply proper design. There is no such possibility in the case of psychological experiments that affect the very psyche of the individual. The very substance of such an experiment is psychological manipulation. Debriefing may well be nothing more than an application of a Band-Aid to a wound that has been artificially inflicted.

This, in turn, points to a fundamental problem for the Tri-Council Guidelines and similar documents. By allowing unconsented-to deception at all, they are in effect saying that if certain data can be obtained only by violating the Principle of Autonomy and Respect for Persons and the Principle of Fidelity, then it is permissible to do so—as long as the risk is minimal.

Debriefing does not change the situation. In fact, to appeal to debriefing as, so to speak, ethically sanitizing the situation is to be logically confused. Even assuming that debriefing works, it amounts to saying that ethical principles have not been violated because one has not produced any harm. That, however, confuses violating a right with taking corrective action once the right has been violated. To draw an analogy—which admittedly is somewhat extreme but will serve to illustrate the point—it would be like saying that it was ethically defensible to non-consensually kill someone for the sake of science if that person could be brought back to life and receive an apology and handsome settlement. The very act itself would still be unethical. The issue is not the correction of a deliberately inflicted harm but the violation of a right.

Consent and Autonomy: The Problem of Incompetent Persons

That leads to another issue. Ironically, strict adherence to the requirement of informed consent by research subjects would constitute discrimination. To put this into context, recall that incompetent persons cannot give consent. That is why, in the therapeutic setting, society has developed substitute decision-making lest incompetent patients be deprived of their right to health care because of their disability. However, a just society must not only ensure that its members have equitable access to the health care that is available but also that appropriate health care is available in the first place.

That poses a problem with children and with adults who are incompetent, when the latter's incompetence is caused by a disease process or condition. As was mentioned, children metabolize drugs differently from adults, their bodies respond differently to surgical and other interventions, and psychiatric interventions for adults are inappropriate for children. The only way to develop appropriate therapies for them is to perform scientifically valid experiments and use them as research subjects. Otherwise, all pediatric therapy would amount to uncontrolled experimentation. As to incompetent adults who suffer from senile dementia, Alzheimer's disease or Parkinsonism—indeed, from any kind of illness that compromises their decision-making capacity—they also will not receive appropriate therapy unless they are involved in research projects that specifically target their conditions.

The strategy for dealing with this issue that has been developed by the Canadian research community and that is endorsed by the Tri-Council is an adaptation of the substitute decision-making approach familiar from the therapeutic context—but with a difference. Substitute decision-makers may enrol their incompetent charges in research projects designed to provide therapeutic answers for their condition if, in the case of Phase I trials, it is reasonably certain that the project involves no more than minimal risk. In Phase II and III trials, the risk must again be no more than minimal. Moreover, the project must be specific for their medical conditions and the placebo controls that are used must not be pure placebos if active placebos—i.e., therapies—already exist. It goes almost without saying that the proxy, or surrogate, decision-makers should be given all the relevant information that would normally be revealed to research subjects if they were competent, and that the values used by the substitute decision-makers in reaching their decisions should not be the substitutes' own but those of the objective reasonable person.

And therein lies a problem. Not all objective reasonable persons volunteer for medical research. Is that because there is no duty to participate in medical research, or is it because these individuals are merely objective reasonable persons from a cognitive perspective and not objective reasonable persons in an ethical sense? In short, is there a moral duty to participate in medical research—a duty that an ethically objective reasonable person would try to fulfill? Because if there is, substitute decision-makers, using the objective reasonable person standard in this second, moral sense would have good grounds for making a decision in favour of participation.

The Duty to Participate in Medical Research

Opinion is divided on this issue. Some ethicists have argued that there is no such duty: that such a duty could exist only if health care were a social good—which they deny.[51] Others (who also reject such a claim) have pointed to the fact that most people pay for the medical care they receive either directly on a fee-for-service basis or indirectly through insurance premiums or their taxes. Hence, they reject the claim that those who benefit from medicine without contributing to research are free riders and are acting unfairly.[52]

Some on the affirmative side have argued that the duty follows from the Principle of Beneficence—the duty to help others.[53] Others have argued that people who wish to receive health care but are unwilling to participate in medical research are "free riders."[54] The issue, so they argue, is not whether they are paying for their therapy, because of course in one way or another they do; the issue is the existence of the therapy itself. If research were not done, irrespective of whether it is done in a controlled or an uncontrolled fashion, the therapy would not exist.

Still others have adopted a more mitigated stance. They have argued that, while there is a duty to participate in medical research, this is an imperfect duty. There is no duty to participate in all possible medical research projects, only a duty to participate in research that touches one's own health care needs or condition.[55] A similar conditional stance is taken by those who argue that the duty is conditioned by the social context in which people find themselves.[56]

Clearly, which stance is ethically more defensible largely depends on what perspective one adopts on the right to health care. If health care is a right, participation is a duty, and the only question is how to manage it.[57] If health care is a commodity, there is no such duty. At best, participation is a supererogatory act that deserves praise. Therefore, the question whether substitute decision-makers, using the objective reasonable person standards, would have good ethical grounds for deciding in favour of participation also depends on which of these perspectives one adopts. Chapter 9 will present reasons for saying that health care is a right. Therefore, if that reasoning is sound, there is a duty for even incompetent persons to participate, and substitute decision-makers may decide accordingly. Arguably, however, it would encompass only those research projects that are relevant to the health conditions of the persons in question.[58]

Infants, Incompetent Adults and Phase I Trials

At first glance, the adoption of a rights-oriented approach to health care answers the initial question of whether substitute decision-makers, using objective reasonable person standards, could enrol infants or incompetent persons in medical research. Since some advantage may be gained for them in Phase II and III trials relevant to whatever health conditions they might have (and since active placebos would be used if treatment existed, so they would not be deprived of treatment otherwise available to them), this would closely mirror the objective reasonable person standard for competent persons.

But this only narrows the problem and does not solve it. It does not apply to Phase I trials. Phase I trials involve healthy individuals. Therefore, unless one can show that the average reasonable competent person would enrol in a Phase I trial, one cannot say that substitute decision-makers, who must use an objective reasonable person standard, would be ethically justified in enrolling their charges in Phase I trials—which, in turn, means that if one were to behave ethically, one could never develop scientifically validated therapies for infants and children.

One could of course adopt the more uncompromising of the two positive positions indicated above and say that all competent persons have a duty to volunteer for Phase I trials, that the fact most people don't merely reflects their lack of ethics in this regard, and that an *ethical* objective reasonable person would volunteer if the risk posed by participating is no greater than minimal.

There is an even easier way to deal with the issue. One could simply adopt a (hedonistic) utilitarian ethics. According to this approach, there is no fundamental right to autonomy, and the whole issue of informed consent and of who participates in what research becomes simply a matter of what is most likely to result in the best possible health care for the greatest number of people. That would allow researchers to enrol anyone—including infants, children and the mentally disabled—into any sort of research at any level, as long as doing so was likely to produce the greatest good for the greatest number. However, this solution would invalidate all of the ethical concerns that led to the condemnation of German and Japanese experiments in prison camps, the use of incompetent children in the U.S. Willowbrook experiment or any other research that did not respect fundamental human rights. It would not even be clear that racist and ethnocentric reasons for selecting research subjects would be ruled out—unless one could come up with a way of showing that hedonistic utilitarianism would militate against such selection.

Assent

Another important issue is what significance to attach to an incompetent person's objection to participating in research. Since they lack competence, should their objection be respected?

The answer that has evolved over the years is couched in terms of *assent*. Assent differs from consent in that it is based not on valuational competence and reasoned understanding but on feelings and inclinations, and it may be expressed either verbally or behaviourally. Therefore, the rule is that substitute consent is necessary but not sufficient for including incompetent persons in medical research. Researchers must also obtain the assent of incompetent persons. If assent is lacking or withdrawn—that is to say, if incompetent persons express dissent or show any sign that they do not wish to be enrolled or continue participation—then they may not be enrolled or their participation must cease, as the case may be.[59]

Appearances notwithstanding, this does not contradict the logic of substitute decision-making. Decisions that are made by competent persons are translated into action on the basis of their values, which function as action potentials. (See Chapter 4.) Competent persons, therefore, would never (competently) act on decisions that violated their values. The feelings and inclinations of incompetent persons function as action potentials; they therefore play the same role as the values of competent persons. Consequently, to force incompetent persons to participate in research against their feelings and inclinations would be like forcing competent persons to participate in research against their values. This would violate the Principles of Equality and of non-Malfeasance.

REWARD AND ENTICEMENT

Consent involves understanding and values, but it also involves volition. As Chapters 4 and 5 pointed out, under certain circumstances a patient's will may be overborne, and while the consent may look free and informed, it is actually coerced. In the therapeutic context, power relationships and undue enticement were identified as being of particular concern in this regard.

Overt coercion does not play much of a role in research since the *Nuremberg Code*. However, power relationships may, and Phase I trials frequently offer rewards in the form of payments or gifts in order to encourage volunteers. Since the attractiveness of a reward depends on the situation of the specific individual, it is possible that if the reward is sufficiently large or attractive, some persons may agree to participate who would otherwise have no such inclination. Arguably, therefore, offering such *undue enticement* would amount to overbearing the individual's will, and the person's consent would be volitionally compromised. That is why it has been argued that if someone participates in research solely because of the reward that is offered, and if in the absence of such a reward the person would not consent, then the reward itself must be considered ethically suspect.

However, it has also been argued that this amounts to a limitation of freedom. All of us do things for reward that we would not do if no reward was offered. Working for a living normally falls under this rubric, yet no one would consider it unethical for employers to offer a salary to their workers for doing the work.

A possible way to resolve this disagreement might be found by linking the nature of the reward to the situation of the potential volunteer. Thus, offering a reward would not be unethical in and of itself. It is unethical only if the nature and size of the reward exceeds normal resource availability for individuals in that position. Similar remarks apply to manipulation, the use of authority (for instance, between teachers and students, employers and employees, or persons in a position of power) and the exploitation of trust relationships such as those that exist between physicians and their patients. It is generally agreed that this rule may be breached under certain circumstances in Phase II and Phase III trials. However, there is no definitive or even generally agreed-on analysis of these issues, and even the Tri-Council Guidelines have very little to offer in this regard.

It is important to note that these considerations, as indeed all the conditions on ethically acceptable research, also apply to all research carried out in the Correctional Service of Canada. Commissioner's Directive "009 – Research" explicitly stipulates, under paragraph 9, that research projects must be in compliance "with the Tri-Council's Policy Statement on Ethical Conduct for Research Involving Humans."

CONSENT AND COLLECTIVITIES

The discussion so far has proceeded on the assumption that consent is something that centres in the autonomy of the individual person. However, collectivities such as the Indian, Inuit and Métis peoples of Canada may have consent traditions that differ from that of non-Aboriginal peoples. Moreover, these collectivities may define their identity not simply in terms of historical and cultural parameters but also in terms of genetic and physiological characteristics as expressed in the fluids, tissues and organ systems of their members. It has therefore been suggested that consent to research involving members of these collectivities should not focus solely on the individual to the exclusion of the collectivity—that over and above individual consent, the collectivity's consent must also be obtained.[60]

It is not clear, however, that tradition in itself is sufficient ethical justification for expanding the consent process. There is a difference between something having historical roots and it being ethically acceptable. The question therefore arises whether traditional consent structures as found among First Nations—or, indeed, among any collectivity in Canadian society—that require consent not only from the individual participant but also from the collectivity are ethically defensible and should be incorporated into the consent process for members of such communities.

An important fact to keep in mind when addressing this question is that being a member of a collectivity does not turn an individual into a non-person. The Principle of Autonomy applies to members of collectivities just as much as to anyone else. As persons, therefore, they have the right to choose their values and to subordinate their autonomy to those of others if they so wish—as long as those values are themselves ethically defensible and the subordination does not reduce them to the status of mere objects. Therefore, as the Tri-Council states, while it is ethically appropriate for researchers to familiarize themselves with the traditional consent structures of collectivities and to engage them when enrolling members of these collectivities in their research projects, consent from the collectivity should not be a substitute for consent from the individual members, and the decision of the collectivity should not devalue the individuals as persons.[61]

THE ROLE OF PHARMACEUTICAL COMPANIES

A final word about a player in human research whose role is central but who has been essentially ignored in the discussion so far. Without this player, health research would generally not proceed. That player is the pharmaceutical industry.

Research funding for Canadian universities has steadily declined over the last decades, and researchers have increasingly been forced to look for outside sources of funding. Not surprisingly, the pharmaceutical industry has become an attractive source. Universities have welcomed this. Among other things, it means that they and the researchers may share in the profits from the research as part of the funding arrangement.

Control of Data and Results

However, while benefiting both sides, this arrangement may pose ethical problems. Specifically, academic researchers have a duty not merely to conduct their research in accordance with the Tri-Council Guidelines but also to publish their results in an unbiased and scientifically valid fashion. By contrast, the pharmaceutical corporations have a duty to maximize profits for their shareholders.

In this connection, it is important to keep in mind that pharmaceutical research is not cheap. Estimates for the costs of bringing a new drug to market range from $800 million to $1 billion.[62] It is understandable, therefore, that given their sizable investments, pharmaceutical companies have a vested interest in bringing their research to market. Otherwise, they cannot recoup their expenses. Moreover, therapeutic products and pharmaceuticals may be marketed in Canada only if they have been approved by Health Canada and received a Notice of Compliance.[63] This is contingent on Health Canada vetting the data developed during the research process and finding nothing untoward. Obviously, therefore, it is important for companies to make sure that the information they provide is positive—which makes it tempting to pressure researchers to either withhold negative information or slant it.

Therefore, when the research data are less than stellar or threaten the possibility of certification, pharmaceutical companies may try to exert control over the research, the data and their publication by either threatening to withdraw funding or by claiming that because the research was funded by them, the results are their intellectual property and may be disclosed only as, when and how they see fit.[64]

The ethics of this aspect of industry involvement is fairly clear in at least one regard: Information that has relevance for the certification process of a drug or device should not be "managed" to obscure (or even misrepresent) relevant facts; and neither researchers nor universities should accept research funds if publication control rests with the funding agency. Funding arrangements between industry and academia should include the stipulation that all results of the research project, whether positive or negative, are publishable by researchers after a modest time interval, and that all industry-university contracts and projects should be subjected to ethics review by an independent national body that is constituted and that functions according to Tri-Council REB rules.[65]

Orphan Drugs

But that is not the only ethical issue that arises from industry involvement. Industry functions on a business model. This means that industry will not conduct non-profitable research, because that would waste stockholders' money—which would violate business ethics. This means that drugs that foreseeably will not yield a return for investment—so-called "orphan drugs"—will not be researched and developed. Therefore, unless such research is funded by government, the research will not be done and the drugs will not exist. This, in turn, means that some patients' right to health care will effectively be held subject to profit.

It is easy to say that industry is therefore unethical—but this would be an overhastily made unconditioned claim. It is not the job of industry to make sure that health care is available on an equitable basis to all who need it: That is the role of government. However, one can attribute at least a partial duty to pharmaceutical companies by arguing that, by conducting business in society, they are the beneficiaries of the socioeconomic structure of society itself. Consequently they have a duty, rooted in Beneficence and Justice, to give an equitable return for their ability to operate.

One strategy for satisfying this duty is for industry to pay appropriate taxes. Another strategy is for companies to invest a percentage of their profits in research on non-profitable diseases or to contribute this percentage to a central pool, managed at arm's length by an administrative body that distributes it on a per-need basis to develop drugs where currently none exist. A third strategy, which combines the underlying ideas of both, is for government to identify drugs that should be developed but for which there would be no return on investment and, using tax monies, to fund the research and development of orphan drugs, possibly also giving tax incentives for corporations that engage in such ventures.

The third option is based on the recognition that society also benefits from the development of drugs and that, as a beneficiary, it should also share in the cost of developing them. This last option has been adopted in many jurisdictions, including the U.S.[66] and the European Union[67] through so-called "orphan drug" legislation. Canada is one of the few jurisdictions where nothing like this is in place.

CONCLUSION

Life is full of decision-making. Health care decisions are merely one example. A rational person, when faced with making a decision, will decide on the basis of the best data available and use the best means to achieve the selected end. When no data are available or they are uncertain, or when there are no valid means to achieve that end, a rational person will set out to acquire sound data or to develop such means.

This is the rationale that underlies research in health care. Health care involves making decisions. These decisions can be made rationally only if the data on which they are based are sound and if there are valid means to achieve the desired ends. Research in health care, therefore, is the attempt to acquire sound data and to develop valid means by using scientifically validated methodologies. Necessarily, it involves human subjects; and necessarily, it requires using those subjects not for their own sake but for the good of others. Research with human subjects is therefore an ethically delicate enterprise that requires the balancing of competing ethical principles. The question is, can they be balanced? The preceding discussion has suggested that they can—that Autonomy and Respect for Persons can be balanced with Beneficence, non-Malfeasance and Fidelity—but that any such balancing must be scrupulously vetted, lest the desire to achieve materially satisfactory outcomes sacrifices fundamental principles and expediency trumps rights.

Further Readings

Baylis, F., and J. Downey. "Children and Decisionmaking in Research." *Health Law Review* 8.2 (1999): 3–9.

Berghmans, R.L.P., and R.H.J. Ter Meulen. "Ethical Issues in Research with Dementia Patients." *International Journal of Geriatric Psychiatry* 10.8 (1995): 647–651.

Glass, K.C., and J. Kaufert. "Research Ethics Review and Aboriginal Community Values: Can the Two Be Reconciled?" *Journal of Empirical Research on Human Research Ethics* (2007): 25–40.

Harris, J. "Scientific Research Is a Moral Duty." *J Med Ethics* 31 (2005): 242–248.

Krugman, S. "The Willowbrook Hepatitis Studies Revisited: Ethical Aspects." *Reviews of Infectious Diseases* 8.1 (1986): 157–162.

Largent, E.A., et al. "Is Emergency Research Without Initial Consent Justified? *Arch Intern Med* 170.8 (2010): 668.

Miller, F.G., and H. Brody. "A Critique of Clinical Equipoise: Therapeutic Misconceptions in the Ethics of Clinical Trials." *Hastings Center Report* 33.3 (2003): 19–28.

Olivieri, N.F. "Patients' Health or Company Profits? The Commercialisation of Academic Research." *Science and Engineering Ethics* 9.1 (2003): 29–41.

Schafer, A. "Biomedical Conflicts of Interest: A Defence of the Sequestration Thesis—Learning from the Cases of Nancy Olivieri and David Healy." *J Med Ethics* 30 (2004): 8–24.

Endnotes

1. M.M. Sajadi, D. Mansouri and M.R. Sajadi, "Ibn Sina and the Clinical Trial," *Annals of Internal Medicine* 150.9 (2009): 640–643.

2. Japanese physicians were never put on trial for pragmatic reasons. The U.S. felt that access to the data on biological warfare and related techniques developed by the Epidemic Prevention and Water Purification Department of the Kwantung Army (Code name: Unit 731) was too important to be jeopardized by putting the perpetrators—who refused to divulge the information unless they were granted immunity from prosecution—on trial. For further reading, see S.H. Harris, *Factories of Death: Japanese Biological Warfare 1932–45 and the American Cover-Up* (London: Routledge, 1994); P. Williams, *Unit 731: Japan's Secret Biological Warfare in World War II* (New York: Free Press, 1989); D. Barenblatt, *A Plague Upon Humanity: The Secret Genocide of Axis Japan's Germ Warfare Operation* (New York: HarperCollins, 2004); and T. Tsuchiya, "Why Japanese Doctors Performed Human Experiments in China 1933–1945," *Eubios Journal of Asian and International Bioethics* 10 (2000): 179–180.

3. The so-called Axis powers were not the only ones who performed unethical experiments on human subjects. Canada conducted unethical experiments on human brainwashing and on the effects of toxic chemicals, gases and bacteria on human beings, as did the U.K. and the U.S.

4. United States of America, vs. Karl Brandt, et al. (Case No. I).

5. Available at http://ohsr.od.nih.gov/guidelines/nuremberg.html

6. World Medical Association. *Declaration of Helsinki*, available at www.wma.net/e/policy/b3.htm

7. World Health Organization, *Operational Guidelines for Ethics Committees that Review Biomedical Research* (2000) accessed 20 Jun 2007 at http://who.int/tdr/publications/publications/pdf/ethics.pdf

8. Council for International Organizations of Medical Sciences (CIOMS), *International Ethical Guidelines for Biomedical Research Involving Human Subjects* (2002), available at www.cioms.ch/frame_guidelines_nov_2002.htm

9. Available at http://conventions.coe.int/Treaty/EN/Treaties/Html/164.htm

10. Australia, National Health and Medical Research, *AHEC Guidelines for Research Involving Humans*, 1992, available at www.nhmrc.gov.au/ethics/human/conduct/guidelines/index.htm

11. Canadian Institutes of Health Research, Natural Sciences and Engineering Research Council of Canada, and Social Sciences and Humanities Research Council of Canada, *Tri-Council Policy Statement: Ethical Conduct for Research Involving Humans, December 2010;* accessed 2 May 2011 at www.pre.ethics.gc.ca/pdf/eng/tcps2/TCPS_2_FINAL_Web.pdf

12. U.K. Medical Research Council. *Ethics and Research Governance*, available at www.mrc.ac.uk/PolicyGuidance/EthicsAndGovernance/index.htm

13. Office for Human Research Protections, Policy Guidance, Code of Federal Regulations, Title 45 Public Welfare, Department of Health and Human Services, Part 46, Protection of Human Subjects, available at www.hhs.gov/ohrp/humansubjects/guidance/45cfr46.htm

14. People's Republic of China, *Regulations on Informed Consent and Protection of Human Subjects in Biomedical Studies*, available at www.usembassy-china.org.cn/sandt/PRCpatient-protection.html

15. There is a whole body of opinion that rejects experimentation with non-human animals. For an exposition from a Christian perspective, see D. Yarri, *The Ethics of Animal Experimentation: A Critical Analysis and Constructive Christian Proposal* (New York: Oxford University Press, 2005). For a non-religious perspective, see T. Regan, *The Case for Animal Rights* (Berkeley: University of California Press, 1985). For a critical approach to animal rights, see J.H. Franklin, *Animal Rights and Moral Philosophy* (New York: Columbia University Press, 2005). For a somewhat dated but conceptually insightful analysis from a researcher's standpoint, see B.E. Ehinger, "Animal Experimentation Ethics from an Experimenter's Point of View," *Acta Physiol Scand* Suppl 554 (1986): 69–77.

16. S. Lewis et al., "Dancing with the Porcupine: Rules for Governing the University–Industry Relationship," *CMAJ.* 165.6 (18 Sep 2001): 783–785; C. Martyn, "The Drug Trial: Nancy Olivieri and the Science Scandal that Rocked the Hospital for Sick Children," *BMJ,* 331.7508 (9 Jul 2005): 115; A. Schafer, "Biomedical Conflicts of Interest: A Defence of the Sequestration Thesis—Learning from the Cases of Nancy Olivieri and David Healy," *J Med Ethics* 31 (2004): 8–24.

17. M.F. Fraga et al., "Epigenetic Differences Arise during the Lifetime of Monozygotic Twins," *Proc Natl Acad Sci USA* 102.30 (26 Jul 2005): 10604–10609.

18. CMA Code of Ethics, accessed 28 Apr 2011 at http://policybase.cma.ca/PolicyPDF/PD04-06.pdf

19. Tri-Council Guidelines, p. 10.

20. B. Freedman, "Equipoise and the Ethics of Clinical Research," *New England Journal of Medicine* 317 (1987): 141–145.

21. H. Olson et al., "Concordance of the Toxicity of Pharmaceuticals in Humans and in Animals," *Regu Toxico Pharmaco* 32.1 (Aug 2000): 56–67. See also A. Knight, "Systematic Reviews of Animal Experiments Demonstrate Poor Human Clinical and Toxicological Utility," *Altern Lab Anim* 35.6 (Dec 2007): 641–659.

22. W. Lilienblum et al., "Alternative Methods to Safety Studies in Experimental Animals: Role in the Risk Assessment of Chemicals under the New European Chemicals Legislation (REACH)," *Arch Toxicol* 82.4 (Apr 2008): 211–213; L.G. Valerio, Jr., "In Silico Toxicology for the Pharmaceutical Sciences," *Toxicol Appl Pharmacol* 241.3 (Dec 2009); 356–370.

23. See Tri-Council Guidelines, at 151.

24. P.R. Ferguson, "Selecting Participants When Testing New Drugs: The Implications of Age and Gender Discrimination," *Med Leg J* 70 (2002): 130–134; B. Healy, "The Yentl Syndrome," *New England Journal of Medicine* 325.4 (1991): 274–276; T.D. Keville, "The Invisible Woman: Gender Bias in Medical Research," *Women's Rights Law Reporter* 14.2–3 (1993): 123–142.

25. Guidelines, at 23.

26. Loc. cit.

27. "Vivisectionist Recalls His Day of Reckoning," *Japan Times* (24 Oct 2007): 3; see also Tsuchiya, op. cit.

28. For a defence of the Willowbrook study by one of its researchers, see S. Krugman, "The Willowbrook Hepatitis Studies Revisited: Ethical Aspects," *Reviews of Infectious Diseases* 8.1 (1986): 157–162.

29. The LD50 design was devised in 1927 by J.W. Trevan. See J.W. Trevan, "The Error of Determination of Toxicity," *Proc R Soc Lond B* 101.712 (1 Jul 1927): 483–514.

30. Cf. Guidelines 6.4.

31. Guidelines 2.4.

32. This was the longest study in the history of modern medicine. It took place in Tuskeegee County, Alabama, over a period of 40 years, between 1932 and 1972, and involved observing the course of untreated syphilis to see what would happen. At the beginning of the study, only Salvarsan had been available as treatment for syphilis. Penicillin and other antibiotics became available in the 1940s, and in order not to arouse the suspicion of the participants, they were given subtherapeutic doses of these new drugs. The participants were not informed of the nature of the study, the treatments available or anything else. The incentive was routine medical examination and free burial—both of which constituted tremendous economic expense for uninsured Afro-American field workers.

33. *Project MKULTRA, the CIA's Program of Research into Behavioral Modification. Joint Hearing before the Select Committee on Intelligence and the Subcommittee on Health and Scientific Research of the Committee on Human Resources, United States Senate, Ninety-Fifth Congress, First Session*, accessed 9 May 2011 at www.nytimes.com/packages/pdf/national/13inmate_ProjectMKULTRA.pdf. For an ethics analysis of the case, see E.-H.W. Kluge, Director of Ethics and Legal Affairs, Canadian Medical Association, accessed 9 May 2011 at www.psychrights.org/Research/Digest/Electroshock/PBregginCites/LMacdonaldvHerMajestytheQueen.pdf

34. A. Collins, *In the Sleep Room: The Story of CIA Brainwashing Experiments in Canada* (Toronto: Key Porter Books, 1988).

35. Collins, *In the Sleep Room*, 197 ff, *et pass.*

36. This analysis is in keeping with the public statement of the Board of Directors of the Canadian Psychological Association, Nov. 11, 1990, that "the practices used would not have been acceptable at that time, nor would they be acceptable now." The Canadian Psychiatric Association initially concurred when it said that "it may well be that certain patients admitted to the Allen Memorial Institute in the 1950s and 1960s were not offered sufficient disclosure, even by the current standards then applicable." (Letter of Q. Rae-Grant, Chairman of the Board, CPS, July 6, 1990, to T.R. Berger).

37. The following is a statement by one of the participants in Cameron's research: "[H]is criteria for the selection of patients for these controversial treatments seemed to broaden. By the time I became personally involved with his patients (1961) it was my own view that many of the schizophrenic patients who were 'depatterned' had not had adequate trials of appropriate phenothiazine medications that were then available and many of the psycho-neurotic patients who received hallucinogenic drugs and psychic driving could have been helped by conventional psychotherapy. *Of course, at the time, I was very junior in status and quite inexperienced in psychiatry.*" (Communication by T. Berger, lawyer representing Linda Macdonald in her action against the Canadian Government for funding the Cameron experiment, TAB 11, p. 10; emphasis added).

38. For a critical look at the distinction, see U. Schuklenk and R. Ashcroft, "International Research Ethics," *Bioethics* 14.2 (2000): 158–172. See also R.J. Levine, "The Need to Revise the Declaration of Helsinki," *New England Journal of Medicine* 341 (1999): 531–534.

39. Tri-Council Policy Statement, p. 151.

40. Tri-Council Policy Statement 2, at 151 f.

41. F.G. Miller and H. Brody, "A Critique of Clinical Equipoise: Therapeutic Misconceptions in the Ethics of Clinical Trials," *Hastings Center Report* 33.3 (2003): 19–28.

42. Halushka v. University of Saskatchewan (1965), 53 D.L.R. (2d) 436. This is one of the few legal judgments in North America that deals expressly with informed consent in the non-therapeutic experimental setting.

43. Halushka v. University of Saskatchewan, at 444.

44. It is estimated that smallpox killed 200 to 300 million people in the 20th century alone. See D.A. Koplow, *Smallpox: The Fight to Eradicate a Global Scourge* (Berkeley: University of California Press, 2003). See also "Smallpox," WHO Factsheet, accessed 29 Nov 2010, available at www.who.int/mediacentre/factsheets/smallpox/en/

45. K. Moe, "Should the Nazi Research Data Be Cited?" *Hastings Center Report* 14.6 (1984): 5–7; A. Schafer, "Using Nazi Data: The Case Against," *Dialogue* XXV (1986): 413–419. For a legal discussion, see D.V. MacDougall, "The Exclusionary Rule and Its Alternative—Remedies for Constitutional Violations in Canada and the United States," *The Journal of Criminal Law and Criminology* 76.3 (1985): 603–665.

46. D. Evans, "Ethical Review of Innovative Treatment," *HEC Forum* 14.1 (2002): 53-63.

47. J. Avorn and A. Kesselheim, "A Hemorrhage of Off-Label Use," *Ann Intern Med* 154 (Apr 2011): 566–567.

48. *Tri-Council Policy Statement: Ethical Conduct for Research Involving Humans* (Dec 2010), accessed 2 May 2011 at www.pre.ethics.gc.ca/pdf/eng/tcps2/TCPS_2_FINAL_Web.pdf

49. Loc. cit.

50. Guidelines, pp. 35–39.

51. H. Jonas, "Philosophical Reflections on Experimenting with Human Subjects," *Daedalus* 98 (1969): 219–247; R.R. Sharp and M. Yarborough, "Additional Thoughts on Rethinking Research Ethics," *American Journal of Bioethics* 5.1 (2005): 40–42.

52. F. Allhoff, "Free-Riding and Research Ethics," *American Journal of Bioethics* 5.1 (2005): 50–51; I. Brassington, "John Harris' Argument for a Duty to Research," *Bioethics* 21.3 (2007): 160–168.

53. J. Harris, "Scientific Research Is a Moral Duty," *J Med Ethics* 31 (2005): 242–248.

54. A.L. Caplan, "Is There a Duty to Serve as a Subject in Biomedical Research?" *IRB* 5 (1984): 1–5; H.M. Evans, "Should Patients Be Allowed to Veto Their Participation in Clinical Research?" *Journal of Medical Ethics* 30.2 (2004): 198–203; Harris, op. cit.; R. Rhodes, "In Defense of the Duty to Participate in Biomedical Research," *Am J Bioeth* 8.10 (Oct 2008): 37–38; A. Ho, "Correcting Social Ills through Mandatory Research Participation," *Am J Bioeth* 8.10 (Oct 2008): 39–40.

55. S. Shapshay and K.D. Pimple, "Participation in Biomedical Research Is an Imperfect Moral Duty: A Response to John Harris," *Journal of Medical Ethics* 33.7 (2007): 414–417.

56. I. de Melo-Martin, "A Duty to Participate in Research: Does Social Context Matter?" *Am J Bioeth* 8.10 (Oct 2008): 28–36.

57. See note 54, *supra.*

58. D. Orentlicher, "Making Research a Requirement of Treatment: Why We Should Sometimes Let Doctors Pressure Patients to Participate in Research," *Hastings Center Report* 35.5 (2005): 20–28.

59. Cf. Tri-Council Guidelines 3.10, 4.4, etc.

60. Guidelines 9.

61. Cf. Guidelines 9 and 12.

62. J.A. DiMasi, R.W. Hansen and G.H. Grabowski, "The Price of Innovation: New Estimates of Drug Development Costs," *Journal of Health Economics,* 22.2 (Mar 2003): 151–185.

63. The licensing falls under the *Food and Drugs Act* (R.S.C., 1985, c. F-27). For details of the approval process, see Health Canada, *Access to Therapeutic Products: The Regulatory Process in Canada*, available at www.hc-sc.gc.ca/ahc-asc/alt_formats/hpfb-dgpsa/pdf/pubs/access-therapeutic_acces-therapeutique-eng.pdf

64. For an example of a case where this became problematic, see F. Baylis,"The Olivieri Debacle: Where Were the Heroes of Bioethics?" *J Med Ethics* 30 (2004): 44–49; for a reply, see M. Rowell, "The Olivieri Debacle: Where Were the Heroes of Bioethics? A Reply," *J Med Ethics* 30 (2004): 50. For a general article, see S. Lewis et al., "Dancing with the Porcupine: Rules for Governing the

University–Industry Relationship." *CMAJ* 165.6 (18 Sep 2001): 783–785. The first-hand account of the Olivieri case can be found at N.F. Olivieri, "Patients' Health or Company Profits? The Commercialisation of Academic Research." *Science and Engineering Ethics* 9.1 (2003): 29–41.

65. A. Schafer, "Biomedical Conflicts of Interest: A Defence of the Sequestration Thesis—Learning from the Cases of Nancy Olivieri and David Healy," *J Med Ethics* 30 (2004): 8–24.

66. U.S. Congress, *Rare Diseases Act of 2002*, accessed 11 May 2011 at http://history.nih.gov/research/downloads/PL107-280.pdf

67. European Union, Regulation (EC) No 141/2000 accessed 11 May 2011 at http://eur-lex.europa.eu/LexUriServ/LexUriServ.do?uri=OJ:L:2000:018:0001:0005:en:PDF

SAMPLE CASES

1. Dr. W., a cardiologist at CR hospital, was not convinced that surgical treatment of patients brought into Emergency with heart attacks to restore circulation to their hearts was the best therapy. She believed that streptokinase would dissolve the clots and blockages and would be just as effective and much less intrusive. She therefore asked the staff to randomly divide patients brought in with heart attacks into two groups: those that were treated with streptokinase and balloon catheterization to open occluded blood vessels, and those that were treated surgically. The matter was brought to the attention of the ethics committee of the hospital, which confronted Dr. W. with the fact that the protocol had not been vetted by the hospital's REB, that no informed consent was being obtained from the patients and that Dr. W.'s funding for the study was being underwritten by PGK, a company that had a patent on "clot-busting" medication. Dr. W. replied that consent was not possible because heart attacks were not like scheduled events, that the people brought into Emergency usually came in by ambulance, generally were incompetent to give consent and that substitute decision-makers, if they were available at all, usually were too upset to be relied on to make any competent decisions either. She also pointed out that if she was right, it would benefit future patients, would save the hospital a lot of money, and that there was no other way to obtain the data because with heart attacks, time was of the essence.

2. HIV/AIDS is widespread in Africa. In part, this is due to a persistent male-dominated culture of unprotected intercourse. A pharmaceutical company in South Africa is interested in developing a vaginal gel that can be applied up to a half-hour before intercourse and that, hopefully, would reduce the transmission of HIV/AIDS by up to 85 percent. It therefore advertised for female volunteers to participate in a randomized study to test the effectiveness of their product, promising free medical examination and treatment for conditions other than HIV/AIDS.

Chapter 7
The Ethics of Deliberate Death

All of us die: The question is not whether but how. Will we die a medicalized death—betubed, sedated, glucosed, aerated and wired for everything including sound; or will we die what the poet Rilke called "our own death"[1]—a death of our choosing, based on our life and our values? Of course, death cannot always be arranged. Sometimes it just happens, as in an accident. But sometimes it can be steered. The theme of this chapter is the issue of deliberate death in the health care setting, with particular focus on euthanasia and assisted suicide. The next chapter will deal with abortion.

The chapter begins with a discussion of various conceptions of death and their associated criteria and relates this to current Canadian medical and legal standards. It then turns to euthanasia and considers the distinction between active and passive euthanasia, relates this to the withdrawal of treatment and palliative care, and concludes by looking at assisted suicide. The reason for the title of the chapter is that in each of these instances death is brought about deliberately, in full awareness that a particular action (or inaction) will result in the patient's death. The central issue in all of this is whether to deliberately bring about a patient's death is always the same as committing murder, whether ethics and the law agree in this connection and—if indeed they disagree—what could account for this difference.

Questions to Keep in Mind While Reading this Chapter:

1. What is meant by saying that someone is dead? Why is the question important in health care?

2. What is the difference between a materialistic and a dualistic conception of personhood, and how are they related to criteria for the determination of death?

3. What is euthanasia, and how does this concept relate to the distinction that is sometimes drawn between using ordinary as opposed to extraordinary means to keep someone alive?

4. Is there a difference between active and passive euthanasia, direct and indirect euthanasia, and voluntary as opposed to involuntary and non-voluntary euthanasia? How could these distinctions be defended from an ethical perspective?

5. How does euthanasia relate to the role of health care professionals and their relationships with their patients?

6. What is suicide—and how does it differ from assisted suicide? Does patient capacity always play a role in suicide, or may it be rational to engage in suicide or to request assistance in committing suicide? How do suicide and assisted suicide relate to the role of health care professionals and their relationships with their patients?

7. Is there a place for the notion of quality of life in decisions surrounding deliberate death?

INTRODUCTION

One of the more controversial issues in health care is whether it is ethical to deliberately allow a patient to die or to actively bring about a patient's death. However, before one can meaningfully discuss this, one should really have a clear understanding of what actually counts as death.

THE CONCEPT OF DEATH

At first glance, this statement may seem surprising. After all, with the possible exception of very young children and some mentally disabled persons, everyone knows what death is. People are dead when their heart has stopped beating, they no longer breathe and their body is cold.

Definitions versus Criteria

However, that answer is not only legally wrong, it is also medically wrong—and perhaps most importantly, it confuses what death is with ways of telling whether someone is dead. In other words, it confuses the concept of death with the criteria for its application. By way of illustration, consider the metal gold. The *definition* of gold is that it is a ductile yellow metallic element with the atomic number 79, having six electron shells with 2, 8, 18, 32, 18 and 1 electrons in them respectively, a specific gravity of 19.32 and a melting point of 1337.33 K. However, that information does not tell someone how to determine whether something is gold. For that one needs a rule or test that allows one to tell whether what is in front of us actually is gold: in other words, one needs a *criterion*. In the case of gold there are various criteria. They include applying nitro-hydrochloric acid, determining its density, etc. In other words, while the criteria for finding out whether something is a certain kind of thing are based on the properties that are stated in its definition, logically speaking, the two are not the same.

The distinction between definition and criteria is important in the case of death, because there are two fundamentally distinct definitions of death, reflecting different metaphysical conceptions of personhood, but the criteria used to apply these definitions are the same.

Materialism versus Dualism

That is to say, in general terms, someone is dead when they are no longer a person. That much all definitions of death have in common. The difference comes in regarding what counts as a person. According to *materialism*, persons are identical with their bodies. In other words, materialism defines a person as living human being—i.e., as a living member of the species *homo sapiens*. Correspondingly, it defines death as the permanent and irreversible cessation of the integrated biological functioning of the human body inclusive of the brain. This permanent and irreversible cessation of integrated functioning may take time, because human body cells and human organs cease to function at different rates. For instance, brain cells start to die approximately five minutes after circulation has ceased and (at room temperature) all are generally dead within twenty minutes.[2] Liver cells[3] and heart cells can live much longer.[4] However, once the integrated functioning of the various organs and the brain has irreversibly ceased, the person is dead.

By contrast, *dualism* maintains that a person is an integrated union of a material substance or body and a spiritual substance or soul. The spiritual substance provides the body with life, and the body is merely the biological vehicle that allows the soul to express its mental and spiritual capacities in material terms. It is the soul that grounds personhood and self-awareness. Therefore, in contrast to materialism, dualism maintains that the destruction of the body does not mean the destruction of the person. All it means is that the spiritual substance has separated from the body. Dualists can therefore meaningfully say that a person "has passed away to a better life," whereas for materialists this is merely a *façon de parler*.

Both materialism and dualism require criteria for the application of their respective definitions of personhood. It is here that developments in the history of medicine become important. Originally, the role of the brain was not fully understood. In fact, it was generally thought to be an organ for cooling the blood.[5] Life was thought to depend on the presence of a beating heart and functioning lungs. Not surprisingly, therefore, the absence of a heartbeat and of independent breathing became the original materialist criterion for the determination of death. It was known as the *cardiopulmonary criterion*.

For dualism, the criterion problem was a trifle more complicated. Ideally, the criterion would have involved directly detecting the presence of a soul. However because souls were immaterial, there was no way of doing that. Therefore, the only way to determine whether a particular body still had a soul was to look at how that body functioned. Specifically, it meant that one had to look at whether the functioning of a particular body signalled the presence of the life-giving powers of the soul and of its capacity for sentient cognitive awareness. This, in turn, meant that one had to look at whether the body was biologically alive and whether its biological constitution was sufficiently intact to sustain sentient cognitive awareness.[6] There was no better way of doing that than using the

cardiopulmonary criterion. Therefore, while dualism used the same criterion as materialism, the criterion meant different things.

Cardiopulmonary Criterion versus Brain-Death Criterion

However, the advent of modern medicine made it very clear that someone who met the
cardiopulmonary criterion might not in fact be dead. The absence of discernible heartbeat
or independent breathing, or even the fact that the body was cold, might simply be indicative of severe hypothermia—especially in children. Moreover, the development of life
support and of advanced surgical techniques such as heart and lung transplants forced a
serious re-examination of the criterion. Patients on life support certainly were not yet
dead; and patients undergoing transplant surgery would neither be breathing (being artificially ventilated) nor have a heartbeat (the blood being artificially circulated by a pump),
and their body temperature would be artificially lowered to avoid trauma and tissue damage. Nevertheless, these patients would definitely not be dead, because at the end of their
operations, independent heartbeat, breathing and temperature would be restored.

This suggested to some that the appropriate way to describe these situations was to
say that the person had died but had been brought back to life. (This perspective is still
encountered in media reports which claim that someone "died on the operating table" but
"was brought back to life" through the heroic and concerted efforts of the medical team.)[7]

However, this perspective was not without its problems. Legally, someone who is dead
is no longer a person. Therefore, if the individual actually was dead, then legally all that
person's property would go to that person's heirs. Consequently when such a person was
resuscitated and "brought back to life," that person would be destitute. Moreover, citizenship belongs only to living persons. Therefore, if a person had actually "died on the operating table" and been "brought back to life," he or she would be a stateless person. Et cetera.

Further developments in medical knowledge also made it clear that if what was
definitive of personhood was the capacity for sentient cognitive awareness, then heart and
lungs had nothing to do with that. What was important was the brain. The heart and the
lungs merely functioned in a supportive role in keeping the brain alive, much like the
kidneys and the liver. In other words, it became clear that the cessation of independent
cardiopulmonary activity really was nothing more than the cessation of a bodily function
that was essential to keeping the brain alive, but that this supportive function could
be interrupted and restored under certain circumstances—as well as artificially supplied.
The litmus test of death, therefore, was not the permanent destruction of this supportive
biological machinery but the permanent destruction of the brain. This position was formally presented in the 1968 Report of a Committee convened by the Harvard Medical
School to examine the criteria for the determination of death.[8] As a result, *brain death*
became the definitive criterion of death in the clinical setting. Accordingly, someone is
dead if and only if his or her brain has been irreparably destroyed.

The brain-death criterion has since become accepted in most countries, and it gained legal recognition in Canada with the 1976 case of *R. v. Kitching and Adams.*[9] However, the legal recognition of the brain-death criterion did not do away with the cardiopulmonary criterion. Brain death may be difficult to diagnose directly without sophisticated diagnostic equipment. Therefore, under normal circumstances—which is to say, outside of the sophisticated clinical setting—the cardiopulmonary criterion continues to be used. It is also important to note that the introduction of the brain-death criterion did not signal the abandonment of either the materialist or the dualist conception of personhood (and therefore of death). Both continue to have their adherents.

Whole-Brain versus Cerebral Death

But there is more to the story. Further advances in medical knowledge showed that the capacity for sentient cognitive awareness is not centred in all parts of the brain but only in the cerebral cortex. The other parts of the brain play a supportive role—much like the heart, liver and kidneys. At the same time, the human body may continue to live and even function at a primitive stimulus-response level as long as the brain stem is intact. This is what happens when someone is in a permanent vegetative state (PVS). Such an individual is dead only if personhood is centred in the capacity for sentient cognitive awareness—which is to say, only if one accepts what has sometimes been called a "personalist" perspective of personhood.[10] From a "vitalist" perspective—from the perspective that it is the integrated functioning of the biological organism that counts—such an individual would still be alive and still be a person.

The controversy over whether the brain-death criterion should be refined into a *cerebral-death criterion* or remain with the *whole-brain criterion* has not yet been resolved. Part of the push for acceptance of the cerebral-death criterion is, of course, resource allocation. Thus, it was estimated in 1994 that the total annual aggregate cost for keeping individuals in a permanent vegetative state (PVS) alive in the U.S. is between $1 and $7 billion. In 2011 terms, this would amount to between $1.48 and $10.36 billion, and adjusted to the Canadian context this would translate to between $148 million and $1.036 billion annually. Given a life expectancy of approximately five years for people in a PVS, this would mean a total cost of between $740 million and $5.18 billion to the Canadian health care system. Given that people in a PVS for more than six months have a less than 0.5 percent chance of recovery to any level of sentient cognitive awareness, the proponents of the cerebral criterion argue that retention of the whole-brain criterion is not only outdated but also deprives many patients of appropriate health care.[11]

However, economics is not the main reason why the controversy remains unresolved. The main reason is that what is here at issue is whether the respective metaphysical definitions of personhood should be refined along personalist lines or whether they should remain with the old vitalist perspective. The battle lines here cross the metaphysical divide between materialism and dualism, because whatever is decided has implications for both regarding the ethics of deliberate death. On the personalist interpretation, killing or allowing a cerebrally dead patient to die would not be morally reprehensible, whereas according to the vitalist conception it very well might be.

DELIBERATE DEATH

Which brings the discussion to the issue of deliberate death. Is it ever ethically acceptable for a physician to deliberately bring about the death of a patient or to deliberately allow that death to occur even though it was preventable?

Some Terminology

It is always useful to clarify beforehand what one means before embarking on a discussion of a controversial issue, lest the discussion flounder in a morass of ambiguity. The following are some terms that are frequently encountered in discussions of euthanasia and deliberate death.

Euthanasia itself is usually understood as the deliberate bringing about of the death of a patient in a good or painless manner, with the sole motivation of sparing the patient irremediable pain or suffering, or of shortening that pain or suffering. *Voluntary euthanasia* is often defined as engaging in euthanasia at the voluntary request of a competent patient; correspondingly, *involuntary euthanasia* is defined as euthanatizing a patient against a patient's wishes, whereas *non-voluntary euthanasia* is defined as euthanatizing a patient who has expressed no wish either way. *Direct euthanasia* is understood as the bringing about of a patient's death by an act or omission that immediately leads to the patient's death without any intervening and mediating causal factors, whereas *indirect euthanasia* is understood as the bringing about of a patient's death by an act or omission that leads to the patient's death only because of intervening and mediating causal factors. Finally, *active euthanasia* is generally defined as being the causal agent of the patient's death, whereas *passive euthanasia* is defined as intentionally allowing death to occur. The relationship between these different types of euthanasia is illustrated by the following diagram (Figure 7.1):

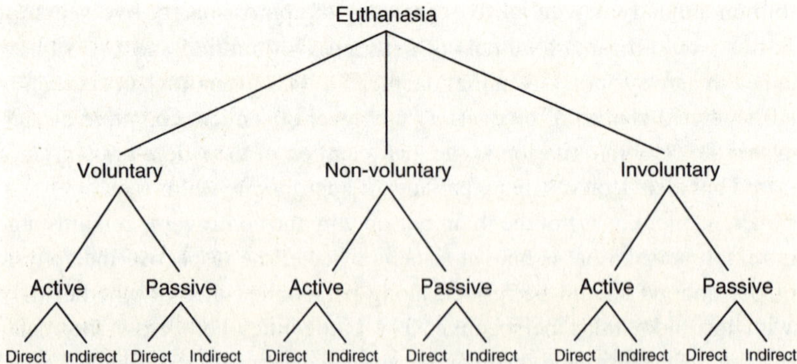

Figure 7.1 Relationship between Different Types of Euthanasia

Over and above these terms, however, one also encounters certain other distinctions in the euthanasia debate. For example, killing is often said to be different from letting die and from palliation and letting nature take its course. Similarly, it is sometimes claimed that there is a fundamental difference between using ordinary as opposed to extra-ordinary means in health care, and that different ethical considerations apply in the respective cases. Since these distinctions are part of the euthanasia debate, they deserve close consideration.

Killing versus Letting Die

To begin with the killing/letting die distinction, is it really true that there is a fundamental ethical difference between killing and letting die? The claim that there is an ethical difference goes back at least as far as Hippocrates. Thus, the Hippocratic tradition made physicians swear that they "will neither give a deadly drug to anybody who asked for it, nor . . . make a suggestion to this effect"[12] but had no problem with physicians allowing patients to die naturally.

Likewise, in the 20th century, the Law Reform Commission of Canada, in its Working Paper 28, *Euthanasia, Aiding Suicide and Cessation of Treatment*,[13] stated that deliberately bringing about the death of a person was murder and reiterated this position in its Report to Parliament, but said that this was different from allowing death to occur.[14] Similarly, the CMA officially endorsed the distinction in 2007 when it said that "Canadian physicians should not participate in euthanasia or assisted suicide,"[15] but that they could ethically allow a patient to die in dignity and comfort when death of the body appeared to be inevitable.[16] This position was echoed by the Ethics Committee of the College of Family Physicians of Canada when it said that the "acts intentionally causing a patient's death either by a physician (active euthanasia) or with a physician's help (assisted suicide) are to be distinguished from the appropriate practice of withholding or withdrawing life-sustaining care."[17] Nor is this stance merely a Canadian phenomenon. It is shared by many medical associations all over the world.[18]

The reasoning underlying this stance is the conviction that allowing death to occur from natural causes is not really an act of deliberate killing and therefore is not really euthanasia. On this understanding, turning off a respirator is ethically distinct from injecting an overdose of morphine into a patient's vein. In the first case, nature is merely allowed to take its course, because the respirator does nothing more than prevent the natural causes of death from taking their effect; in the second case, however, an additional element is added to the causal chain, and it is this additional element that is the real cause of death.[19]

However, it is not at all clear that the distinction between killing and letting die or the distinction between active and passive euthanasia is sound. As James Rachels argued in an article that has become a classic in bioethics,[20] while not doing anything may not be an action in the physical sense of the term, it certainly counts as an action in the moral sense. The difference between the two is merely linguistic—and possibly psychological.

To see why Rachels is correct, and why the distinction between killing and letting die is not really an ethically relevant distinction in the context of health care, it is necessary to take a brief look at the difference between causality and ethical responsibility.

Causality

There is more than one way to determine the outcome of a given causal chain of events. One can determine it either by physically doing something—for instance, by giving a patient a drug such as penicillin to which the patient is allergic, after which the patient dies of an induced allergy reaction; or by not doing something—for instance, by simply standing and, without lifting a finger, watching a patient who has an allergic reaction to a particular medication die. In both cases, the physician is in a position to affect the chain of events, and in both cases the physician is the determinant of outcome: What he or she does or does not do determines what the case will be.

In other words, while a physical cause will always be a determinant of an outcome, the determinant of an outcome will not always be a physical cause. Figure 7.2 illustrates this. The line at the top represents a course of events that reaches a point x, where there are two possibilities. If the established causal flow of events is not interfered with, the outcome will be A; if the established causal flow of events is interfered with, the outcome will be B. In either case, however, the person at x will determine how the causal flow unfolds. Therefore, a failure to act, which has sometimes been called a negative act, can be the determinant of a particular outcome just as much a positive act, that is to say, a physical action.

Physical or positive action, therefore, is not necessary for a person's being the determinant of a particular outcome. The very failure to act may have that effect—and

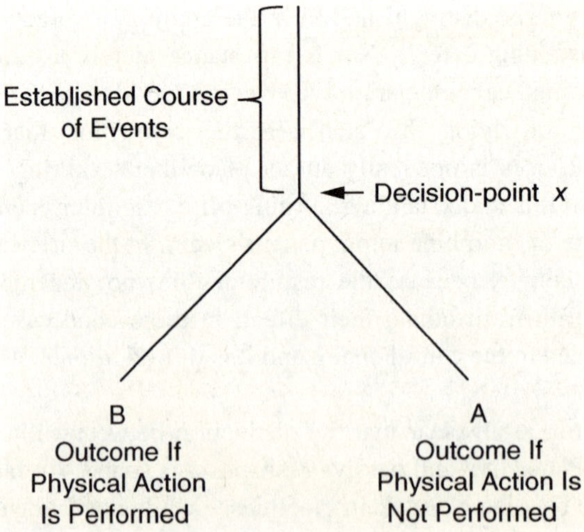

Figure 7.2 Established Course of Events

thereby function as cause. This is what underlies the law of negligence. People who are negligent are considered to be causally responsible for the negative outcome precisely because they did not do anything physically, and by not doing anything physically ensured that the chain of events would unfold causally in a particular direction.

Ethical Responsibility

Put simply, to be the determinant of a particular outcome is to be responsible for that outcome. However, that says nothing about whether being thus responsible is an ethically good or bad thing. That depends on what one's obligations are at that point in time. If one has an obligation to make sure that the causal chain unfolds in a certain direction and does not do it, then one has failed in one's duty—and that is ethically a bad thing. Conversely, if one has an obligation to make sure that the causal chain unfolds in a certain direction and does that, then one has fulfilled one's duty—and that is ethically a good thing. In other words, the ethically relevant question is not the manner of determining how the causal chain unfolds but whether one has a duty to ensure that it unfolds one way rather than another and whether one actually does so. In other words, as Rachels rightly observed, the distinction between active and passive euthanasia is a morally bogus distinction, because it confuses a matter of physics with a matter of ethics. In each case, the physician is responsible for the death of the patient.

To put this into the context of health care, let us consider the 1935 case of *Mulloy v. Hop Sang*[21] that was discussed in Chapter 4. Dr. Mulloy saved Mr. Sang's life by amputating his gangrenous right hand, despite Mr. Sang's explicit wishes not to have his hand amputated. At that time—antibiotics not yet having been developed—there was no other way of dealing with the gangrene. Dr. Mulloy was certainly responsible for saving Mr. Sang's life. However, it would be nonsense to say that Dr. Mulloy was guilty for having done that. What Dr. Mulloy was guilty of, both ethically and legally, was failing in his duty to follow Mr. Sang's competent wishes. In other words, he was guilty because he failed in his duty to respect Mr. Sang's competent and informed consent.

The point is important because it goes to the very heart of the question of whether allowing a patient to die or killing a patient is ethically defensible. One is guilty of something only if one has a responsibility and did not fulfill it. Therefore, someone can be guilty for killing a patient or for letting a patient die only if there was a duty to do one's best to prevent the patient's death. However, just as a right is not an abstract and absolute thing, so a duty is not an abstract and absolute thing either. Both always hold *prima facie*. (See Chapter 1, "Deontological Theories.") They are always conditioned by the facts of a given situation and by whatever other rights or duties that obtain.

Therefore, even when there is a duty to try to save a patient's life, that duty is conditioned by the facts of the situation—where these include the availability of the means necessary for saving the patient's life such as surgical tools, medications, operating space, etc.—and by whatever other duties that hold in the case in question. If the means are not available, then the physician who does not save the patient's life is not guilty of anything. The Principle of Impossibility exculpates the physician. And if the patient has competently refused the relevant interventions, then the physician's duty to follow the informed and competent consent of the patient[22] trumps the duty to save the patient's life. Therefore, while Dr. Mulloy had a *prima facie* duty to save Mr. Sang's life, that duty was trumped by his duty to follow Mr. Sang's competently expressed wishes not to have his hand amputated. To reiterate, Dr. Sang was both ethically and legally guilty, not because he saved Mr. Sang's life but because his duty to try to save the latter's life had been conditioned—had been trumped—by his duty to follow Mr. Sang's informed consent.

The Ethics of "Letting Nature Take Its Course"

This takes the discussion to the claim that letting nature take its course absolves the physician of responsibility for the death of the patient and should not be called euthanasia. It is simply letting nature take its course. Nature is here the dominant agent and really bears the blame.[23]

However, this is really to obfuscate the issue. Nature *always* takes its course. An injection of morphine, for example, or of penicillin will not work unless there are laws of nature. Likewise, pulling the plug on life support will not lead to the death of the patient unless the standard and familiar laws of nature hold sway. And they always do. No one and nothing can violate the laws of nature. They are always present, whether the stance one adopts is active or passive.

So, pointing to the fact that nature is dominant does not settle the issue of responsibility and of praise or blame. Nature is always the dominant cause. That dominance is inherent in the laws of nature themselves, and without it, medicine itself would be impossible. The real question is not one of dominance or physical activity but of responsibility and control. Moral responsibility is assigned only on the assumption that one has the power to determine how a causal chain of events unfolds. In any given instance, therefore, the first question to ask is whether the voluntary agent—in this case the physician—is in a position to determine how the causal chain of events unfolds. If the answer is in the negative, the ethics of the situation is settled. Neither praise nor blame attach to the physician. On the other hand, if the answer is in the affirmative, it then becomes important to ask whether the physician has a duty to determine the unfolding in one direction rather than another.

This leads to a further observation. The picture of certain possibilities being left open by a passive (non-active) stance and of the future being left uncertain when one does not act in a physical or positive fashion is really quite illusory. Responsible medical decision-making does not occur in a vacuum. It takes place in the context and against the backdrop of the physician's knowledge and training. These allow the physician to form an opinion—an informed opinion—about the status of the patient.

Therefore, when a physician decides to "let nature take its course," that decision is not made in isolation. It is made on the understanding that *because* the condition of the patient is what it is, *because* the nature of the disease or condition is such and so, and *because* the medico-social circumstances are what they are, *therefore* death is expected to occur if treatment is suspended. To put it bluntly, the physician who makes such a decision expects that only a miracle could alter the chain of events, which foreseeably will lead to death. However, the expectation that only a miracle will change the expected outcome is the very same sort of understanding that the physician who acts positively has. In either instance, the physician expects that, except for a miracle, the laws of nature will yield a fatal outcome.

Therefore, the decision to let nature take its course is made in a climate of relative diagnostic and prognostic certainty. Otherwise, the physician could not even talk meaningfully about letting nature take its course. The situation would be different if physicians approached the future not as governed by the laws of nature but rather as a series of unpredictable, random or chaotic events. That sort of perspective, however, cannot be reconciled with what is called scientific medicine. While the physician might feel emotionally more comfortable about the death of the patient because he or she did not physically do anything, that really has nothing to do with the ethics.[24]

Palliation versus Euthanasia

This also shows why palliation is ethically distinct from euthanasia, whether that be understood in the active or the passive sense. There is no question that by merely palliating a patient, the physician is allowing the causal chain of events to unfold in such a way that it leads to the patient's death. However, this would be ethically objectionable only if it were possible to try to save the patient's life *and* if there were a duty to try to keep the patient alive—for instance, if the patient had insisted on being treated or there were other clear reasons (for instance, an advance directive) to believe that the patient wanted the effort to be made. On the other hand, if the patient is competently refusing any intervention and has opted for palliation, or if there is an advance directive that is reasonably available at this point in time and applies to the specific context—or, failing the availability of such an advance directive, if a duly empowered substitute decision-maker is reasonably available to make a decision for the patient—then merely palliating the patient and allowing the patient to die would be ethically appropriate. (See Chapter 5.) In fact, to try to save the patient under such circumstances would be wrong.

This conclusion is not mere theory. It finds reflection in Canadian law. The *Criminal Code* stipulates that once a health care professional has begun to deliver health care, he or she has the duty to continue that care if failing to do so threatens the life of the patient.[25] However, that legal duty is conditioned by the overriding legal duty to respect any competently expressed wishes of the patient (or of the duly empowered substitute decision-maker). This was clearly expressed in the case of *Starson v. Swayze*, when the Supreme

Court stated that "[the] right to refuse unwanted medical treatment is fundamental to a person's dignity and autonomy"[26] and characterized the right to refuse such treatment as falling within the right to liberty and security of the person as guaranteed by section 7 of the Canadian Charter of Rights and Freedoms.

A case that clearly illustrates how this works when there is an advance directive is that of *Malette v. Shulman.*[27] Here the court ruled that even though Dr. Shulman saved Mrs. Malette's life by giving her a blood transfusion, what otherwise would have been his duty in acting in a medically appropriate fashion[28] was trumped by her refusal of consent, because she carried a signed card that explicitly and clearly stated that she did not want any blood or blood products. Therefore, if Dr. Shulman had followed that directive and not given Mrs. Malette a transfusion and she had died, he would have done the ethically correct thing and would not have been found guilty *even though he would have been responsible for her preventable death.* The outcome would have been tragic, but Dr. Shulman would have acted in an ethically and legally appropriate manner.

Moreover, the *Criminal Code* distinguishes between culpable and non-culpable homicide.[29] It defines culpable homicide as death that is brought about either through negligence in carrying out one's duty or by performing an unlawful act. Since neither of these would be the case in consented-to palliative care, such care may be (indirect) euthanasia but it would not be legally actionable. Therefore, ethics and law agree.

Right to Life versus Duty to Life

These conclusions seem to run head on into the claim that the health care professional's duty to try to keep patients alive is not a merely *prima facie* duty, conditioned as it were by the equal and competent other duties that may exist in a given situation, but an absolute duty. This is frequently expressed in religious terms by saying that life is a gift from God, and that to not try to preserve life is disrespectful towards God and violates God's explicit command not to engage in murder.[30]

However, it is not at all clear that this position has much relevance for the Canadian legal context. Section 15 of the Charter stipulates that any law or public policy that is based on religious considerations is *ultra vires* the powers of Parliament. Therefore, even if God's command were interpreted as entailing that life-saving or -sustaining measures are always obligatory—a point to which we shall return in a moment—there could not be a legal duty to this effect in Canada.

In addition, while the claim that there is an absolute duty to preserve life may be true for religious believers, it cannot be true from a purely ethical perspective, because it confuses a right with a duty. In ethics, it is generally agreed that there is a right to life. As we saw in Chapter 1, a right is a justified claim that we may exercise if we wish, but we don't have to. In other words, a right involves choice on the part of the right-holder. By contrast, a duty is something that one has to do if the enabling conditions are met. If the conditions that trigger the duty are met, there is no choice. That means that the person who has the right to life—that is to say, the patient—may choose not to exercise that right. Consequently, the claim that health care professionals have an absolute duty to try to keep all patients alive even against their competently expressed wishes would mean that patients do not have a choice in the matter—which, in turn, means they do not have a right to life but a duty.

Moreover, nowadays most organized religions have come to accept that while there is a right to life and that this right should be exercised responsibly, this does not mean treating life as though it were an absolute good. When keeping a patient alive serves no purpose beyond saving that patient's life, and when that life lacks all moral or ethical content or the possibility for sentient cognitive awareness, then the patient need not accept life-saving or -sustaining care, and the physician's duty to keep the patient alive ceases to be a duty. This is perhaps most clearly expressed in the following statement by Pope Pius XII:[31]

> Natural reason and Christian morals say that man (and whoever is entrusted with the task of taking care of his fellow man) has the right and duty in the case of serious illness to take the necessary treatment for the preservation of life and health . . . But morally, one is held to use only ordinary means—according to the circumstances of persons, places, times and cultures—that is to say, means that do not involve any grave burdens for oneself or another. A more strict obligation would be too burdensome for most men and would render the attainment of a higher, more important good too difficult.

Ordinary versus Extraordinary Means

The passage just quoted introduces another distinction that is often encountered in the euthanasia debate: the distinction between ordinary and extraordinary means. While at first glance this is a reasonable distinction, some people have argued that one really cannot distinguish between medical procedures and regimens in this fashion.[32] Whether a particular intervention is ordinary or not is not something that is inherent in the technique or the procedure. It depends on the context. For example, an appendectomy under primitive conditions in a camp in Nunavut by medically untrained geologists would definitely have to be considered extraordinary treatment, whereas an appendectomy performed by properly trained medical staff in a well-equipped Toronto hospital would be quite ordinary. Likewise, a corneal transplant for an otherwise healthy forty-five-year-old person would generally be considered ordinary, whereas the same procedure for a forty-five-year-old terminal AIDS patient who has only about three weeks to live might well be considered extraordinary; and so on. In other words, it has been argued that taking the distinction as absolute commits the *fallacy of isolation*.

However, the fact that what counts as ordinary as opposed to extraordinary depends on the situation does not undermine the validity of the distinction, any more than the fact that what counts as just as opposed to unjust depends on the particulars of a given case. Therefore, it does allow health care professionals to say that their duty to sustain life has limits: that it extends only to using means that could reasonably be considered ordinary—that is to say, means that are standard and established therapy in that kind of situation—and that it does not extend to using means that would have little chance of success and would seriously interfere with the ability to provide standard and necessary care for other patients. Thus, the ordinary–extraordinary distinction is tenable, but can legitimately be used by health care professionals only in gauging the extent of their duty in a given setting.

Direct versus Indirect Euthanasia

Another distinction that is sometimes encountered in discussions of deliberate death is the distinction between direct and indirect euthanasia, as was mentioned in the beginning.[33] An example of direct euthanasia is the case of the Montreal physician who injected potassium chloride into a terminal AIDS patient at the patient's request.[34] The patient's death was the immediate and unmediated result of the potassium chloride stopping the heart. An example of indirect euthanasia would be the palliative care physician who gives increasing doses of opioids to manage the pain of a terminal cancer patient, thereby hastening the patient's death.[35] The direct–indirect distinction is represented graphically in Figures 7.3, 7.4 and 7.5.

While the direct–indirect distinction is valid from a purely causal perspective—the causal structure in direct euthanasia is much simpler than in indirect euthanasia—it has little, if any, ethical relevance. As was already pointed out, medical decisions are made not in isolation but in context, and the context always includes the duties of the physician and the rights of the patient—whereby the former are always conditioned by the latter. If the patient has competently consented to life-shortening palliative measures, then whether the causal structure that leads to the end of that life is long or short is really irrelevant. What is important from an ethical perspective is neither the length of the causal chain nor its complexity. What is important is whether the professional involved in structuring the flow of causal events leading to the patient's death has a duty to try to structure the causal flow in another direction.

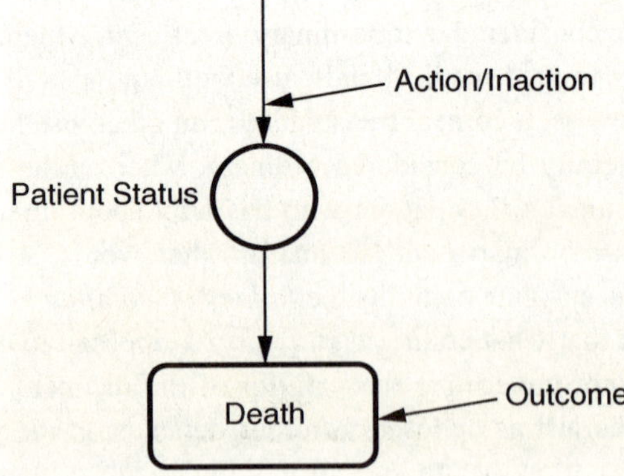

Figure 7.3 Direct Euthanasia

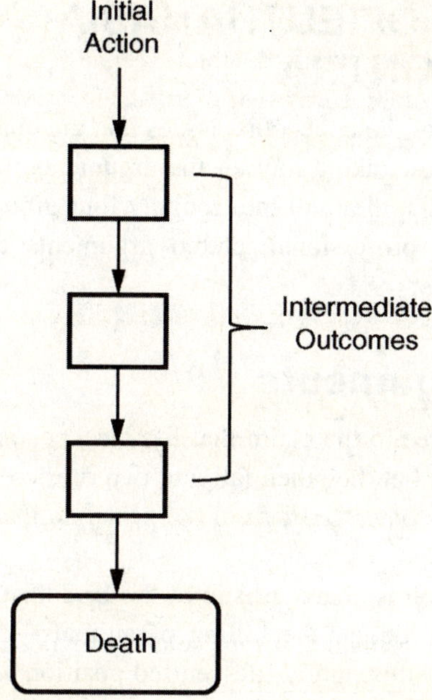

Figure 7.4 Indirect Euthanasia

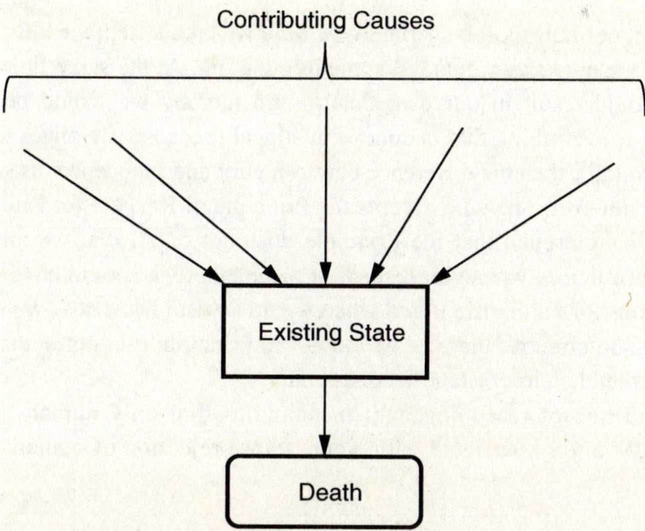

Figure 7.5 Indirect Euthanasia

THE MORALITY OF EUTHANASIA: ARGUMENTS CONTRA

Having disentangled some of the conceptual issues that are commonly encountered in the euthanasia debate, let us now take a look at the arguments themselves. Beginning with arguments against euthanasia, they fall into roughly four groups: life-centred arguments, person-centred arguments, professional-centred arguments and pragmatic arguments, each with its own subgroups.

Life-Centred Arguments

Life-centred arguments agree in the claim that life has special value and that to deliberately end a life is unethical, but they then fall into two rubrics. Some maintain that all life must be respected, whereas others start from the principle that only human life has such special status.

The first sort of position is characteristic of the Buddhist tradition. It tends to characterize killing—and in particular the killing of animals—as having negative karmic implications.[36] In the West, this purely life-centred position was part of the Manichaean creed[37] (which disappeared in the Middle Ages) and made a resurgence in the 20th century with people such as Albert Schweitzer, who maintained that "the ethics of respect for life . . . admits as good only the preservation and advancement of life. All destruction and harming of life, no matter what the circumstances under which it may occur, it designates as evil."[38]

It is not clear, however, that one can ground a workable ethics on such a value position, because it guarantees that no matter what we do, we shall be morally guilty. Every time we breathe, our lungs kill bacteria; every time we take a step, we kill minute animals; and every time we digest, our guts kill some living thing. At the same time *not* to breathe, eat or drink would result in our own death—and thereby we would become guilty as well. However, if everything that is done is unethical (because it violates the fundamental injunction not to kill), then the difference between guilt and innocence disappears.

Of course, not everyone who accepts the Principle of Respect for Life has gone quite this far. Some have argued that the Principle does not entail that we may not take life under any circumstances whatever. Instead, it means that we should have good and overwhelming reasons for taking life if and when we do so. But because it would allow taking a life under certain circumstances, it would not in principle rule out euthanasia. It would merely require that the circumstances be special.

The second line of reasoning, which maintains that only human life has a privileged position, is often associated with Kant, whose rejection of euthanasia and suicide is classic:[39]

> If, in order to escape from some burdensome circumstances, we were to kill someone
> or he asked to be destroyed, we—and he as well—would be using a person merely as
> a means to maintaining a tolerable condition to the end of life. Man, however, is not a

thing, and therefore not something that may be used merely as a means, but in all acts must forever be considered an end in itself.

Arguably, however, the claim that human beings are ends in themselves does not establish the conclusion that euthanasia would be unethical under all circumstances. Certainly, it would allow euthanasia when the individual was in a PVS. After all, what allegedly makes human beings ends in themselves is not the fact that they are biologically alive but that they are sentient beings with will and understanding. When that very capacity is gone, what makes them ends in themselves has also disappeared. To treat the organism that housed this capacity as special simply because the individual is alive is to confuse biological life with personal life; in other words, it is to simply assert the correctness of the vitalist position.

Person-Centred Arguments

Another common argument against euthanasia is based on the claim that everyone has an obligation to develop his or her potentials. It is encountered both in religious and non-religious contexts,[40] and Kant also maintained such a stance. As he put it in his *Metaphysics of Morals*, we have a self-regarding duty to develop our human capacities, and these involve not only intellectual capabilities but also personal ones such as perseverance, humility and so on. Therefore, to end a life that affords the possibility of realizing these potentials is to fail to rise to the challenge of what can make us human in the fullest possible sense.

However, one could reasonably ask whether it even makes sense to talk about self-realization when the quality of life that someone experiences or that lies in store for that person makes it impossible to enjoy cognitive sapient awareness, socialization and emotional interaction with others. As to the possibility that others—onlookers or participants in the drama, as it were—might benefit and realize *their* personal potentials, that would be to degrade the individual to the status of a tool for the benefit of others. If the sole purpose of keeping someone alive is that others may achieve their humanity, then something has gone drastically wrong. In principle, such a perspective would allow any kind of action, so long as others benefited as persons. Ethically, this is disturbing. And ironically enough, this very stance would also allow euthanasia in those cases in which the sufferer's circumstances no longer offered the possibility of self-improvement, either for the sufferer or for others.

Professional-Centred Arguments

Another kind of anti-euthanasia argument appeals to the rights and duties of physicians. The central claim here is that the very nature of medicine rules out participation in euthanasia. As was mentioned in the beginning, this stance is closely associated with the Hippocratic Oath, which requires that an ethical physician will "never administer a poison to anybody when asked to do so, nor . . . suggest such a course."

But like other traditions, this one has not gone unchallenged. For instance, the medical professions in the Netherlands and Belgium have gone on record as saying that under certain circumstances it is a physician's duty to assist a patient in dying,[41] and the medical profession in Switzerland has long accepted that under certain circumstances a physician may have a duty to bring about deliberate death at the request of the patient.[42] They have justified this by means of what has been called a *force majeure* argument.[43] It begins with the claim that physicians have not one duty but two: to try to keep the patient alive (if the patient so requests) and to alleviate pain and suffering. At times, the two conflict. Under those circumstances, the second duty takes priority.[44] It is interesting to note that the medical professions of other countries are slowly changing their traditional perspective in this regard as well.[45]

Furthermore, there are cases where there is no hope of cure or improvement—even of stabilization—for a patient and where the only reasonable option is palliation. In such cases it may happen that the medications necessary to produce a proper palliative effect also shorten the life expectancy of the patient who receives them. Strictly speaking, the physician who embarks on such palliative actions becomes an agent of death. After all, death could be staved off a little longer if the physician were to employ the means that are available to sustain life. However, the fact that this may occur does not mean that the conscientious physician should not engage in purely palliative care, even though the outcome is an accelerated death. Therefore, to say, as does the Canadian Medical Association, that the physician must never be an agent of death is simply to *define* such practices as not being euthanasia. But that is merely to insist that there is a distinction between good medical practice and euthanasia, where in fact there is none.

The Doctrine of Double Effect The claim that life-shortening palliation is not euthanasia is sometimes defended by the argument that only the palliative effect is intended and that death is merely the unfortunate side effect. This line of reasoning uses what has come to be called the *doctrine of double effect*. The doctrine was originally developed by St. Thomas Aquinas in the Middle Ages to explain why it was morally acceptable to kill in self-defence,[46] and it was later adapted by the Catholic Church to deal with interventions that would save the life of a pregnant woman but would kill the fetus.[47] The doctrine itself states that it is permissible to engage in an act that has both a negative and a positive outcome if there are serious reasons for engaging in the act, if considered in itself the act is not morally bad, if the bad outcome is not a necessary temporally prior means to achieving the good outcome and if the agent intends only the good outcome and not the bad.

However, as has been variously pointed out, the doctrine amounts to no more than a psychological ploy to hide from the fact that such palliative actions do involve a knowing and deliberate shortening of life.[48] The physician cannot intend only the good (palliative) effect without at the same time foreseeing the negative outcome (death of the patient). By intending the good effect *while foreseeing the negative outcome, which is an integral and ineluctable part of the scenario*, the physician is also willing that negative outcome. To try to separate the two would require an impossibly tortuous feat of self-deception and selective memory. What the physician does is to will the good effect *despite* the fact that it will hasten the patient's death.[49]

The point to keep in mind is that being a determinant of death is not necessarily ethically reprehensible: It all depends on the circumstances. Once that is recognized, there is no need to hide behind psychological manoeuvres in order to come to terms with a deliberate death.

Pragmatic Arguments

Of course, not all arguments against euthanasia are grounded in purely ethical considerations. Some are pragmatically orientated. They tend to fall into three groups: arguments from the *difficulty of legislation*, the so-called *wedge or slippery-slope* arguments, and the argument from *brutalization.*

The argument from difficulty of legislation centres in the claim that it is impossible to construct a law that would legalize euthanasia, because one cannot spell out sufficient safeguards to prevent misuse. In the Canadian context, this consideration was argued by several intervenors in the case of *Rodriguez. v. British Columbia*[50] and in submissions to the Special Senate Committee on Euthanasia and Assisted Suicide.[51]

The slippery-slope argument does not question the possibility of drafting appropriate legislation but contends that once deliberate death has been legally sanctioned in any context, no matter how carefully circumscribed, it is only a small step to allowing society to kill unwanted population. Yale Kamisar brilliantly summarized this perspective in his classic 1958 article when he said that "Miss Voluntary Euthanasia is not likely to be going it alone for very long. Many of her admirers . . . would be neither surprised nor distressed to see her joined by Miss Euthanatize the Congenital Idiot and Miss Euthanatize the Permanently Insane and Miss Euthanatize the Senile Dementia."[52] He argued that this "parade of horrors" argument cannot be dismissed lightly, because this is precisely what took place in Germany in the 1930s and '40s. While euthanasia was originally intended for incurable German patients who led a life "not worth living," it soon became a tool for killing Gypsies, Jews, Jehovah's Witnesses and politically troublesome persons.

The message of the argument from brutalization is equally simple: Legally sanctioning euthanasia will lead to an erosion of public sensitivity and to a brutalization in the face of suffering.[53] Suffering deserves our compassion and should evoke a helping response. Once euthanasia is legislatively permitted, that response will disappear, to be replaced by a response that treats those who suffer like troublesome objects that no longer meet our expectations. The value of human life will become measured in QALYs and DALYs, and it will be only a short step from this to the position that human life must be evaluated in terms of social utility.

Clearly, these arguments merit serious consideration. However, this does not mean that they are trenchant. For instance, the difficulty-of-legislation argument can easily be countered by pointing to the fact that both the Netherlands[54] and Belgium[55] have had euthanasia legislation since 2002. There is no reason to suppose that similar legislation could not be developed in Canada.

As to the slippery-slope argument, it would be foolish to deny either the fact that euthanasia legislation has been misused in the past or that it might not be misused in the future. However, that does not establish the validity of the argument. As David Hume pointed out years ago,[56]

> There is no method of reasoning more common, and yet none more blamable, than. . .
> to endeavour to refute any hypothesis by pretext of its dangerous consequences. . .
> When an opinion leads to absurdity, 'tis certainly false; but 'tis not certain an opinion
> is false because 'tis of dangerous consequences.

Like all slippery-slope arguments, the euthanasia slippery-slope argument is only as strong as the comparison on which it is based.[57] The Canadian socio-legal context is entirely different from that of Nazi Germany. Moreover, as was just pointed out, euthanasia has been legal in the Netherlands and Belgium since 2002, yet no slippery-slope scenario has developed. This suggests that any slippery slope could easily be avoided by following the Dutch and Belgium models of legislation.

Finally, it is not at all clear that the brutalization argument has it right. In point of fact, the opposite conclusion seems more appropriate. To save or maintain a patient at all cost—betubed, sedated, glucosed, aerated and wired for pace-making and monitoring devices of all sorts without reasonable expectation of improvement, so full of narcotics and analgesics as to be non-cognitive in any real sense, vegetating until the final systemic collapse occurs—seems more brutal than to make for "a fair and easy passage."[58] Likewise, to force a congenitally and severely deformed and disabled neonate to live by dint of technology and professional determination; to save or sustain a radical burns victim with no reasonable hope of recovery, or someone with incurably metastasized cancer, and so on, seems less humane and less respectful of human dignity than to allow an earlier but easier death.

Another well-known argument against euthanasia is presented by Leon Kass. Like Kamisar, Kass argues against the legalization of euthanasia on a combination of logical, ethical and pragmatic grounds. Even though most of Kass's arguments are addressed throughout this chapter, it may be worth considering them together as an example of an anti-euthanasia position as advanced by a philosopher who is also a physician.[59]

He begins with the claim that the request to be euthanatized is actually not a request to be killed but a cry for help. What patients who request euthanasia really want, he argues, is to be free from pain and suffering, and the fact that sometimes they cannot be helped because there is no effective means for dealing with their condition does not mean that they should therefore be killed. Instead, society should spend more resources to develop an appropriate means of treatment. Moreover, given their condition, it is highly unlikely that the patient is competent to make such a request in the first instance.

Moreover, so he continues, if euthanasia were ever legalized, it would be impossible to confine it to those who freely and knowingly request it. It would be the beginning of a slippery slope that would ultimately see irremediably and incurably ill patients killed. Patients would be persuaded to ask for death because they are inconvenient burdens, and patients unable to ask for death would simply be killed, to relieve not merely them but also their families and significant others of the further stress of their disease and dying.

Kass also maintains that it is a logical mistake to present death as a benefit for those who would be euthanatized. Logically, something can be a benefit for someone only if that someone exists. Therefore, the claim that euthanasia would be a benefit for the irremediably and incurably suffering person is simply logically fallacious. As to the claim that euthanasia allows the patient to die a death with dignity, this is based on a radical misunderstanding of what dignity is all about. Dignity does not mean shortening the dying process but allowing patients who are dying to face death with virtue and courage. For those who surround dying persons, it does not mean getting rid of the objects of their compassion and their grief but being with them, and refusing to treat them like mere animals that will be "put down" once their physical existence has reached a certain state.

Kass also considers the nature of the physician–patient relationship and the consequences of turning physicians into agents of death. *First* of all, so he argues, for physicians to become agents of death is contrary to the Hippocratic Oath and the Hippocratic tradition that has characterized medicine since its beginning. *Second*, it would change the physician–patient relationship from one of trust, where patients can trust that physicians will always do what is in the patients' best interests, to one of uncertainty and mistrust: Patients can then no longer be certain that physicians, acting in a patriarchal manner, will not kill them—or try to persuade them that death is in their best interests.

Finally, Kass asks a very fundamental ethical question, one not about the morality of deliberate death itself but about the extent of the Principle of Autonomy: Do those who advocate legalizing euthanasia go too far in the direction of patient autonomy? Just because a patient wants to die does not mean that someone has a duty to act on that request. If one were to put Kass's point here into the Canadian setting, one could argue that Canadian law recognizes that there are limits to autonomy, because it stipulates, in section 14 of the *Criminal Code*, that "no person is entitled to consent to have death inflicted on him, and such consent does not affect the criminal responsibility of any erson by whom death may be inflicted on the person by whom consent is given."

Law is not identical with ethics, and the real question is whether Kass is correct in his reasoning. The slippery-slope argument was already discussed when dealing with Kamisar's arguments and therefore needs no further discussion. As to the claim that euthanasia violates the Hippocratic ethics of the medical profession, the medical associations of several countries—here the Netherlands, Belgium and Switzerland are the best-known examples—have officially stated that euthanasia is not against either the Hippocratic Oath or medical ethics, and that there are circumstances when it is, in fact, the physician's duty to euthanatize a patient if the patient competently requests death.

Nor do these medical associations agree that a request for euthanasia is always a cry for help or the result of pressure being brought to bear on the patient, or that a patient who asks for death is incompetent—and the legislative bodies in their respective countries agree with them in their assessment of the situation. Finally, the argument that it is illogical to consider death a benefit because the alleged beneficiary no longer exists because she is dead, is itself guilty of a logical mistake. The benefit does not redound— and is not intended to redound—to the dead person: it redounds to the living person who is relieved of her suffering. That the relief of suffering occurs during the dying process and as a result of being killed does not change the fact that, during the dying process, the patient no longer suffers. Therefore, the beneficiary of the relief from suffering does exist. It is the dying patient. The fact that the end of the process of alleviating the suffering is also the end of the sufferer's existence does not entail that there has been no beneficiary.

Moreover, it is at least arguable that Kass's claims about dying with dignity and courage are based on a valuational framework that ultimately places human life above all else. Thus, it is not at all clear in any objective sense that dying in irremediable agony and completely nauseous is a dignified end. Nor is it clear that not taking steps to end one's life (or to ask it to be ended) is indicative of a lack of courage. It all depends on how dignity and courage are defined—and here there are no objective standards.

Finally, Kass's appeal to the Hippocratic Oath ignores one important fact: All specific clauses in the Hippocratic Oath, such as the prohibition of abortion, euthanasia or performing surgery for gallstones, are governed by the Oath's initial and overarching clause which states "that I will fulfil this oath and this covenant *according to my ability and judgment.*"[60] Logically, this means that if physicians who have taken the Oath think that it is appropriate to assist patients in dying or to euthanatize patients, their actions would in fact not violate the Oath at all. After all, they would be acting on the basis of their professional judgment as physicians.

THE MORALITY OF EUTHANASIA: ARGUMENTS PRO

However, showing that an argument is invalid or does not establish its alleged conclusion is not the same as showing that the opposite of what that argument is trying to establish is true. Therefore, the thesis that euthanasia is ethically acceptable has to be argued on its own terms.

Autonomy-Based Arguments

There are several ways in which one could ground such an argument. A common way is to appeal to autonomy, that is to say, to the right to self-determination. As a matter of ethics and law, everyone has the right to accept or reject any intervention. (See Chapter 4.) That includes life-saving or -sustaining interventions. This, in turn, means that health care professionals have a duty to respect a patient's decision to reject life-saving or -sustaining interventions. However, by acting in accordance with such a wish and refraining from providing life-saving or -sustaining interventions, the health care professional is engaging in passive euthanasia. As the discussion at the beginning of this chapter has made clear, the distinction between actively bringing about the deliberate death of a patient—by physically doing something and not adopting a passive stance—as opposed to allowing it to occur through inaction is not an ethically relevant distinction. In either case, the professional will be the causal determinant of the patient's death. What is ethically important is whether the professional has a duty in this matter, and what that duty is. If the patient has competently requested death, the ethics of informed consent entails that the professional has a corresponding duty to respect that wish, and passive euthanasia is ethically acceptable.

This conclusion can be strengthened further by arguing that health care professionals may have a duty to not only engage in passive euthanasia, but even physically and actively bring about the patient's death. The argument here is based in Fidelity. If the professional has a duty of fidelity towards the patient—and as was shown in Chapter 3, this is what the fiduciary relationship between health care professionals and patients is all about—then the professional has the duty to fulfill that obligation to the best of her or his ability. Therefore, if the professional has a duty to structure the causal flow of events in such a way that the patient dies, the question becomes what the best way of fulfilling this duty is.

Here the values of the patient move to centre stage because they are relevant to assessing what counts as the best quality of life while dying—or, to put it differently, what constitutes the best quality of dying—in keeping with the patient's fundamental values. If the only way these values can be honoured is to administer lethal medication, then Fidelity entails that the professional has the duty to employ such means. On the other hand, if the patient's fundamental values would not be violated by allowing death to occur in a more protracted manner—i.e., through appropriate palliation and "allowing nature to take its course"—then the focus shifts to the professional's values. Under these circumstances, if the professional's values militate against engaging in active means, then the professional has the option of allowing the dying process to proceed at its own pace.

It is important to note, however, that an autonomy-based argument would be unsuccessful in concluding that *every* health care professional—and in particular, that *every* physician—therefore has a duty to act either as an active or as a passive determinant of death. Health care professionals are also persons, and as such have a right to have their fundamental values respected. Therefore, if being the active or passive causal determinant of a patient's death conflicts with the professional's fundamental values, then the professional has the right to be excused from the case. However, as was pointed out in Chapter 3, the professional has a duty to make such compunctions clear to the patient and other relevant parties before the inception of the health care professional–patient relationship, and must take appropriate steps that some other professional will act in the appropriate manner. Otherwise, this would amount to an unethical abandonment of the patient.

Equality and Justice–Based Arguments

One can also construct an argument in favour of euthanasia based on the Principle of Equality and Justice. Such an argument would begin with the fact that some patients—for instance, those who are quadriplegic and ventilator dependent—cannot be the agents of their own death. This was the case with Nancy B.[61] Someone in her position could not be an agent of her own death because she was being kept alive by mechanical ventilation. After having lived for several years thus ventilator dependent, she wished to die. However, she could not herself translate that wish into reality, because she was paralyzed. If someone else had not turned off her ventilator and thereby killed her, she would have continued to be treated, but against her consent. This would have constituted discrimination on the basis of disability, thereby violating Equality and Justice. (See Chapters 3 and 4.) Equality and Justice therefore entailed that someone had to turn off her ventilator—which, in fact, is what happened. With due alteration of detail, this reasoning can be generalized for every other similarly placed disabled person.

One might try to counter this reasoning by saying that the person who turns off the ventilator (or does something similar) is not really the agent of death. Here, death is caused by the patient's underlying condition, and one is really dealing with passive rather than with active euthanasia, which is why this would be perfectly in keeping with the CMA policy.

However, such a counterargument would not be cogent. As has already been pointed out, the active–passive distinction is ethically irrelevant. *How* the death is brought about is not what makes it euthanasia: it is the fact *that* death is deliberately brought about by ensuring that the causal flow of events unfolds in a certain way. Moreover, such a counterargument would not invalidate the claim that the reason the death is brought about through the actions of someone other than the patient is because the patient cannot perform the act him- or herself. And that, in turn, is to recognize the relevance of the Principle of Equality and Justice in such situations.

Beneficence and Non-Malfeasance–Based Arguments

Finally, one could also construct an argument based on the Principles of Beneficence and of non-Malfeasance. In contrast to arguments that are based on Autonomy (which focus on the right of the patient to make a decision) or on arguments that are based on Equality and Justice (which focus on the right of the patient to have that decision carried out if the patient is unable to do so him- or herself), this sort of argument would address itself to the manner in which such a decision would be effected.

In more concrete terms, it would focus on the fact that not all dying is qualitatively the same. Some dying involves not only pain, nausea, etc., but also a physical and mental decline, which causes suffering to the patient because it violates the patient's fundamental values and sense of dignity. To instill suffering, or not to prevent suffering when it is possible to do so, is to cause harm. Therefore, if there is a duty to advance the good of the patient and a corresponding duty to prevent harm (where the nature of the good and the harm is defined by the patient's values),[62] then under certain circumstances there may lie a duty for the professional to engage in active euthanasia.

A possible reply to this would be to argue that all that is really necessary in these sorts of cases is to palliate patients, so that they are unaware of this violation of their sense of dignity and their fundamental values. However, this would be both illogical and morally perverse. Palliation is appropriate for dealing with physical pain and discomfort. It cannot deal with a violation of dignity and of fundamental values.

Or more correctly, it can deal with this only by sedating sufferers to the point that they are no longer aware that their values and their dignity are being violated. That, however, is not to deal with the violation of dignity and of fundamental values that gave rise to the suffering. To say that it did would be like saying that making someone unaware of being discriminated against but leaving the fact of discrimination intact is dealing with the harm of discrimination. The ethically appropriate way to deal with discrimination is to remove the discrimination itself. The only way to deal with the violation of fundamental values and the affront to personal dignity caused by a particular manner of dying is to change that manner of dying. This means that, under certain circumstances, active rather than passive euthanasia is appropriate. This is one of the reasons why both the Netherlands and Belgium crafted their euthanasia legislation in such a way as to allow physicians to be the active agents of deliberate death when the patient's dignity and fundamental values are violated by their manner of dying.

As an aside, and as a concluding note on euthanasia, it is interesting that while most medical associations (including the Canadian Medical Association, the American Medical Association and the British Medical Association) have gone on record as condemning euthanasia as murder and as unethical, none have gone on record as condemning the Royal Dutch Medical Society and the Belgian Association of Medical Unions, which sanction their respective national euthanasia laws, for condoning murder. This may be either an oversight—which seems hardly likely, given the prominence of the issue of euthanasia in the professional and public spheres—or a matter of definition, because the Associations simply define the active killing of a terminal patient by means of relevant drugs as "terminal sedation."

ASSISTED SUICIDE

Assisted suicide differs from euthanasia in that the patient is the agent of death and merely—as the phrase suggests—has the assistance of a second party.

Suicide is not illegal in Canada. The law prohibiting suicide was repealed in 1972. Anything that is not legally prohibited is legally allowed. This effectively makes suicide what is called a freedom right—which means that everyone is free to commit suicide and may not be interfered with on pain of assault and battery unless there are reasonable grounds to suppose that the person is incompetent.

The immediate temptation is to say that the intention to commit suicide is always and in itself an indication of incapacity and mental imbalance. However, that is not correct. There are cases—the case of Sue Rodriguez is probably the best-known Canadian example—in which a psychiatric assessment of a patient may bring back a verdict of "suicidal but competent."[63] These are cases where the manner of dying violates the patient's sense of dignity and fundamental values, or where continued life is experienced as merely protracted, irremediable and incurable suffering.

It is tempting to argue that patients can always kill themselves. They can leap from buildings, use firearms, hang themselves or use overdoses of readily available poisons—and if all else fails, they can always starve themselves to death. However, as will be apparent by now, none of these ways of dying may be consonant with the patients' fundamental values. Alternatively, patients may wish to live as long as possible and die only when they have reached this final stage of valuational dissonance, but at that point no longer be in the position to kill themselves, because they will have lost the ability to bring about their own death. This was the case with Sue Rodriguez, who suffered from ALS. Therefore, the argument that it is always possible for patients to kill themselves may be correct in principle—we will return to exceptions in a moment—but its application may involve paying for that agency with the coin of fundamental values.

With due alteration of detail, therefore, the arguments that support the duty to engage in (active or passive) euthanasia can be used to support the claim that under certain circumstances there may lie a duty to assist a patient in committing suicide. Such arguments can be particularly focused on physicians by pointing to the fact that only physicians can legally prescribe the necessary medication.

Therefore, there may be cases in which physicians have a duty to assist their patients in committing suicide. However, assisted suicide is prohibited by section 241(b) of the *Criminal Code*. (Incidentally, this section of the Code is unique in that it makes it a criminal offence to assist another person in doing something that is legal.) This poses a serious dilemma for Canadian physicians. On the one hand, the ethics of the fiduciary physician–patient relationship suggests that physicians have a duty to help their patients in dying; on the other hand, the law seems to suggest that if they fulfill this duty, they will be liable to prosecution. This dilemma clearly illustrates that while law and ethics may coincide, this will not always be the case. It also illustrates that there may be occasions when acting ethically may be dangerous to one's social well-being.

EUTHANASIA AND BRAIN DEATH

One of the key presumptions underlying the discussion so far has been that the individuals in question are persons. However, when the patient is decerebrate, the presumption of personhood becomes questionable. The patient—if that is still the right term—is then what one theologian has described as a living human body. Does a physician therefore still have a duty to keep that individual alive?

At first glance, the answer appears to depend on the criterion of death. From the whole-brain perspective it seems to be in the affirmative; from the cerebral perspective it seems to go the other way. Legally, of course, the answer is simple. Only a whole-brain dead individual has no more right to health care—but that does not really address the ethics of the situation.

However, the issue may not be as clear as all that. Every right and every duty is conditioned by the competing rights and duties of others—and at this point resource allocation begins to raise its head. If the figures mentioned at the beginning of this chapter are correct, then in Canada the aggregate cost of keeping all Canadian patients who are in a PVS alive would range from $148 million to $1.036 billion annually. Given a life expectancy of approximately five years for individuals in a PVS, this would mean a total cost between $740 million and $5.18 billion to the Canadian health care system. Individuals who are in a PVS for more than six months have a less than 0.5 percent chance of recovery to any level of sentient cognitive awareness. Providing them with sustaining care seriously erodes the accessibility of ordinary patients to the health care they need.

The question that now arises, therefore, is whether the rights of ordinary patients take precedence over the commitment to keep individuals in a PVS alive. And if the answer is that they do, then it becomes relevant to ask whether it is ethically more appropriate to bring about the death of individuals in a PVS through inaction—which leads to a dying process that also consumes resources—or to bring it about directly by active means.

VOLUNTARY VERSUS NON-VOLUNTARY EUTHANASIA

Finally, the discussion so far has not dealt explicitly with the distinction between voluntary and non-voluntary euthanasia that was mentioned at the beginning of this chapter. Voluntary euthanasia, it will be recalled, is usually understood as the euthanatizing of a patient at his or her own request, whereby, of course, it is assumed that the patient who makes this request is competent at the time of making it. Non-voluntary euthanasia, on the other hand, is usually understood as the euthanatizing of a person without that person having expressed such a wish.

The reason why this distinction has not been explicitly addressed is not that the distinction is not valid but that, in a sense, the whole discussion has really dealt with some aspect of it or other. One can therefore sum up the tenor of what has been said so far as follows: All other things being equal, voluntary euthanasia is ethically defensible. The only real question is whether anyone has a duty to act on a voluntary request for euthanasia if the patient is no longer capable of killing him- or herself by committing suicide. And here we have also suggested an answer.

As for non-voluntary euthanasia, the discussion implies that under certain circumstances it, too, is ethically defensible. For instance, it is ethically defensible in the case of congenitally incompetent persons who have never been in a position to formulate any values, let alone express wishes, and when the continuation of their lives would amount to unmitigated and unrelenting torture. People who are in such a position should not be treated worse than people who have the good fortune to be able to make their own decisions. The rights of the incompetent should not be less than the rights of the competent solely because of their incompetence! That is why duly empowered substitute decision-makers should be allowed to make the relevant decision on their behalf.

However, at this point Yale Kamisar's impassioned argument against euthanasia comes back to haunt us. Kamisar is right: There is the danger that, once accepted in principle, non-voluntary euthanasia will become the justification for killing unwanted population, for emptying hospital beds or for ridding ourselves of people whom we consider undesirable. That must not be allowed to occur. Therefore, any move to give legal recognition to euthanasia must provide some mechanism that would rule this out. This could be done by enacting legislation similar to what is in effect in the Netherlands and Belgium. Alternatively, it could be done by placing the power to make such a decision into the hands of the courts. The courts, exercising their *parens patriae* powers, could then reach a decision on the basis of argumentation on both sides of the issue and after an examination of all appropriate evidence. Under such circumstances, non-voluntary euthanasia would be acceptable, not because the legal decision would make it ethically acceptable, but because the legal process would provide the safeguard that what is ethically acceptable *per se* would not be misused.

CONCLUSION

If the discussion in this chapter is correct then, under certain circumstances, euthanasia and assisted suicide are ethically acceptable. However, the question of whether something is ethically acceptable is different from the question of whether it should be allowed by law. It is here, as was noted, that the slippery-slope argument comes into its own. Whatever its logical cogency, it is certainly correct in arguing that there is a dimension in human beings that allows them to depart from what is ethical. And the argument is surely justified in pointing to the danger this may pose. The historical facts are incontrovertible.

The question therefore is whether, given these facts, and given this potential for unethical behaviour, euthanasia and assisted suicide should be legalized. Arguably, the answer still is a qualified yes. Since health care professionals in general and physicians in particular are currently caught in a dilemma between ethics and law, and since finessing the law (as is currently done) carries its own ethical dangers, it seems appropriate to solve the problem by amending the *Criminal Code*. The Appendix contains a suggestion as to how this might be effected.

It is interesting to note that the attempts to change to the *Criminal Code*'s prohibition of assisted suicide under section 241(b) have recently been re-opened with the case of *Taylor v. Attorney General of Canada*.[64] The plaintiff in this case, Ms. Gloria Taylor, suffers from ALS, as did Sue Rodriguez. Since the matter had already been considered— and decided—in *Rodriguez*, the Court would have refused to hear the application unless the case could be distinguished from that of *Rodriguez*. The application by Ms. Taylor therefore includes the submission that the prohibition of assisted suicide violates section 7 of the Charter, which guarantees the right to life, liberty and security of the person. Specifically, section 7 stipulates that

> Everyone has the right to life, liberty and security of the person and the right not to be deprived thereof except in accordance with the principles of fundamental justice.

The claim that is being made in this case, therefore, is that the interpretation of section 7 rights has evolved to the point to where it is now understood to encompass the right to be free from excruciating physical pain and agony, as well as to be free of the mental suffering caused by a violation of fundamental values. At time of writing, it is unclear what the ultimate decision in this case will be or whether, in case the application fails, Ms. Taylor will receive leave to appeal the matter to the Supreme Court which, absent Parliament striking down section 241(b), has the final authority in the matter.

Further Readings

Douglas, C., I. Kerridge and R. Ankeny. "Managing Intentions: The End-of-Life Administration of Analgesics and Sedatives, and the Possibility of Slow Euthanasia." *Bioethics* 22.7 (Aug 2008): 388–396.

Jansen, L.A. "Disambiguating Clinical Intentions: The Ethics of Palliative Sedation." *J Med Philos* 35.1 (Feb 2010): 19–31.

Jones, G. "The Problematic Symmetry between Brain Birth and Brain Death." *Journal of Medical Ethics* 24 (1998): 237–242.

Kamisar, Y. "Some Non-Religious Objections against Proposed Mercy-Killing Legislation." *Minnesota Law Review* 42 (May 1958): 969–1042.

Kass, L.R. "Neither for Love Nor Money: Why Doctors Must Not Kill." *Public Interest* 94 (Winter 1989): 25–46.

Kass, L.R. "I Will Give No Deadly Drug: Why Doctors Must Not Kill" in *The Case Against Assisted Suicide: For the Right to End–of-Life Care*, ed. K. Foley and H. Hendin (Baltimore: The Johns Hopkins University Press, 2002), 17–40.

Miller, F.G., R.D. Truog and D.W. Brock. "Moral Fictions and Medical Ethics." *Bioethics* 24.9 (Nov 2010): 453–460.

Pabst-Battin, M. *Ending Life: Ethics and the Way We Die* (Oxford and New York: Oxford University Press, 2005).

Prado, C.G. *Assisted Suicide: Canadian Perspectives* (Ottawa: University of Ottawa Press, 2000).

Puccetti, R. "Does Anyone Survive Neocortical Death?" in *Death: Beyond Whole-Brain Criteria*, ed. R. Zaner (Dordrecht, NL: Kluwer, 1988): 75–90.

Qill, T.E., R. Dresser and D. Brock. "The Rule of Double Effect: A Critique of Its Role in End-of-Life Decision Making." *New England Journal of Medicine* 337.4 (1997): 1768–1771.

Rachels, J. "Active and Passive Euthanasia." *New England Journal of Medicine* 292.2 (9 Jan 1975): 78–80.

Special Senate Committee on Euthanasia and Assisted Suicide. "On Life and Death: Final Report," available at www.parl.gc.ca/Content/SEN/Committee/351/euth/rep/lad-e.htm

Endnotes

1. R. Rilke, "About Poverty and Death," *The Book of Hours*.

2. P. Lipton, "Ischemic Cell Death in Brain Neurons," *Physiological Reviews* 79 (1999): 1431–1568; accessed 9 Jan 2011 at http://physrev.physiology.org/content/79/4/1431.full

3. S. Todo et al., "Extended Preservation of Human Liver Grafts with UW Solution," *Journal of the American Medical Association* 261.5 (Feb 1989): 711–714.

4. N. Mendler, "The Meta-Physiology of Organ Preservation," *J Heart Lung Transplant* 11(4 Pt 2) (Jul–Aug 1992): 192–195.

5. Aristotle, *de Anima*, Book II.

6. For a classic discussion of this issue, see St. Thomas Aquinas, *Summa contra gentiles* II:83:10, II:85:35, IV:84:4 and II:89:3. St. Thomas expressed the issue in terms of whether a soul could be united to something that was not its "proper matter"—i.e., to a body that could not allow the soul to fulfill its "proper function," which he identified as sentient cognitive awareness.

7. K. Roche, "No Legs but Standing Tall" *Ottawa Sun*, Sunday, 9 Jan 2011; accessed 9 Jan 2011 at www.ottawasun.com/news/ottawa/2011/01/08/16813276.html

8. "A Definition of Irreversible Coma: Report of the Ad Hoc Committee of the Harvard Medical School to Examine the Definition of Brain Death," *Journal of the American Medical Association* 205.6 (5 Aug 1968): 337–340. (No authors listed.)

9. R. v. Kitching and Adams, [1976] 6 WWR 697.

10. For a discussion of the distinction between a personalist and a vitalist conception and its implications for abortion, see G. Jones, "The Problematic Symmetry between Brain Birth and Brain Death," *Journal of Medical Ethics* 24 (1998): 237–242.

11. R. Pucetti, "Does Anyone Survive Neocortical Death?" in *Death: Beyond Whole-Brain Criteria*, ed. R.M. Zane (Dordrecht: Kluwer Academic Publishers, 1989), 75–90.

12. From *The Hippocratic Oath: Text, Translation, and Interpretation*, by Ludwig Edelstein (Baltimore: Johns Hopkins Press, 1943).

13. Law Reform Commission of Canada, Working Paper 28, *Euthanasia, Aiding Suicide and Cessation of Treatment* (Ottawa, 1982).

14. Report 20, *Euthanasia, Aiding Suicide and Cessation of Treatment* (Ottawa: Minister of Supply and Services, 1983).

15. CMA Policy: *Euthanasia and Assisted Suicide* (Update 2007) available at http://policybase.cma.ca/dbtw-wpd/Policypdf/PD07-01.pdf

16. Canadian Medical Association, "Canadian Physicians and Euthanasia," 1993, 19.

17. Ethics Committee of the College of Family Physicians of Canada, "Statement Concerning Euthanasia and Physician-Assisted Suicide" (2010) available at www.cfpc.ca/English/cfpc/communications/health%20policy/2000%20statement%20concerning%20euthanasia/default.asp?s=1

18. Cf. American Medical Association, *Code of Ethics*, Opinion 2.21. "Euthanasia" available at www.ama-assn.org/ama/pub/physician-resources/medical-ethics/code-medical-ethics/opinion221.shtml; British Medical Association (2007), "Euthanasia and Physician Assisted Suicide—Do the Moral Arguments Differ?" available at www.bma.org.uk/ethics/end_life_issues/Euthanasiaphysicianassistedsuicide.jsp; World Medical Association, *Declaration on Euthanasia*, adopted by the 39th World Medical Assembly, Madrid, Spain, October 1987, and reaffirmed at the 170th Council Session, Divonne-les-Bains, France, May 2005, accessed 10 Jan 2011 at www.wma.net/en/30publications/10policies/e13/index.html

19. D. Walton, *On Defining Death: An Analytic Study of the Concept of Death in Philosophy and Medical Ethics* (Montreal: McGill-Queen's University Press, 1979), 170. See also T.L. Beauchamp, "A Reply to Rachels on Active and Passive Euthanasia," in *Ethical Issues in Death and Dying*, ed. T. Beauchamp and S. Perlin (Englewood Cliffs, NJ: Prentice Hall, 1978), 246–248.

20. J. Rachels, "Active and Passive Euthanasia," *New England Journal of Medicine* 292.2 (9 Jan 1975): 78–80. See also R. Macklin, *Mortal Choices* (New York: Pantheon Books, 1987), 78 ff.

21. Mulloy v. Hop Sang [1935] 1 W.W.R. 714.

22. Or, in the case of an incompetent patient, of the competently expressed wishes of the duly empowered substitute decision-maker.

23. Cf. D.N. Walton, *On Defining Death: An Analytic Study of the Concept of Death in Philosophy and Medical Ethics* (Montreal: McGill-Queen's University Press, 1979), 96 f. See also T.L. Beauchamp, "A Reply to Rachels on Active and Passive Euthanasia," in *Ethical Issues in Death and Dying*, eds. T. Beauchamp and S. Perlin (Englewood Cliffs, NJ: Prentice Hall, 1978), 246–248; and P. Foot, "Killing and Letting Die" in *Abortion: Moral and Legal Perspectives*, ed. J.L. Garfield and P. Hennessey (Amherst: University of Massachusetts Press, 1984), 177–185.

24. F.G. Miller, R.D. Truog and D.W. Brock, "Moral Fictions and Medical Ethics," *Bioethics* 24.9 (Nov 2010): 453–460.

25. S. 217. "Every one who undertakes to do an act is under a legal duty to do it if an omission to do the act is or may be dangerous to life."

26. Starson v. Swayze (2003), 225 D.L.R. (4th) 385 (S.C.C.), at 412.

27. Malette v. Shulman (1987), 47 D.L.R. 4th 18 (Ont. H.C.), affirmed (1990). 67 D.L.R. (4th) 321 (C.A.).

28. See *Criminal Code of Canada*, s. 217.

29. Loc. cit., s. 222.

30. In the Talmudic, Orthodox, Anglican, Reformed and some other Christian traditions this is the sixth commandment. In the Islamic tradition, this is expressed slightly differently in the Qur'an in Surah Al-Isra' 17:33: "Nor take life—which Allah has made sacred—except for just cause." *The Holy Qur'an: English Translation of the Meanings and Commentary*, revised and edited by The Presidency of Islamic Researchers, IFTA. See also Surah Al-An`am 6:151.

31. "Prolongation of Life: Allocution to an International Congress of Anesthesiologists," 24 Nov 1957; Pope Pius XII, *Osservatore Romano* 4 (1957). For a more recent restatement of this position, see *Sacred Congregation for the Doctrine of the Faith*, Declaration on Euthanasia, Vatican City, 1980; available at www.vatican.va/roman_curia/congregations/cfaith/documents/rc_con_cfaith_doc_19800505_euthanasia_en.html. For a similar position in Islam, see N. Sarhill et al., "The Terminally Ill Muslim: Death and Dying from the Muslim Perspective," *American Journal of Hospice and Palliative Medicine* 18.4 (Jul–Aug 2001): 251–255; and correspondingly for Judaism, Rabbi J. David Bleich, "In Support of H.R. 2260, the Pain Relief Promotion Act of 2000," testimony before the U.S. Senate Judiciary Committee, 25 Apr 2000; H.L. Gordon, *Questions and Answers about Jewish Tradition and the Issues of Assisted Death* (New York: Union of American Hebrew Congregations, 1998).

32. See R. Veatch, *Death, Dying, and the Biological Revolution: Our Last Quest for Responsibility* (New Haven and London: Yale University Press, 1970), 106. For a somewhat different discussion, see S.D. John, "Ordinary and Extraordinary Means," in *Principles of Health Care Ethics*, ed. R.E. Ashcroft, A. Dawson and H. Draper (Sussex, U.K.: John Wiley & Sons, 2007), 269–272.

33. A.B. Shaw, "Two Challenges to the Double Effect Doctrine: Euthanasia and Abortion," *J Med Ethics* 28.2 (Apr 2002): 102–104. For an interpretation that identifies indirect euthanasia with palliative care, see "Direct v. Indirect Euthanasia," *Canadian Medical Association Journal*, accessed 12 Jan 2011 at http://findarticles.com/p/articles/mi_7490/is_200902/ai_n32203969/ and N. Tanida, "The View of Religions toward Euthanasia and Extraordinary Treatments in Japan," *Journal of Religion and Health* 39.4 (Winter 2000): 339–354.

34. *Calgary Herald*, 20 Jun 1992; *Montreal Gazette,* 19 and 20 Jun 1992.

35. D.M. Sawyer, J.R. Williams and F. Lowy, "Canadian Physicians and Euthanasia: 2. Definitions and Distinctions," *Canadian Medical Association Journal* 148.9 (1993): 1463–1466.

36. See P. Harvey, *Introduction to Buddhist Ethics* (Cambridge: Cambridge University Press, 2000).

37. G. Widengren, *Mani and Manichaeism* (London: Weidenfeld and Nicholson, 1965).

38. A. Schweitzer, *Kultur und Ethik* (Bern: Paul Haupt, 1923), 339, author's translation.

39. Immanuel Kant, *Foundations of the Metaphysics of Morals* (New York: Bobbs-Merrill, 1959), 47 (B422).

40. Anglican Church of Canada, *On Dying Well* (Toronto: Anglican Church Information Office, 1975); C.A. Campbell, *Moral Intuition and the Principle of Self-Realization* (Oxford: Oxford University Press, 1948). For a traditional Christian perspective on the point of suffering, see St. Augustine, *City of God*, Book XIX, 25. For a detailed analysis of the notion, see E.-H.W. Kluge, *The Ethics of Deliberate Death* (Port Washington: National University Publications, 1980), 38 f.

41. K. Chambaere et al. "Trends in Medical End-of-Life Decision Making in Flanders, Belgium 1998–2001–2007." *Med Decis Making*. (29 Dec 2010), Epub ahead of print.

42. S. Burchardt et al., "Euthanasia and Assisted Suicide: Comparison of Legal Aspects in Switzerland and Other Countries," *Medicine, Science and the Law* 46 (2006): 287–294.

43. H.J. Leenen and C. Ciesielski-Carlucci, "Force Majeure (Legal Necessity): Justification for Active Termination of Life in the Case of Severely Handicapped Newborns after Forgoing Treatment," *Cambridge Quarterly of Healthcare Ethics* 2 (1993): 271–274; E. Vermeersch, "The Belgian Law on Euthanasia: The Historical and Ethical Background," *Acta chirurgica belgica* 102 (2002): 394–397, accessed 17 Jan 2011 at www.belsurg.org/uploaded_pdfs/102/102_394_397.pdf

44. F.G. Miller, R.D. Truog and D.W. Brock, "Moral Fictions and Medical Ethics," *Bioethics* 24.9 (Nov 2010): 453–460.

45. "One in Three Doctors Support Euthanasia," *London Telegraph*, accessed 17 Jan 2011 at www.telegraph.co.uk/health/healthnews/5044885/One-in-three-doctors-support-euthanasia.html; W.J. Stronegger et al., "Changing Attitudes towards Euthanasia among Medical Students in Austria," *J Med Ethics* (1 Dec 2010), Epub ahead of print.

46. Thomas Aquinas, *Summa Theologiae* II, Q. 64, Art. 7.

47. See P. Foot, "The Problem of Abortion and the Doctrine of Double Effect," in *Ethical Theory: An Anthology*, ed. R. Shafer-Landau (Oxford: Blackwell, 2007), 582–589.

48. C. Douglas, I. Kerridge and R. Ankeny, "Managing Intentions: The End-of-Life Administration of Analgesics and Sedatives, and the Possibility of Slow Euthanasia," *Bioethics* 22.7 (Aug 2008): 388–396.

49. See Foot, op. cit. See also P. Allmark et al., "Is the Doctrine of Double Effect Irrelevant in End-of-Life Decision Making?" *Nursing Philosophy* 11.3 (Jul 2010): 170–177; and T.E. Qill et al., "The Rule of Double Effect: A Critique of Its Role in End-of-Life Decision Making," *New England Journal of Medicine* 337.4 (1997): 1768–1771. For an opposing view, see L.A. Jansen, "Disambiguating Clinical Intentions: The Ethics of Palliative Sedation," *J Med Philos* 35.1 (Feb 2010): 19–31.

50. Rodriguez v. British Columbia (Attorney General) [1993] 3 S.C.R. 519.

51. Special Senate Committee on Euthanasia and Assisted Suicide, *On Life and Death: Final Report*, accessed 22 Jan 2011 at http://dsp-psd.pwgsc.gc.ca/Collection-R/LoPBdP/CIR/919-e.htm

52. Y. Kamisar, "Some Non-Religious Objections against Proposed Mercy-Killing Legislation," *Minnesota Law Review* 42 (May 1958): 969–1042.

53. A. Schafer, "The Great Canadian Euthanasia Debate," *Globe and Mail* (5 Nov 2009), accessed 17 Jan 2011 at www.theglobeandmail.com/news/opinions/the-great-canadian-euthanasia-debate/article1353068/

54. *Termination of Life on Request and Assisted Suicide (Review Procedures) Act*, available at www.academiavita.org/english/AltriDocumenti/org_int/OLANDA/Testo%20legge%20olandese%20eutanasia%5B1%5D.pdf

55. *The Belgian Act on Euthanasia of May 28th, 2002*, available at www.kuleuven.be/cbmer/viewpic.php?LAN=E&TABLE=DOCS&ID=23

56. D. Hume, *Treatise on Human Nature*, ed. L.A. Selby-Bigge (Oxford: Clarendon Press, 1967), s. VIII, "Of Liberty and Necessity," Part 2, para. 1.

57. J.A. Burgess, "The Great Slippery-Slope Argument," *J Med Ethics* 19.3 (Sep 1993): 169–174.

58. Francis Bacon, *The New Atlantis* (London, 1627).

59. L.R. Kass, "Neither for Love Nor Money: Why Doctors Must Not Kill," *Public Interest* 94 (Winter 1989): 25–46; and L.R. Kass, "I Will Give No Deadly Drug: Why Doctors Must Not Kill" in *The Case Against Assisted Suicide: For The Right to End–of–Life Care*, ed. K. Foley and H. Hendin (Baltimore: The John Hopkins University Press, 2002), 17–40.

60. See note 12, *supra*.

61. Nancy B. v. Hôtel-Dieu de Québec et al. (1992), 86 Dominion Law Reports (4th) 385 (Quebec Superior Court).

62. Before taking on the case of Sue Rodriguez, the author asked for two independent assessments of Sue Rodriguez. The assessments came back as "suicidal ideations but competent."

63. See note 62, *supra*.

64. Carter, Johnson, Shoichet, The British Columbia Civil Liberties Association and Taylor v. Attorney General of Canada, Supreme Court of B.C. No. S I 012688 (Vancouver Registry). At time of writing, the case had not been decided.

SAMPLE CASES

1. Aristotle J. has had a severe stroke, and has been brought to the emergency department of Our Lady of the Sorrows Hospital. He is being maintained on a ventilator, but it is clear to the emergency room physician and the rest of the staff that he will not recover to any level of sapient cognitive awareness. The next-of-kin have been made aware of the current status of Mr. J. After consultation with the attending physician and the chaplain, they decide that continuing treatment would be pointless. They therefore authorize the physician to cease all efforts. The physician has some qualms about doing so, because on one level she feels that to turn the ventilator off is to kill the patient. However, after some reflection, she decides that she would not be the primary and direct cause of Mr. J.'s death. Her causal involvement would be indirect only, since the direct causal agent would be the disease process that has brought Mr. J. to this state. She therefore turns off the ventilator, confident in the opinion that no real responsibility for Mr. J.'s death falls on her.

2. Arthur Q. had been admitted to hospital with a diagnosis of cancer of the lung. A lobectomy had been recommended and he had agreed to it. In fact, he had been a most cooperative patient. He followed the prescribed regimen faithfully, and it looked as though the surgery had been successful. Three months later, a checkup revealed that not all had gone as hoped. The cancer had metastasized into the liver, and several other metastases were noted. The other lung also was affected. Considered opinion was that the best that could be done for Arthur Q. was to give him

palliative care. Arthur Q. accepted this. When the pain became too great and he could no longer eat, he was hospitalized. He grew steadily weaker—and the pain control regimen had to be increased steadily. After several weeks in hospital, he conferred with his attending physician and his nurses and told them that he did not want any more visits from his grandchildren and his next-of-kin. He had fought the good fight, and he felt that he now deserved to die. He had informed his family of his decision. While they had difficulty facing it, they respected it as his right. Arthur Q. was a proud man. He was a veteran—a CF-18 pilot who had seen action in Afghanistan, had been decorated and was a war hero. He wanted to die while he still had a shred of dignity left. He had no firearm—and in any case he was convinced that if he were to kill himself by such means, his family and, above all, his grandchildren would be deeply shocked. He therefore asked the physician to give him something that would allow him to die painlessly, peacefully and in his sleep.

Medical practitioner not required to provide treatment when a person competently requests non-treatment or cessation of treatment

217.1 Nothing in sections 14, 45, 215, 216 and 217 and other relevant sections of the Criminal Code shall be interpreted as

(a) requiring a qualified medical practitioner to initiate or to continue surgical or medical treatment to a person who competently requests that such treatment not be commenced or continued;

(b) requiring a qualified medical practitioner to initiate or to continue surgical or medical treatment to a person who has previously made a competent determination that such treatment not be commenced or continued and who has not revoked such determination;

(c) requiring a qualified medical practitioner to initiate or to continue surgical or medical treatment to a person when a duly empowered proxy decision-maker of that person, using appropriate standards of proxy decision-making, formally requests that such treatment not be commenced or continued; or

(d) preventing a qualified medical practitioner from initiating or continuing palliative care and measures intended to eliminate or relieve the suffering of a person solely for the reason that such care or measures will or are likely to shorten the life expectancy of the person, except where

    (i)   that person competently requests or has competently requested that such measures not be undertaken if these measures have a life-shortening effect; or

    (ii) the duly empowered proxy decision-maker of that person, using appropriate standards of proxy decision-making, requests that such measures not be undertaken if these measures have a life-shortening effect.

No offense committed when medical practitioner does not provide treatment at the request of the person

xxx.1 Notwithstanding anything in sections 14, 45, 215, 216, 217 or any other relevant section, no qualified medical practitioner commits an offence set out in those sections where the practitioner

(a) does not initiate or continue to administer

    (i)   surgical or medical treatment to a person who competently and formally requests that such treatment not be commenced or continued;

    (ii) surgical or medical treatment to a person who has previously made a competent determination that such treatment not be commenced or continued and who has not revoked such determination;

(iii) surgical or medical treatment to a person when a duly empowered proxy decision-maker of that person, using appropriate standards of proxy decision-making, formally requests that such treatment not be commenced or continued;

or

(b) commences or continues to administer palliative care and measures intended to eliminate or relieve the suffering of a person for the sole reason that such care or measures will or are likely to shorten the life expectancy of the person, except where

(i) that person competently requests or has competently requested that such measures not be undertaken if these measures have such a life-shortening effect, or

(ii) the duly empowered proxy decision-maker of that person, using appropriate standards of proxy decision-making, requests that such measures not be undertaken if these measures have a life-shortening effect.

Palliative care and shortening of life expectancy

xxx.2 In the event that the life of the person will or is likely to be shortened by the use of palliative measures involving medications or similar means, and the time span of this shortening exceeds what would normally be expected using appropriate and recognized palliative measures, the case shall be subject to review by an independent body consisting of a physician having no connection with any party involved in the case, a member of the Attorney General's Department of the jurisdiction in which the death has occurred, and an independent member of the public having training in ethics.

xxx.3 If this independent body finds that the event was not in accordance with the competently expressed wishes of the patient or in accordance with appropriate standards of proxy decision-making, as the case may be, the otherwise relevant provisions of the Criminal Code shall apply.

Voluntary euthanasia and assisted suicide: Application by competent persons on their own behalf

yyy.1 If a person suffers from an incurable and irremediable disease or medical condition, and if that person experiences the disease or condition as violating the fundamental values of that person, then

(a) that person may make application to a superior court for permission to request the assistance of a physician in terminating his life as quickly and as painlessly as possible in keeping with the fundamental values of that person; and

(b) on presentation of evidence by an independent psychiatrist and the attending physician that the person making the request is competent to do so, the court shall hear such a request as expeditiously as possible.

yyy.2 The court, upon due consideration of the mental and physical state of the person requesting permission under yyy.1, and of that person's fundamental values; and taking due account of the medical nature of the affliction of the person requesting such assistance, may grant such an application.

yyy.3 Any permission granted under sec. yyy.2

(a) shall be registered with the regional coroner of the relevant jurisdiction;

(b) shall be for a period of six months; and

(c) shall include an order that there shall be due notification of the coroner if such a permission has been acted upon.

yyy.4 Any physician acting upon a permission under sec. yyy.2 and in accordance with the wishes of the person making the request under yyy.1, shall use such measures as he deems, upon due consideration, to be appropriate for terminating the life of that person as quickly and painlessly as possible.

yyy.5 Any physician acting upon a permission granted under secs. yyy.2, yyy.3 and yyy.4, and acting in accordance with the provisions set out therein, shall be deemed not to have committed an offence within the meaning of this Act.

yyy.6 Any revocation of a request made by a competent person under sec. yyy.1 shall take immediate effect and shall be deemed to render null and void any previous request made by that person under sec. yyy.1

Euthanasia: Application on behalf of an incompetent person.

zzz.1 Any person who suffers from an incurable and irremediable disease or medical condition, and who, by reason of incompetence, is unable to make application to a court as allowed under sec. yyy.1, may have such application made for him by a duly empowered proxy decision-maker using appropriate standards of proxy decision-making.

zzz.2 Any application brought under sec. zzz.1 shall be treated by the court as though it were an application brought by the incompetent person on his own behalf.

zzz.3 In considering an application brought under sec. zzz.1, the court shall have due regard to the previous, competently expressed wishes and values of the now incompetent person, if that person was previously competent.

zzz.4 In the event that such values cannot be satisfactorily ascertained, the court shall use the values and standards currently accepted by Canadian society, where the nature of these values and standards shall be determined by the court in consultation with

(a) a duly empowered representative of an association for disabled persons;

(b) a practising physician;

(c) a practising nurse;

(d) a person having expertise in biomedical ethics; and

(e) a member of the public at large.

zzz.5 In the event that an application brought under sec. zzz.1 is on behalf of a person who has never been competent, the court shall use the values and standards currently accepted by society, where these values shall be determined as under sec. zzz.4.

zzz.6 Any revocation of a request brought under sec. zzz.1 by a duly empowered proxy decision-maker using appropriate standards of proxy decision-making shall take effect immediately and shall be deemed to render null and void any previous request made by that person under sec. zzz.1.

Amendment to Section 241.

241. (b) This Section is struck down.

Chapter 8
Abortion

One of the more controversial issues in biomedical ethics is abortion. Not only are there different ethical opinions, there are also different legal perspectives. Some countries treat abortions as medical procedures to be decided on by a woman in consultation with her physician; others agree that abortions are a medical matter but allow a woman to have an abortion only when her health is at risk or the child will be severely "malformed" and disabled.[1] Still other countries insist that an abortion must be performed in an accredited hospital after three medical specialists have agreed that the abortion is medically necessary for the health of the woman, and the woman's husband or guardian has to agree to the procedure.[2] Canada is unusual in that it has no law on abortion. To some, this is worrisome. They believe that the deliberate killing of a human being at any stage of development is murder. To others this is appropriate. They believe that fetuses are not persons and that therefore abortion has no ethical implications except for informed consent on the part of the pregnant woman.

This chapter begins with a brief look at the evolution of Canadian abortion law, so as to provide a context for the discussion. It then opens the ethical analysis with a look at the status of the human fetus and its relationship to the pregnant woman, turns to the issues of fetal, maternal and paternal rights and concludes with a closer look at some of the more representative arguments on both sides of the abortion debate.

Questions to Keep in Mind While Reading this Chapter:

1. What does it mean to say that the fetus is or is not a person? Why is this question important? Is there any ethically relevant difference between saying that the fetus is a person and saying that it is a human being?

2. If a fetus is a person, does this mean that abortion is ethically unacceptable?

3. What about the rights of the mother in the abortion context? Of the father? Of society? How can we explain this in terms of one of the ethical systems sketched in the preceding sections?

4. Is there an ethical difference between types of abortions?

INTRODUCTION

Not all human pregnancies go to term. It is estimated that approximately 31 percent end in spontaneous abortions. Over half of these occur before the woman has even realized that she was pregnant.[3] Miscarriages or spontaneous abortions, therefore, are not at all uncommon. Furthermore, there is usually a good medical reason why they occur. In about 54 percent of spontaneous abortions, the fetus is found to be physiologically abnormal—usually to a degree incompatible with what is considered to be a reasonable and acceptable quality of life. Spontaneous abortions, therefore, might be called nature's way of correcting mistakes.

However, not all terminations of pregnancy are spontaneous. From early times, people have terminated pregnancies deliberately by inducing abortions. This is true in all cultures, all countries and all religions,[4] whether in the historical past or at the present time.[5]

Some Historical Background

Of course, induced abortions have not always been judged in the same way. Not even in religious contexts. Christianity provides a good example. If we can take the writings of St. Augustine (5th century C.E.) and St. Thomas Aquinas (13th century C.E.) as representative, early and medieval Christianity did not condemn all abortions as murder. Instead, it maintained that there is a difference between the early and the late stages of fetal development. This reasoning was based on an acceptance of the dualistic conception of personhood already discussed in the preceding chapter. According to this conception, killing is murder only when what is killed is a human person—and something is a human person only if it has a human soul. As far as St. Augustine and St. Thomas were concerned, a fetus does not have a human soul from the beginning. It acquires a human soul only after the fetal body has developed sufficiently to be capable of sensation and mental activity. Therefore, until that point has been reached, abortion is not murder.[6] While this was the position of the Catholic Church until the end of the Middle Ages, it has since changed. The current position is that the human fetus is a person from conception on, and therefore to kill it intentionally is to commit murder.[7] Other religions have (and always have had) a more liberal stance. Islam allows abortions for medical reasons,[8] as does Judaism;[9] and while Buddhism appears to reject it, its rejection is phrased in terms of karmic guilt incurred by those who kill the fetus. It does not, therefore, have anything specifically addressed to abortion.[10]

The legal position of Western culture has also changed over the years. In Roman and Greek times, the law permitted abortion at the behest of the head of household.[11] In English-speaking countries, this was also law in the Middle Ages[12] and persisted until the end of the 17th century. According to Blackstone, it did not matter who performed the abortion or at whose instigation it was done, nor did it matter whether the abortion was induced before or after "quickening." An induced abortion was simply a misdemeanour.[13] As time went on, inducing an abortion became an increasingly serious matter until in the 19th century it became characterized as murder.[14]

Canadian law initially followed English law in this matter. It classed induced abortions as murders until the proclamation of section 251 of the *Criminal Code*. That section allowed abortions, but only under certain conditions: It had to be approved by ". . . the therapeutic abortion committee for [an] accredited or approved hospital, by a majority of the members of the committee and at a meeting of that committee at which the case of such female person has been reviewed;"[15] and the committee had to certify in writing that in the opinion of the committee ". . . continuation of the pregnancy of such female person would or would be likely to endanger (the woman's) life or health."[16]

In 1988 the Supreme Court, in the case of *R. v. Morgentaler*[17] struck down section 251 as unconstitutional. In giving its reasons, the Court focused on the requirement of an abortion committee that was stipulated in section 251. It rejected this requirement as imposing an unequal burden on women living in isolated and rural parts of the country. It also stated that[18]

> [f]orcing a woman, by threat of criminal sanction, to carry a fetus to term unless she meets certain criteria unrelated to her own priorities and aspirations, is a profound interference with a woman's body and thus an infringement of the security of the person.

This ruling left Canada without any federal legislation targeted specifically at abortion. Sections 45, 215 to 217, 222 to 226 and 229 of the *Criminal Code* did remain in force; however, they dealt with medical practice in general: i.e., the duties of physicians towards their patients, use of surgical procedures, duty of care and so on.[19] There were provincial restrictions. However, these focused on funding, not criminality, and regulated access under the provincial health insurance plans. (See Chapter 9, concerning provincial health insurance plans.)

Even though the Court struck down section 251 as unconstitutional, it did not rule out the right of the federal government to pass a law specifically aimed at controlling abortion.[20] The only requirements the Court suggested was that such a law would have to allow for the "priorities and aspirations" of women and could not impose undue and unequal burdens with respect to access.

In 1989, the issue of abortion once more came before the courts. This time, however, the focus was not the right to have an abortion but the right to prevent an abortion. In the leading case of *Tremblay v. Daigle*,[21] the biological father alleged not only that as biological father he had the right to be consulted about an abortion, but also that a fetus was a human being and therefore had a right to life. The Supreme Court unanimously rejected the claim that a biological father had a right to be consulted about an abortion. However, it refused to rule on the status of the human fetus. It said that the fetus had no standing in current law, and that it was up to Parliament and not the Court to change the situation:[22]

> The respondent's argument is that a fetus is an *être humain*, in English "human being," and therefore has a right to life and a right to assistance when its life is in peril. In examining this argument it should be emphasized at the outset that the

argument must be viewed in the context of the legislation in question. The Court is not required to enter the philosophical and theological debates about whether or not a fetus is a person, but, rather, to answer the legal question whether the Quebec legislature has accorded the fetus personhood . . . The Court's task is a legal one. Decisions based upon broad social, political, moral and economic choices are more appropriately left to the legislature.

On November 3, 1989, driven by public pressure and by the perceived political need to remove the issue from the federal scene, the federal government introduced Bill C-43, "An Act Respecting Abortion." The stated intent of that bill was threefold: to fill the legislative void created at the federal level by the 1988 *Morgentaler* decision, to "protect the fetus" and to provide uniformity throughout the provinces.[23] The effect of Bill C-43 would have been to make abortion a matter of medical judgment by individual physicians. Bill C-43 was passed by the Commons but went down to defeat in the Senate because the Canadian Medical Association urged the Senate to reject re-criminalization of any aspect of abortion.[24] The matter has not been before Parliament since.

FRAMING THE ABORTION ISSUE: SOME INTRODUCTORY CONSIDERATIONS

Canadian law, therefore, is silent on abortion itself. However, abortion is more than a legal issue. The fact that something is permitted or enjoined by law (or that the law is silent) says nothing about the ethics, nor do the policies of medical associations—including the Canadian Medical Association[25]—settle the matter. It simply entails that in the eyes of the law and of organized medicine, abortion is an acceptable practice. Both the law and organized medicine, however, ignore the question that arguably lies at the heart of the abortion controversy: "What is the ethical status of the human fetus?"[26] If the fetus is a person, then to kill it intentionally, i.e., to perform an abortion, is to engage in intentional homicide, and serious ethical consequences follow. If the fetus is not a person, then ethically the matter is moot—at least as far as homicide is concerned. The only issue that might arise is whether ethical considerations that apply to non-human animals also apply to human animals.

Several distinct ethical positions have been advanced in the debate over the status of the human fetus.[27] At one extreme is the view that a fetus is a person from the moment of fertilization and therefore enjoys the same fundamental rights as other persons.[28] Among other things, this implies that preventing the implantation of a fertilized ovum is ethically questionable and that abortions have to be rejected except when they are done for the sake of the fetus itself[29] or, in certain cases, when the life of the mother is threatened. (For a discussion of the Doctrine of Double Effect, see Chapter 7.)

An intermediate position is that the human fetus acquires personhood at some time in its development, and that it is only after this stage has been reached that abortion has ethical implications. Traditionally, and from a dualistic metaphysical perspective, this was known as the doctrine of *mediate animation*.[30] From a materialist perspective it has become known as *gradualism*.[31] The position allows for some variations in the exact point when the crucial developmental stage has been reached. Twelve and twenty weeks of gestation are the most common variants. The most important implication of this stance is that any constraints on the treatment of the fetus prior to reaching that stage must be anchored in the interests and rights of members of society. However, once the fetus has developed sufficiently to count as a person, its rights and interests must be taken into account and balanced against the rights of all other relevant persons.

Another position holds that a fetus is a person only after it has been born and has acquired self-awareness and the ability to formulate life plans.[32] According to this view, abortion would be ethically permissible at any time. Infanticide would also be permissible until the child has attained self-awareness and has acquired the ability to formulate life plans.

A still more extreme position maintains that the fetus is simply a part of the mother and has no ethical standing until it has been born. This position finds its most radical expression in statements like the following:[33]

> A woman is her fetus. Until the fetus is born, there is only one person, the mother . . .
> say "no" to fetal personhood. Trust your instinct and assert your womanhood. Let us
> reestablish organic unity between the fetus and the mother through the recognition of
> only one person prior to childbirth, the mother.

A still different view holds that personhood is a social construct and must be defined in terms of interactions and relationships with others.[34] From this perspective, a fetus has personhood only if it is part of a web of social relations of which the pregnant woman is the primary focus. This means that fetal personhood takes its cue from the maternal relationship to it and depends on the woman's social role and embedding.

Is the Fetus Ever a Person?

There are other positions, but this will give some indication of the range of perspectives on fetal personhood. The only way to decide which of these positions—if indeed any—is correct is to go back to basics. This means going back to the notion of personhood itself and asking whether the concept can ever legitimately apply to a fetus. And here the discussion in the previous chapter becomes relevant. The reason is that the question of whether the fetus is ever a person is really the question of whether there is a stage in the development of a member of the species *homo sapiens* before it is born when it satisfies the criteria for personhood. That, however, is the flip side of the question of whether there is a stage in the life of a member of the species *homo sapiens* when it no longer satisfies that criterion. The two are opposite sides of the same coin.

The previous chapter had identified two distinct metaphysical positions on personhood—the dualistic and the materialistic position—but had made it very clear that both of them used the same type of criterion: namely that of brain death. The chapter had also made it clear that both metaphysical positions had to decide what was important about the brain: whether it was the whole brain or only the cerebral cortex. The vitalist perspective said that a functioning brain stem was sufficient. In other words, it opted for the whole-brain criterion. The personalist perspective, however, said that this was insufficient. Instead, the individual had to have a (minimally) functioning cerebral cortex. This meant that it opted for the cerebral death criterion.

Not surprisingly, when one applies these considerations to the issues of fetal person-hood, one gets two distinct answers. From the vitalist perspective the fetus is a person just as soon as it has a functioning brain stem. In other words, the fetus becomes a person at some time around the twelfth week of gestation.[35] From the personalist perspective, however, the fetus is a person just as soon as it has a functionally developed cerebral cortex, which means that it becomes a person around twenty weeks gestation.

Therefore, this does not rule out either the gradualistic perspective or that of immediate animation. All it means is that if one wants to be consistent, one cannot use one conception of personhood in the case of fetuses and another in the case of human beings that have already been born. That is to say, one cannot be a vitalist in one context and a personalist in another—unless, of course, one does not mind being inconsistent and begging the question.

By the same token, similar considerations apply to the notion of personhood as a social construct. If one says that personhood is a social construct in the case of the fetus, consistency in the use of the notion demands that one must also say that it is a social construct in the case of other human beings. Correspondingly, if one wants to say that personhood is not a social construct in the case of other human beings, then one cannot consistently treat it as a social construct in the case of fetuses.

Moreover, it is important to note that however one understands the notion of person-hood, it is not always clear whether a biologically human entity is a person. There are always borderline cases. Therefore, whether a fetus is a person is not always a clear-cut matter and easy to decide—any more than it is always clear-cut and easy to decide whether any other member of the species *homo sapiens* is a person. Thus, whether one adopts a vitalist or a personalist perspective, there will always be cases in which one is unsure whether the individual is a person, because both the whole-brain and the cerebral criterion may give ambiguous answers in borderline cases. This is true whether one is dealing with fetuses or with people who are dying. With due alteration of detail, there will also be borderline cases if one adopts a social-construct perspective.

Potentiality

The discussion so far has ignored what has sometimes been called the argument from potentiality. The argument here is that the fetus is a potential person, and that if it is allowed to develop it will become an actual person. Therefore, the biological continuity of the fetus during its gestational development means that it should count as a person from the moment of its origin as a biological human being.[36] This stance is then com-bined with an argument that connects the continued biological history and identity of the developing human being with the interests it has as a developed human being, in order to show that abortion at any stage is unethical. It would, so the argument goes, violate the interests that this human being has, irrespective of whether its potentialities are mere potentialities or are in fact actualized, because these interests are grounded in its nature as a human being. Exceptions are then made in cases in which the fetus's interests in continued life are not considered overriding because this life would be filled with serious, incurable and irremediable congenital disabilities involving only pain and suffering.

A variant on this position is that the development of the fetus is inherent in its very DNA, and that its actualization is merely an unfolding of what is already there.[37] The child that is born is numerically the very same entity that was the fetus. The two differ only materially as to the complexity of their organ systems. Therefore, if the child is a person and as such should not be killed, it would be unethical to kill the very same entity earlier in its biological career.[38]

While the argument from potentiality has some intuitive appeal, it ultimately fails in both of its versions. To begin with, it fails logically because it assumes that a potential *x* is ontologically or otherwise the same as an actual *x*. That, however, is not the case precisely because it is *potential*. Moreover, it assumes that a potential *x* has the same standing as an actual *x*—and that is also false. A Nobel Prize winner has a certain standing and is entitled to certain respect that the very same individual did not have (or deserve) before becoming an actual Nobel Prize winner. Similarly, someone who potentially is a physician does not yet have the duties that actual physicians have, even though the earlier person is numerically the same as the later person. The same holds true for any other potentiality. Or, perhaps a closer analogy would be an acorn. An acorn is a potential oak, but it would be sheer nonsense to say that it has the same standing as an actual oak; and the forester who sued a pig farmer for thousands of board feet of oak because the farmer's pigs had eaten the acorns would be laughed out of court. Potential and actual simply are not the same. So the argument from potentiality simply begs the question.[39]

As to the argument based on interests, this encounters two problems. First, the claim that a fetus has interests needs to be supported by data. If "interests" is understood in terms of cognitively meaningful desires, this is simply false. Fetuses have no cognitively meaningful desires. If, however, "interests" is meant in an instinctive sense, this needs further argument to show that anything that has an instinctive desire thereby has an ethical right to what it instinctively desires. In the absence of such an argument, the argument from interests simply assumes that the fetus's instinctual interests are ethically relevant, and that is to beg the question.

The Fetus as a Dependent Being

It is also important to note that the question of whether the fetus is a person is independent of where the fetus is or how it is kept alive.

To begin with the issue of location, the question of the ethical status of the human fetus is the question of whether the fetus, as a biologically human entity, ever meets the criterion of personhood—whichever criterion that may be. Logically, therefore, whether the fetus is in an artificial incubator or in a natural one—which is to say, whether it is in a machine specifically designed to keep fetuses (premature babies) alive or in a uterus—has nothing to do with its ethical status. It may affect whether the rights it has as a person have the same strength as the rights that are had by other persons, but that is another issue. Therefore, the argument that a fetus *in utero* is ethically different and not a person because it is *in utero* simply assumes that where something is defines what it is. It therefore also begs the question.[40]

The following case illustrates the point at issue.[41]

> A seven month-old fetus at L.L. hospital has been diagnosed by sonogramme as having a surgically correctable spina bifida. The paediatric surgical team is prepared to correct the malformation by removing the fetus from the uterus, performing the necessary repair, and then returning it to the uterus once again. The team performs the operation, returns the fetus to the uterus, and the fetus continues to develop normally until it is born two months later.

If where a fetus is determines its ethical status, then the fetus in this case would not be a person prior to the operation, would be a person during the operation because it was outside the uterus, would once again not be a person when it was returned to it, and finally would be a person when it was born. Such a stance would be bizarre, to say the least.

Legally, of course, the analysis would be different. According to current Canadian law, a fetus does not become a person until ". . . it has proceeded, in a living state, from the body of its mother whether or not (a) it has breathed, (b) it has an independent circulation, or (c) the navel string is severed."[42] Therefore, according to current Canadian law the fetus would have become a person once it had emerged from the uterus because of the operation. However, it would then stay a person *even after it had been replaced* when the operation was finished because once it has become a person, it would have to meet the criteria for death in order to stop being a person. That would mean that a fetus that had been removed from the uterus and then replaced would be a person, whereas a fetus who had not been removed (because it did not need surgery, or whatever) would not be a person, even though it was at the very same (or even greater) stage of development as the one who had been removed. In other words, legally speaking, the one fetus would count as a person simply because it had briefly changed its place of residence, while other fetuses that had remained where they were would not, even though they would otherwise be identical in development and constitution. However, these are purely legal considerations, have nothing inherently to do with ethics and only underline the insufficiency of Canadian law as it stands.

As to the issue of how the fetus is kept alive, the point to keep in mind here is that how something is kept alive is irrelevant to the question of whether it meets the vitalist or the personalist criterion of personhood. How it is kept alive may have implications for the strength of its rights. That, however, says nothing about the issue of rights itself. The issue of strengths of rights has to be considered independently and on its own terms.

One final remark on the issue of fetal personhood. As was seen above, the law as to when a fetus becomes a "human being"—which is legalese for "person"—is that it becomes a person when it has proceeded alive from the body of its mother. This definition is seriously outdated. As will be discussed more fully in Chapter 12, reproductive technology is making such great strides forward that an artificial uterus (which currently is being developed on animal "models") may soon be a reality.[43] If this technology is used for human beings—and women who have had their uteruses removed for medical reasons may want to take advantage of this possibility—it would mean that a fetus who was gestated in such an artificial uterus would never legally be a person because it would never "proceed alive from the body of its mother."

FETAL RIGHTS

Both the vitalist and the personalist positions entail that the fetus becomes a person at some time in its development. This moves the question of whether the fetus has an ethical right to life, and the question whether it has the right to a certain type of treatment, to centre stage.

The two questions are closely connected but logically independent of each other. Beginning with the right to life, the Principle of Equality and Justice entails that all persons, insofar as they are persons, are equal and have the same rights. Therefore, both the vitalist and the personalist position entail that at some stage in its development, a fetus will have the right to life.[44]

However, that does not entail that this right will be absolute. As was explained in Chapter 1, all rights are conditioned by the equal and competing rights of others.[45] Therefore, if the right to life of the fetus conflicts with the right to life of some other person— the pregnant woman would be an obvious contender in this regard—it becomes appropriate to ask whose right to life takes priority.

Moreover, conflicts of rights are not limited to rights of the same kind. Thus, the right to freedom of speech may conflict with the right to security of the person. As one jurist famously put it, "The most stringent protection of free speech would not protect a man falsely shouting fire in a theater and causing a panic."[46] The question, therefore becomes whether the conflict of competing fetal and maternal rights must always involve competing rights to life, or whether considerations that involve other rights may be relevant.

Maternal–Fetal Conflict

Some Preliminary Considerations It would be an understatement to say that the answer to these questions is far from simple. But it would also be disingenuous to overplay the difficulties of the issue. Many of the difficulties that arise in this context derive not from the ethics but from the socio-political and psychological contexts in which the questions are normally asked. These contexts tend to colour the analysis. However, if one abstracts from these parameters and focuses only on the ethics, the following considerations seem relevant.

First, the Principle of Equality says that all persons have the same ethical standing insofar as they are persons. Therefore, if the fetus is a person, then it cannot be a foregone conclusion either that the rights of the fetus take priority over those of the woman or that the rights of the woman take priority over those of the fetus. If either takes priority, that has to be grounded in some ethically relevant difference.

Second, the fact that something is not allowed or forbidden by an ethical principle does not mean that there are no other parameters that constrain the relevant action. The ability to formulate a workable social policy may play an important role as to which rights are protected by law. After all, not everything that is ethically appropriate can be or should be protected by legislation. Lying is a case in point. While lying is generally considered unethical, it would be inappropriate to pass a law that condemned it.

Third, one should always be careful to distinguish between what one would like to see happen in terms that are emotionally acceptable or that fit a particular agenda, and what is defensible in ethical terms.

With this in mind, and on the assumption that the fetus is a person at some stage or other in its development, let us return to the question "What is the relationship between the right of the fetal person and the rights of the pregnant woman?" The answer is that one cannot tell *a priori*. It depends on the nature of the circumstances, the strength of the competing rights and the values that are involved. What one can say is that when there is a conflict, one should approach the situation as free of emotional predispositions as possible and try to resolve the situation in ethical, not emotional terms.

However, although one cannot give a general and universal answer *a priori*, there are some general considerations that seem to be relevant. For example, it seems safe to say that the balancing process that was spoken of a moment ago is different in the various stages of fetal development. Thus, if one adopts a gradualist perspective, then in the early stages when the fetus has not yet become a person in either the vitalist or the personalist sense, it is more appropriate to describe it as a balancing of the value of respect for the life of the fetus as against the claim of autonomy and the right to self-determination of the woman. In other words, in the early stages of pregnancy, when the fetus meets neither the vitalist nor the personalist conception of personhood, it is not really a balancing of competing rights. However, as the pregnancy progresses and the fetus becomes a person, it becomes a genuine balancing of competing rights.

At the same time, this notion of balancing should not be approached in too restrictive a fashion, either from the side of the fetus or from the side of the woman. As Edward W. Keyserlingk put it in 1984,[47]

> two extremes must be avoided. One is that only the pregnant woman's health and welfare should count, but not that of the unborn child, the latter classified as simply a

biological extension of the woman with no rights of its own. The other extreme to be rejected is that only the unborn child's health and welfare should count, but not that of the pregnant woman, the latter considered as essentially and only the incubator or support system for the unborn child, her own rights and health taking second place. . . Both are (or should be) patients, but neither of them in an absolute or unqualified sense.

Moreover, it is also important to remember that whether a given right is claimed depends on the values of the individual whose right is at issue. Since whether a right is claimed depends on the values of the individual, this means that when it comes to balancing competing rights, the nature and strengths of the respective values also have to be taken into account. The more strongly a value is held, the more likely that the person who holds it will want to insist that it be observed.

This in turn creates a twofold problem: *First*, a fetal person cannot claim a right. It lacks the cognitive and physiological ability to do so. Therefore, it follows that if the fetus is ever a person, and if the rights of the fetal person are to be translated into practically meaningful terms, there has to be a surrogate or proxy who exercises the right for the fetal person. *Second*, a fetus does not have values. Therefore, a surrogate will have no basis on which to decide whether to exercise a particular right for a fetal person, let alone in what direction. All of this presents a dilemma.

A possible solution to the dilemma lies in the fact that a fetus has instinctive drives that it shares with all other human beings. In an inchoate form, these drives correspond to the values that function as motivational gradients in the case of otherwise full-fledged persons. These are similar to what were identified as values in Chapter 1. This means that in the context of decision-making for fetuses, the drives take the place of the values that determine the actions of ordinary persons, and can therefore be used as values by the proxy decision-makers when deciding what to do. The estimated strength of these drives will govern the rigidity with which the surrogate has to insist on the relevant rights of the fetal person, and their nature will determine the direction in which the decisions should be made. Since these drives become stronger and more defined as the fetus develops, this would be expressed as a corresponding increase in insistence on fetal rights as the pregnancy progresses.

One can therefore make some practical sense of the notion of fetal rights. What is more, one can talk about them in essentially the same terms as the rights of all other persons. One can even talk about balancing rights claims by taking into account the strengths of the values that are relevant to a particular rights claim. This also allows one to make sense of the direction given by the General Council of the CMA in 1989 to the Committee on Ethics, which was that it incorporate into its policy development regarding abortion the proposition that "in the decision concerning an abortion, both parties must consider the existence of the unborn child and respect its rights."[48]

Balancing of Rights   As to how this balancing of fetal versus maternal rights may be achieved, some insight may be gained by looking at one of the more famous arguments that have been raised in this connection. It contends that casting the issue of abortion as one of balancing competing rights is fundamentally mistaken. The right to life is logically distinct from the right to use someone's body.[49] Therefore, even if fulfilling the right to life necessitates the use of *a* body, depriving someone of the use of *a particular* body is not to deprive that individual of the right to life. According to this argument, therefore, the fetus does not have the right to force the woman in whose uterus it is and who has, so to speak, provided this venue out of kindness, to continue providing this particular means of fulfilling the fetus's right to life.[50] In fact, there is no right that the fetus can legitimately address to a particular woman.

However, this reasoning ignores several important facts. The *first* is that under the Principle of non-Malfeasance, everyone has the duty to prevent harm to another person if it is possible to do so without causing undue harm to oneself. (See Chapter 1.) This is not merely a matter of ethics. In many jurisdictions[51]—including Quebec[52]—it is also the law. Therefore, if one accepts the Principle of non-Malfeasance, then ethically speaking, if the fetus's right to life can be fulfilled only by the use of the woman's uterus and that use does not endanger the life or welfare of the woman, she has an ethical duty to allow that use. The crucial issue here, of course, is what constitutes endangering the welfare of the woman. However, mere lifestyle convenience and similar considerations would probably not meet that condition.

Second, as we shall discuss further in Chapters 9 and 10 when dealing with the right to health care and resource allocation, persons are responsible for the reasonably foreseeable consequences of their voluntary actions. Therefore, if the pregnancy is the result of voluntary intercourse and, moreover, if the pregnancy was allowed to progress to the point where the fetus satisfies the criterion for personhood, then the woman is responsible for the existence of these rights. This entails that she in fact has abrogated her right to autonomy and to the integrity of her body in this regard. Under these circumstances, continuation of the pregnancy is not a matter of kindness but a matter of having acquired a duty through an action—or, in this case, an inaction.[53]

Moreover, even if one maintained that a pregnant woman owes no duty to the fetus and has the right to remove it from her uterus, this does not mean that she has the right to have it killed. That would have to be established on other grounds. And failing such grounds, there would be a duty to use only such methods of abortion as would maximize the fetus's chances of staying alive. It would also entail that once the fetus has been aborted, every attempt would have to be made to keep it alive.

Finally, if the fetus ever has a right to life (alternatively—if the fetus is ever a person), then how the fetal person came into existence—for instance, through rape—has nothing to do with whether the fetal person has a right to life or whether its right to life is outweighed by the woman's right to self-determination. If it were otherwise, then pediatric persons—that is to say, children—who had been born as a result of rape could also be killed if their continued life interfered with their mother's autonomy. And here it would be unacceptable to reply that the case of such children would be different because they already exist and, moreover, are not in their mother's body. In the first place, the assumption that underlies the whole debate is that the fetus is a person. Without that assumption there is simply nothing to debate. In the second place, as was pointed out in the previous section, the argument assumes that *where* something is alters the strength of its rights. That may be a legitimate claim, but it is one that has to be argued on its own merits. It cannot simply be asserted as an intrinsic truth.

The upshot of all of this is that insofar as abortion is an ethical issue at all, it is correctly structured as an issue of balancing conflicting rights. Moreover, it follows that when the conflicting rights are otherwise equal, then how the conflict came about is relevant to identifying whose rights take priority. For instance, if the fetal right to life exists only because of some voluntary action (or inaction) on part of the woman, then *prima facie* the woman's rights have lower priority, because she is responsible for the foreseeable consequences of her voluntary actions.

Awareness and Social Embedding Yet there seems to be something intuitively troublesome about the thesis that the issue of abortion is an issue of balancing competing rights. One is tempted to argue that the woman is a fully conscious being with interests, desires and life plans, and that she is embedded in a social context of rights and expectations that involve other persons. None of this is true of the fetus. Therefore, the rights of the woman should take priority over the rights of the fetus as a matter of general principle, and this is especially true when it comes to the right to life.

However, if one were to accept the premise that underlies this argument, one would also have to say that it is ethically acceptable to engage in early infanticide (say, within the first six months after birth) or to kill mentally severely disabled persons if their needs interfered with our own. Of course, these implications do not logically disprove that the complexity of awareness and of social relations determines the strength of rights. However, they certainly encourage further reflection on the acceptability of the premise. In this connection the following comments of Abraham Lincoln are surely germane:[54]

> If A can prove, however conclusively, that he may, of right, enslave B—why may not B snatch the same argument, and prove equally, that he may enslave A? You say A is white, and B is black. It is color, then; the lighter, having the right to enslave the darker? Take care. By this rule, you are to be slave to the first man you meet, with a fairer skin than your own. You do not mean color exactly? You mean the whites are intellectually the superiors of the blacks, and, therefore have the right to enslave them? Take care again. By this rule, you are to be slave to the first man you meet, with an intellect superior to your own. But, say you, it is a question of interest; and, if you can make it your interest; you have the right to enslave another. Very well. And if he can make it his interest, he has the right to enslave you.

The Doctrine of Double Effect One of the classic arguments in the abortion debate makes use of the Doctrine of Double Effect. The Doctrine, as was pointed out in the previous chapter, was originally developed by St. Thomas Aquinas in the Middle Ages to explain why it was morally acceptable to kill in self-defence.[55] It was later adapted by the Catholic Church to deal with interventions that would save the life of a pregnant woman but kill the fetus.[56]

The general difficulties that beset the Doctrine have already been discussed in Chapter 7, "The Ethics of Deliberate Death," and need not be restated here. However, when the Doctrine is used to justify the unintended but unavoidable killing of the fetus to save the life of the woman, it runs into a problem that is unique to the context of abortion. To be usable here, it not only has to deal with the issue of foreseeable but unintended outcomes, it also has to structure the problem as one of balancing maternal versus fetal rights. However, the Doctrine will lead to the conclusion that it is ethically acceptable to kill the fetus only if it *assumes* that the woman's right to life automatically outweighs that of the fetus. And that begs the question.

That is to say, it makes sense to appeal to the Doctrine only if both the fetus and the woman are considered to be persons. But if both are persons, then the Principle of Equality and Justice entails that both have equal rights. Logically speaking, the Doctrine as such is neutral as to whose right to life takes priority (and therefore should be saved), because it states only the conditions that must be met for a negative consequence to be acceptable when an action has both a negative and a positive outcome. This means that if one wants to use the Doctrine to show that it is all right to kill the fetus by doing something that saves the woman's life, one has to assume the additional premise that the woman's right to life has greater weight than that of the fetus. Otherwise, why not argue that it is all right to let the woman die by doing something that saves the fetus's life?

One might reply by saying that if the pregnant woman dies, the fetus will die as well. However, that is not necessarily the case. For instance, suppose the woman has an aggressive cancer that has to be treated with chemotherapy and radiation if the woman is to survive—where such treatment will, of course, kill the fetus. If one did not automatically assume that the right to life of the woman took priority over that of the fetus, one could use the Doctrine to argue that one should refrain from treating the pregnant woman's cancer for as long as it takes the fetus to mature to the point where it can survive in an incubator once it is removed from her body—by which point it will be too late to treat the cancer and save the woman's life.

Therefore, at best, the Doctrine can be used only when the fetus cannot be saved under any circumstances. In that case, however, the Doctrine is unnecessary, because the very impossibility of doing anything to save the life of the fetus absolves the professional from trying to save it. One cannot have a duty to try to do the impossible. Hence, futility itself entails that efforts should be concentrated on saving the pregnant woman. The issue of balancing—and hence use of the Doctrine—does not arise.

One could, of course, try to save the Doctrine by saying that the woman's life is richer, that it is more fully developed, etc. That, however, would run into the very same objection that was pointed out a few paragraphs ago. That premise would also justify the killing of mentally severely disabled persons in favour of those who are not thus disabled. While that may be impeccable as a logical inference, it is questionable whether it would satisfy the Principle of Equality and Justice.

THE ETHICAL RELEVANCE OF METHODS OF ABORTION

So far, the issue of abortion has been framed as the question of balancing rights. However, there is an entirely different question, also ethically relevant, that has received relatively little attention in the literature. It is the question whether the method used to abort a fetus should be correlated with its developmental status. The reason the issue has not received much attention is the general assumption that because the fetus lacks consciousness, how it is aborted is really irrelevant. After all, if something cannot experience pain and suffering, the question which method of abortion produces the least amount of pain and suffering is ethically moot.

However, this reasoning may not be all that secure. It ignores the fact that the notion of pain experience may be understood in two ways: as pain perception at the punitive level (sometimes called nociception) and as pain perception at the cognitive level (sometimes called pain perception in the full sense of that term). Nociception is "the neural process of encoding and processing noxious stimuli."[57] It is present whenever there are appropriate neural receptors. By contrast, pain perception in the full sense of that term requires not merely the encoding and processing of neural stimuli in various neural receptors but also their integration in a central neural receiving and processing structure.[58] All animals that have neural receptors capable of signaling injury, trauma or stress are capable of nociception; however, only those animals that have, in addition to such structures, the equivalent of a spinal medulla, brain stem and telencephalon are capable of pain perception.[59]

It has been known since the 1970s that the human fetus has nociceptive sensory receptors surrounding the mouth by the seventh week of gestation, that the distribution of these receptors spreads to the face, the palms of the hands and the soles of the feet by the eleventh week, to the trunk and proximal parts of the arms and legs by the fifteenth week, and that they are present in all cutaneous and mucous surfaces by the twentieth week of gestation.[60] These data clearly establish that the human fetus is capable of nociception from very early in the pregnancy. As to the capacity to experience pain in the full sense of that term, this overlaps with nociception. Evidence shows that the development of the neocortex begins by the eighth week of gestation and is structurally complete by the twentieth week.[61] Therefore, the integrated neural structures that are necessary for pain perception in the full-blooded sense of that term are present by the twentieth week of gestation. These data suggest that the method by which a fetus is aborted should be a matter of ethical concern.

Not only that: As we have seen, at some stage in its development—the precise stage depending on whether one accepts a vitalist or a personalist account—the fetus satisfies the brain-based criterion for personhood. Therefore, even if one maintains that abortion is ethically defensible, the Principles of Beneficence and non-Malfeasance entail that, minimally, how one aborts a fetus should be attuned to when the fetus becomes a person and to its capacity to have nociception or pain perception. From a vitalist perspective, nociception is the key; from a personalist perspective, pain perception.

In theory, once could go even further. One could argue that the human fetus is an animal. As such, it should have the same rights as all other animals. In particular, it should have the right to be killed as quickly and humanely as possible. Consequently, so the argument would continue, how a fetus is aborted is always relevant after it has developed the capacity for nociception—even if it does not yet satisfy the vitalist criterion of personhood. However, such an argument would depend on the thesis that all animals have rights—and that is an issue that transcends the present context.

ARGUMENTS FOR AND AGAINST ABORTION

Given these considerations, the arguments both for and against abortion really require little discussion, because most of them ignore one or more of the points that have been raised. However, for the sake of clarity it may be useful to give a brief sketch of the more common arguments and then make some summarizing remarks, because the arguments themselves tend to fall into readily identifiable patterns.

Arguments Pro

On the affirmative side, there is a whole series of arguments that find their focus in the claim that a woman has a fundamental and inalienable right to self-determination. The argument that is encountered most often in this connection is that a woman has a right to her own body. Pregnancy is a condition of her body. Consequently a woman has the right to terminate her pregnancy. Otherwise the right to her own body would be empty.

Then there are arguments based on the premise that every woman has the right to shape her life according to her wishes and aspirations. After all, women are not mere fetal containers.[62] An unwanted pregnancy, however, would make the attainment of her life goals impossible. Therefore, the Principle of Autonomy and Respect for Persons entails that she should be able to have an abortion if she so wishes. This sort of reasoning finds clear support in the Supreme Court judgment of *Morgentaler v. the Queen*, where Chief Justice Dickson and Mr. Justice Lamer stated that[63]

> Forcing a woman, by threat of criminal sanction, to carry a foetus to term unless she meets certain criteria unrelated to her own priorities and aspirations, is a profound interference with a woman's body and thus an infringement of the security of the person.

Some arguments focus on how the pregnancy came about. For example, there is the argument from contraceptive failure. Even though both the woman and her partner may have taken due care to prevent pregnancy, contraceptive methods sometimes do fail.[64] Not to allow an induced abortion in such cases would be to punish the woman for something that is not her fault. The argument from rape goes in a similar direction. A wrinkle is introduced by the argument from incest. It contends that abortions have traditionally been allowed in such cases. Therefore, to forbid them now would be to fly in the face of what society has always accepted.[65]

Health reasons have also been thought to provide legitimate grounds for permitting abortions. When the health or life of the woman is threatened by a continuation of the pregnancy, an abortion should be permissible. Conditions such as Eisenmenger's syndrome come to mind in this context, as do progressive renal failure and similar conditions. Unless the woman herself has clearly understood the danger of the risks associated with pregnancy and has given a voluntary, competent and informed consent to its continuation, the fact that her health and life are threatened is sufficient to guarantee her the right to an abortion. Both the old section 251 and the new section 287 of the *Criminal Code* explicitly recognize such factors, and confer a legal right. A variant of this kind of argument focuses on the threat to the pregnant woman's psychological well-being and maintains that if her "mental or psychological health" is threatened or if she is likely to commit suicide in desperation, an abortion would be legitimate no matter what the stage of fetal development.[66]

Some arguments maintain that abortions should be allowed not only when the woman's health and life are in danger but also when the health or welfare of the as-yet-unborn child are at risk. Prenatal diagnosis can sometimes show that the child-to-be would suffer from a congenital defect such as Tay-Sachs disease, hemophilia, spina bifida, cystic fibrosis, etc. Conditions such as these, it is argued, would justify an abortion for the sake of the child.[67] A variant on this theme is the claim that sometimes a pregnant woman is—or is perceived to be—a bad risk as a mother because she has a track record of abusing or neglecting her children. Severe maternal mental handicap has also been of special concern in this connection.[68] In these cases, so the argument goes, it would be better for the child to be aborted before it is born than to be born and become a grim statistic.

The fetus has also been described as an "unjust pursuer."[69] The thrust of this observation is that abortion should therefore be allowed at any stage of fetal development, because it simply amounts to self-defence.

Lastly, although by no means finally, there is the argument that abortion is acceptable because the fetus is not a person. It therefore poses no ethical problem whatever.[70]

Arguments Contra

The arguments against abortion are equally varied. For instance, it has been said that abortion is ethically indefensible because the fetus is a person. As we have seen, for the logic of this argument it is irrelevant whether the fetus is a person from the moment of conception[71] or only after it has passed a certain stage of development. On either perspective, there is some stage in the fetus's development when it has right to life. At that point—whenever it may be—its right to life trumps all quality-of-life–related rights of the woman, because the right to life always trumps the right to a certain quality of life.

A slightly different argument focuses not on any interplay of rights but on the notion of helplessness and dependence. It postulates the premise that utter helplessness demands utter protection.[72] It then points out that the fetus is utterly helpless and utterly dependent. On that basis, it concludes that it would be unethical to abort the fetus—not because its rights are violated but because the fundamental premise of helplessness demands it. This argument is sometimes varied by adding the premise that all life has intrinsic value, and that this applies in particular to human life.[73]

Another line of argumentation against abortion adopts a still different tack. Instead of advancing a positive thesis, it seeks to invalidate the arguments that have been advanced in favour of abortion. For example, some of the arguments in favour of induced abortion are based on the contention that abortions may be necessary to protect the mental health of the pregnant woman. These latter arguments point to figures that suggest that between 85 and 95 percent of all abortions in Canada are done for psychiatric reasons, ostensibly to protect the mental health of the pregnant woman.[74] However—so this anti-abortion line of reasoning claims—not only are the majority of so-called psychiatric indications for abortions spurious or even manufactured,[75] but women who have had abortions for psychiatric reasons have done either no better[76] or actually worse than those whose requests for abortions were refused.[77]

In fact, some versions of this argument claim that from a purely prudential perspective—and possibly as a matter of a self-regarding duty as postulated by Kant—it is better not to have an abortion because there is evidence showing that women who have had abortions have a small but statistically significantly higher risk of subsequent mental disorders or mental illnesses.[78] They may also claim that post-abortion trauma can manifest itself years after the abortion has occurred.[79] Consequently, abortions should be avoided as a matter of duty not to injure oneself.

Still other arguments against abortion maintain that to allow abortions results in the brutalization of our society,[80] whereas a philosophically more sophisticated rejection of abortion under most circumstances is grounded in a neo-Aristotelian virtue ethics approach, which centres in the attainment of happiness and a good life. Hursthouse's analysis is particularly noteworthy in this connection.[81]

Finally, one of the more interesting attempts to show that abortion is immoral, and one that is worth consideration in its own right, is presented by Don Marquis.[82] Marquis divorces the issue of abortion from the issue of the status of the human fetus and instead looks at the nature of the act: not at the mechanics of the act, however—at how the abortion is performed—but at its implications for the fetus. His reasoning begins from the fact that, biologically, a fetus is a human being and that abortion is an act of non-consensually killing a fetus. To kill something, so he continues, is to end the life of that being and thereby to deprive it of its future. Fetuses, being human, are like adult humans in that they have a "future of value" or, as he also calls it, a "future like our's." Deliberately killing adult humans non-consensually is immoral because it non-consensually deprives them of a future of value; by the same token, therefore, abortion is also immoral because it non-consensually deprives fetuses of their future (of value). This reasoning, so he contends, has several advantages. It not only sidesteps the whole issue of the status of the human fetus, it also does not apply to gametes—and thereby does not rule out contraception—and it allows for consensual active euthanasia. Moreover, it is not "specieistic" but in principle holds for all living things that have a "future of value."

Closer consideration, however, shows that this argument is not quite as trenchant as it seems at first glance, because it contains several crucial ambiguities and ultimately begs the question. If the notion of a future of value is understood as a future that is valued by the individual whose future it is, then a fetus does not have such a future because a fetus has no values. On the other hand, if it is understood in some absolute sense, then the argument has to assume that all human futures have value—which is not true. For example, a child's future as a sex slave to be killed when no longer considered suitable for that role, or one of pure agony as a subject in vivisection experiments, are futures that have no absolute value. The only way to give value to all human futures, including those of sex slaves or vivisection subjects, is to say that it is the very fact of being a living human that has value—but that is the very question at issue. Moreover, if one admits that different types of human lives are valuationally different, then this legitimates abortions not only when fetuses have incurable and serious medical problems that lead to a life of suffering, but also if the fetuses face a bleak and irremediable future in non-medical terms.

Moreover, even if we accept Marquis's premises, it does not follow that we can say that a *particular* abortion is immoral. That would follow if, and only if, there were a decision procedure that allowed us to determine whether the fetus in question actually had a future. There is no such decision procedure. It is estimated that between 34 and 50 percent of all pregnancies end in a miscarriage or spontaneous abortion[83], 80 percent of which occur in the first three months of pregnancy and 15 percent after the woman has recognized that she is pregnant. This does not include stillbirths at full term. It follows that unless one can identify with certainty that a particular pregnancy will not end in a miscarriage or a stillbirth, one cannot say with certainty that a particular fetus has a future, let alone a future of value. Therefore, even if one accepted Marquis's premise, it would not allow one to say that a particular abortion is immoral. At most, one could say that it is *possible* that a particular abortion is immoral—but that is a far cry indeed from showing that all abortions are immoral.

Finally, one of the key claims that Marquis makes is that his argument holds only for non-consensually imposed death; that if competent persons do not see their futures as having value, then they may agree to be euthanatized. However, what is sauce for the goose is sauce for the gander. In other words, using Marquis's own premise, it follows that the same consideration must apply to fetuses. However, analogous to the point just made, there is no way of finding out whether any fetus sees its future as having value. In fact, the very notion of a fetus having any considerations about its future, value or otherwise, is simply contradicted by the fact that fetal neurological development is insufficient for it to have any considerations of value at all. Therefore, the moral basis of Marquis's claim—that it is the *non-consensual* deprivation of a future of value—cannot be operationalized in the case of a fetus. This would hold true even if, in keeping with the discussion in Chapter 5, one appointed a substitute decision-maker for the fetus, and this substitute decision-maker used objective reasonable person values. It would be appropriate to appoint a substitute decision-maker only if one had already decided on other grounds that the fetus had rights—but that is the very point at issue.

CONCLUSION

It may be tempting to say that in the end, all of the argumentation pro and con does not really matter. What matters are the facts of life. Abortions have always been performed and always will be, if not legally, then illegally—and women whose lives could have been saved by legal abortions will die when abortion becomes an illegal practice. Moreover, the status of the fetus is irrelevant to all of this, because fetuses will die no matter what. The key issue is harm reduction. Therefore, while the abortion debate may be an interesting intellectual exercise, it cannot form the basis of social policy. The function of social policy is to regulate human interactions in such a way as to maximize the good and minimize the harm, and to provide everyone with the greatest possible opportunity to realize his or her legitimate desires and potentials.

There is no denying the emotional strength of this reasoning. Moreover, the phenomenon of the identified victim lends it tremendous appeal. (For more on the phenomenon of the identified victim, see Chapter 10.) We know the woman who wants a abortion; we don't know the fetus who is to be aborted. Considerations that touch the former therefore have much greater appeal than considerations that touch the latter. And if what one wants from a social policy is for it to make for smooth social interactions and to justify existing practices, then ethical considerations drop out of the picture altogether.

It is at this juncture that one has to decide whether one wants to be practical and do what works, or whether one wants to be ethical. If one only wants to be practical, then one simply crafts a social policy that reduces preventable female deaths and that causes the minimum of friction. From that perspective, it is unnecessary for Canada to promulgate any laws or establish any regulations if there is no practical need.

On the other hand, if one wants to be ethical, then one has no choice but to consider the ethical status of the human fetus, whether the fetus ever has rights, what they might be and how they would stack up against the rights of the mother. That may lead to emotionally unappealing conclusions. It may also lead to social policies that conflict with existing practice; and it may even result in a series of otherwise preventable female deaths. However, that would not change the ethics of the situation. Nor should it lead to the conclusion that one should tailor one's ethics to one's emotions or adjust social policy to remove the possibility of conflict. Quite the reverse. It should lead to the conclusion that one should tailor one's emotions to one's ethics, and that one should adjust social policy and practice in a way that minimizes the perceived need to behave unethically.

In this context, it may be appropriate to recall the words of the Supreme Court in *Morgentaler*. Although the Supreme Court of Canada carefully avoided making any pronouncement on the ethical status of the human fetus, it did look at the ethics, and on that basis came up with the following consideration:[84]

<blockquote>
Section 1 of the *Charter* authorizes reasonable limits to be put upon the woman's right having regard to the fact of the developing fetus within her body . . . The value to be placed on the fetus as potential life is directly related to the stage of its development during gestation. The undeveloped fetus starts out as a newly fertilized ovum; the fully developed fetus emerges ultimately as an infant. A developmental progression takes place between these two extremes and it has a direct bearing on the value of the fetus as potential life. Accordingly, the fetus should be viewed in differential and developmental terms. This view of the fetus supports a permissive approach to abortion in the early stages where the woman's autonomy would be absolute and a restrictive approach in the later stages where the state's interest in protecting the fetus would justify its prescribing conditions. The precise point in the development of the fetus at which the state's interest in its protection becomes "compelling" should be left to the informed judgment of the legislature which is in a position to receive submissions on the subject from all the relevant disciplines.
</blockquote>

—an "informed judgment" which, in the eyes of the Court, should not ignore the ethics.

What would that mean in real terms? The preceding discussion suggests some considerations. To begin with, it would mean that abortion is ethically defensible, but only within certain limits. These limits are reached when the fetus has become a person. Until that point has been reached, abortion will not violate any fetal rights because until the fetus has reached that stage, it has no rights. At least, not ethical ones. The only ethical protection the fetus has prior to becoming a person derives from our society's fundamental value of respect for human life and the rights of others not to be psychologically assaulted. However, these values and rights may be overruled by the right to self-determination of the pregnant woman. That right, in turn, is basic because it derives from the Principle of Autonomy and Respect for Persons.

But here one has to be careful. As the Supreme Court pointed out, and as has been argued in Chapter 1, no right is absolute. Every right is constrained by the conditions under which it arose and under which it is claimed. It is also subject to the equal and competing rights of others. The right to self-determination, therefore, is not the right to license. Neither is it the right to offend the sensibilities and values of others if there are reasonable alternatives available: alternatives that allow the woman to retain her autonomy and satisfy her life plans within the context of society's values. If there are such alternatives, then the weight of this right will have to be balanced against the alternatives that are thus open to the woman.

What this means is that it is relevant to ask whether the pregnancy is the result of the woman's competent and voluntary behaviour; whether society has made it possible for her to avoid becoming pregnant by providing appropriate access to early abortions or to contraceptives and other appropriate methods of birth control; furthermore, whether society makes it possible for the woman to pursue her life plans without abortion by offering her a reasonable alternative that does not amount to punishing her in an unjust fashion. The answers that one gives to these questions have a bearing on the ethical acceptability of the social policy that is crafted.

However, these conditions are seldom met at the present time. Arguably, it would be unjust to deny women who have taken due care to avoid pregnancy, but who nevertheless find themselves pregnant, the right to an abortion. Arguably, therefore, an ethical society would make abortions readily accessible in the early stages of pregnancy and would fund them as insured services within the twenty-week time frame. In fact, since an abortion would be a medical service, society would also defray the costs that are incurred by a woman who tried to avail herself of this right. Travel and accommodation costs to the nearest facility that provides abortion services would here be implicated as well. Economic status should not be allowed to invalidate a right to health care.

As to the twenty-week limit on induced abortions, once this limit has passed the only exceptions would be fetal indications. It would be discriminatory to suggest that a fetal person must await the onset of an unbearable existence before a decision to end that life could be made. The law against suicide has been repealed for decades. While the decision to end one's life may be viewed with awe, concern or even misgivings, a competent person has the right to commit suicide before an incurable cancer, Huntington's chorea or other extremely debilitating diseases overtake him or her. The repeal of the suicide clause from the *Criminal Code of Canada* was at least partly based on recognition of this fact. Ethically speaking, an incompetent person should not be placed in worse straits. "The rights of the incompetent should not be less simply because of the fact of their incompetence."[85]

In other words, what traditionally have been called medical indications in favour of abortion—that is to say, medical indications from the side of the fetus—would seem to be entirely appropriate. They merely empower the woman or other appropriate proxy decision-maker to use the qualitative criteria that are appropriately applied by competent decision-makers in their own case. The argument here is relatively straightforward. Once the fetus has become a person, it is still an incompetent one. That fact of incompetence, however, does not entail that it has no rights. It merely means that these must be administered by proxy. Proxy decision-makers, however, as we have seen in Chapter 5, must use an objective reasonable person standard when administering the individual's rights, unless they are faced with a previous competent indication by the now-incompetent person, which in this case clearly does not apply. (See Chapter 5.)

Objective reasonable person standards involve quality-of-life considerations. Medical prognosis, etc., clearly enter in. Therefore, if according to the best data available under the circumstances, the quality of life that the fetal person can expect will be so irremediably low as to not be worth living—Tay-Sachs, severe neural tube defects, congenital abnormalities inconsistent with cognitive sapient and pain-free existence, for example, come to mind here—the proxy decision-maker would have a strong obligation to prevent such a life from materializing. Abortion in as painless a manner as possible should therefore be considered.

Of course, it is also true that under certain circumstances, a woman simply does not have access to an abortion until the stage of fetal personhood has been passed. This is particularly true in rural areas. However, if the fetus ever becomes a person *in utero*, this would not constitute an ethically defensible reason for extending the period within which abortions are defensible. What it does show is that society has an obligation to make sure that these circumstances do not arise.

Finally, there are cases in which continuing the pregnancy foreseeably will result in the death of the mother. It might be thought that in such cases abortion would be acceptable as a matter of the woman's right even after the fetus has become a person. But, as was seen above, this is not necessarily true. Once the fetus has become a person, the only way of justifying a preference for the woman's life is by showing that fetal and maternal life are not on a par. To be sure, the woman is more fully conscious, she has more fully developed life plans, her life includes lines of obligations towards others that are not present for the fetal person, and so on. However, in the end all this means is that the fetal person has not yet had opportunity to make such connections. Lack of opportunity does not change one's ethical status. Furthermore, it may be argued that by allowing the pregnancy to progress to the point where the fetus has become a person, the woman has subordinated her rights to the rights of the fetus. Therefore, once the fetus meets the conditions that are otherwise accepted as definitive of personhood, the life of the mother does not automatically take priority. A genuine balancing process must occur.

At the same time, just as the woman's right to life does not automatically overrule the fetus's right to life once it has become a person, so the fetal person's right to life does not automatically overrule the woman's right to life. The Principle of Fidelity therefore entails that one should do the best possible for each as person. That may result in a tragic outcome for either party. However, not everything that is tragic is unethical—and tragic outcomes should not be avoided by unethical means.

Further Readings

Boonin, D. *A Defense of Abortion* (Cambridge: Cambridge University Press, 2003).

Dworkin, R. *Life's Dominion: An Argument about Abortion, Euthanasia, and Individual Freedom* (New York: Random House, 1994).

Hedayat, K.M., P. Shooshtarizadeh and M. Raza. "Therapeutic Abortion in Islam: Contemporary Views of Muslim Shiite Scholars and Effect of Recent Iranian Legislation." *Journal of Medical Ethics* 32.11 (2006): 652–657.

Hursthouse, R. *Beginning Lives* (Oxford: Basil Blackwell, 1987).

Lecso, P.A. "A Buddhist View on Abortion." *Journal of Religion and Health* 26.3 (1987): 214–218.

Marquis, D. "Why Abortion Is Immoral." *Journal of Philosophy* 86 (1989): 183–202.

Sacred Congregation for the Doctrine of the Faith. *Declaration on Procured Abortion*, available at www.vatican.va/roman_curia/congregations/cfaith/documents/rc_con_cfaith_doc_19741118_declaration-abortion_en.html

Schiff, D. *Abortion in Judaism* (Cambridge, MA: Cambridge University Press, 2002).

Sherwin, S. "Abortion through a Feminist Lens." in *Readings in Biomedical Ethics: A Canadian Focus*, ed. E.-H. Kluge (Toronto: Pearson, 2005): 339–352.

Sumner, W. "Toward a Credible View of Abortion." *Canadian Journal of Philosophy* 4 (1974): 163–181.

Thomson, J.J. "A Defense of Abortion." *Philosophy and Public Affairs* 1.1 (1971): 47–66.

Endnotes

1. For instance, Germany has such a law. See D. Reitz and G. Richter, "Current Changes in German Abortion Law," *Cambridge Quarterly of Healthcare Ethics* 19 (2010): 334–343.

2. *Population Policy Data Bank*, maintained by the Population Division of the Department of Economics and Social Affairs of the United Nations, accessed 27 Jan 2011 at www.un.org/esa/population/publications/abortion/doc/saudiarabia.doc

3. A.J. Wilcox et al., "Incidence of Early Loss of Pregnancy," *New England Journal of Medicine* 319.4 (28 Jul 1988): 189–194. Compare H. Pilpel, "Personhood, Abortion and the Right to Privacy" in *Defining Human Life: Medical, Legal and Ethical Implications*, ed. M. Shaw and A. Doudera (Ann Arbor: AUPHA Press, 1983), 154; and J.B. Henry, *Clinical Diagnosis and Management by Laboratory Methods*, 18th ed. (Philadelphia: W.B. Saunders, 1991), 478, for somewhat different figures.

4. Compare I. Makdur, "Sterilization and Abortion from the Point of View of Islam" in *Islam and Family Planning*, Vol. 2 (Beirut, 1972), 271; see also A.R. Omran, "Abortion in the Natality Transition in Moslem Countries," in the same text, 70.

5. See B. Dickens, "Comparative Legal Abortion Policies and Attitudes Towards Abortion," in Shaw and Doudera, ref. note 3.

6. See J. Donceel, S.J., "Abortion: Mediate vs. Immediate Animation," *Continuum* 5 (1967): 167–171; J. Donceel, S.J., "Immediate Animation and Delayed Hominization," *Theological Studies* 31 (1970): 776–805. See also E.-H. Kluge, "St. Thomas, Abortion and Euthanasia," *Philosophical Research Archives*, 1981/82.

7. Sacred Congregation for the Doctrine of the Faith, *Declaration on Procured Abortion*, accessed 27 Jan 2011 at www.vatican.va/roman_curia/congregations/cfaith/documents/rc_con_cfaith_doc_19741118_declaration-abortion_en.html

8. F. Rahman, "Birth and Abortion in Islam," in *Abortion: A Reader*, ed. L. Steffen (Cleveland, OH: The Pilgrim Press, 1996), 202–211.

9. I. Jakobovits, *Jewish Medical Ethics* (New York: Bloch Publishing, 1959).

10. P. Harvey, *Introduction to Buddhist Ethics* (Cambridge: Cambridge University Press, 2000).

11. See Dickens, op. cit.

12. Henry de Bracton [c. 1250], "The crime of homicide and the divisions into which it falls" in *On the Laws and Customs of England*, Vol. 2, ed. G.E. Woodbine and trans. S.E. Thorne (1968), 341.

13. Dickens, op. cit., 242.

14. Lord Ellenborough's Act, June 24, 1803, accessed 27 Jan 2011 at http://web.archive.org/web/20070918233015/http://members.aol.com/abtrbng/lea.htm

15. *Criminal Code of Canada*, s. 251 (4).

16. *Criminal Code of Canada*, s. 251 (4)c.

17. R. v. Morgentaler [1988] 1 S.C.R. 30, 63 O.R. (2d.) 281, 26 O.A.C. 1, 44 D.L.R. (4th)385, 82 N.R. 1, 3 C.C.C. (3rd)449, 62 C.R. (3rd) 1, 31 C.R.R.

18. Loc. cit.

19. This has sometimes been represented as leaving Canada without any laws governing abortion. As should be clear from the articles of the *Criminal Code* that we have just cited, this was not exactly the case.

20. That statutory interference, however, would have to follow the principle of the least intrusive alternative as underlying the *Canadian Human Rights Act* S.C. 1976–7, c. 33; appealed to in *Re Eve* (1987), 31 D.L.R. (4th) 1 (S.C.C.) 2 S.C.R. 388; *Re Infant K*, Supreme Court of B.C. Jan. 30, 1985, Vancouver Registry A 842 616. See also D. Chambers, "The Right to the Least Restrictive Alternative" in *The Mentally Retarded Citizen and the Law*, ed. M.I. Kindred et al. (New York: Free Press, 1976), 93, which says that when government does have a legitimate communal interest to serve by legislating human conduct, it should use methods that curtail individual freedom to no greater extent than is essential for securing that interest.

21. Tremblay v. Daigle, 62 D.L.R. (4th) 634. For a parallel case that never reached the Supreme Court, see Murphy v. Dodd et al., 70 O.R. (2d) 681.

22. Tremblay v. Daigle, S.C.R. 21533, 18–19.

23. "[Bill C-43] has as its overriding objective the balancing of interests: the rights and interests of women, and Society's interest in the protection of the foetus" and went on to say that "there is a

clear policy decision to protect the interests of the foetus throughout the pregnancy." (Notes for an Address by the Honourable Douglas Lewis, Minister of Justice and Attorney General of Canada to the House of Commons on Second Reading, Bill C-43, *An Act Respecting Abortion*, 2nd Session, 34th Parliament, 38 Elizabeth II, 1989).

24. Brief to the Standing Senate Committee on Legal and Constitutional Affairs Re: Bill C-43, *An Act Respecting Abortion* submitted by the Canadian Medical Association, Ottawa, Ontario, 13 December 1990, presented by E.-H. Kluge, Director of Ethics and Legal Affairs, CMA.

25. CMA Policy Summary on Induced Abortion, *CMAJ* 1176A (1988), available at http://policybase.cma.ca/PolicyPDF/PD88-06.pdf

26. Cf. M.A. Warren, "On the Moral and Legal Status of Abortion" in *Biomedical Ethics*, 4th ed., ed. T.A. Mappes and D. DeGrazia (New York: McGraw-Hill, 1996), 434–440. For a view that dismisses the question of the status of the fetus as irrelevant, see R. Hursthouse, "Virtue Theory and Abortion," *Philosophy and Public Affairs* 20.3 (1991): 223–246, at 236.

27. See Tri-Council Policy Statement, *Ethical Conduct for Research Involving Humans*, available at www.umanitoba.ca/research/media/TCPS_gov_canada_statement.pdf

28. See Pope Paul VI, Encyclical Letter "Humanae Vitae," *Acta Apostolicae Sedis* LX: 9 (1968).

29. We will address this issue later, from the perspective of therapeutic abortions to prevent what Engelhardt has called "the injury of continued existence."

30. See St. Thomas Aquinas, *supra*.

31. W. Sumner, *Abortion and Moral Theory* (Princeton, NJ: Princeton University Press, 1981).

32. M. Tooley, *Abortion and Infanticide* (New York: Oxford University Press, 1984).

33. Federation of Medical Women of Canada *Newsletter*, 1 (Oct 1989): 1. For a similar position, see C. Overall, "Selective Termination of Pregnancy and Women's Reproductive Autonomy," *The Hastings Center Report* 20 (1990): 6–11.

34. Cf. S. Sherwin, "Abortion through a Feminist Lens," in *Ethical Issues: Perspectives for Canadians*, ed. E. Soifer (Peterborough, ON: Broadview Press, 1999).

35. See R.R. Llinas (ed.), *The Biology of the Brain from Neurons to Networks* (New York: H.W. Truman, 1989).

36. M. Lockwood, "Warnock versus Powell (and Harradine): When Does Potentiality Count?" *Bioethics* 2.3 (1988): 187–213. For a reply, see R.M. Hare, "When Does Potentiality Count? A Comment on Lockwood," *Bioethics* 2:3 (1988): 214–226. See also D. Marquis, "Why Abortion Is Immoral," *Journal of Philosophy* 86 (1989): 183–202.

37. P. Singer and K. Dawson, "IVF Technology and the Argument from Potential," *Philosophy and Public Affairs* 17 (1988): 89. Singer and Dawson reject this argument. For similar rejections, see also E.-H. Kluge, *The Practice of Death* (New Haven, CT: Yale University Press, 1975) and J. McMahan, *The Ethics of Killing: Problems at the Margins of Life* (Oxford: Oxford University Press, 2002).

38. J. Stone, "Why Potentiality Matters," *Canadian Journal of Philosophy* 17.4 (Dec 1987): 815–829. Stone correctly points out (p. 816) that Sumner's extreme version of the potentiality argument in *Abortion and Moral Theory*, at p. 104 (see ref note 31) to include gametes misses the point, because the zygote is not numerically identical with the gametes.

39. Cf. Warren, op. cit.; Kluge, op. cit.; McMahan, op. cit. For more on this, see the analysis of Marquis's argument, *infra*.

40. It is important to note that, with due alteration of detail, similar considerations apply to the claim that the fetus is not a person because it is dependent on the mother. How something is kept alive is logically distinct from what it is.

41. Based on a case available at www.med.umich.edu/fdtc/diagnoses/fetal_surgery/index.shtml

42. *Criminal Code of Canada*, s. 223 [206].

43. M. Sakata et al., "A New Artificial Placenta with a Centrifugal Pump: Long-Term Total Extrauterine Support of Goat Fetuses," *J Thorac Cardiovasc Surg* 115 (1998): 1023–1027; N. Unno et al., "Development of Artificial Placenta: Oxygen Metabolism of Isolated Goat Fetuses with Umbilical Arteriovenous Extracorporeal Membrane Oxygenation," *Fetal Diagnosis and Therapy* 5.3–4 (1990): 189–195.

44. The law may wish to accord a fetus statutory rights. The judgment in *Morgentaler* suggests as much. That, however, is a function of what lawmakers consider appropriate. It says nothing about the ethics.

45. For a legal reflection of this ethical principle, see *R. v. Oakes* [1986] 1 S.C.R. 103, where the Supreme Court of Canada established the Oakes test, which allows reasonable limitations on rights and freedoms if this can be shown to be necessary for a free and democratic society.

46. Schenck v. United States, 249 U.S. 47 (1919).

47. E.W. Keyserlingk, "Fetal Surgery: Establishing the Boundaries of the Unborn Child's Right to Prenatal Care," in *Biomedical Ethics and Fetal Therapy*, ed. C. Nimrod and G. Griener (Waterloo, ON: Wilfrid Laurier Press, 1988), 81–105, at 102.

48. CMA, Resolutions of General Council, Quebec City, 1989.

49. J.J. Thomson, "A Defense of Abortion," *Philosophy and Public Affairs* 1.1 (1971): 47–66, at 55.

50. Thomson, at 63.

51. For example, Austria, *Criminal Code* §95 StGB; France, *Criminal Code* §63(2); Germany, *Criminal Code* §323c.

52. *Revised Statutes of Quebec,* c. C-12, Charter of Human Rights and Freedoms (1975), c. 6, s. 2: "Every human being whose life is in peril has a right to assistance. Every person must come to the aid of anyone whose life is in peril, either personally or calling for aid, by giving him the necessary and immediate physical assistance, unless it involves danger to himself or a third person, or he has another valid reason."

53. The reply to Thomson's argument, therefore, is that the fetus can be construed as an invader only if the woman does not, so to speak, adopt it by allowing it to stay in her uterus long enough to become a person.

54. A. Lincoln, "Fragment on Slavery," in *Abraham Lincoln: Speeches and Writings 1832–1858*, D.E. ed. Fehrenbacher (Library of America, 1989).

55. Thomas Aquinas, *Summa Theologiae*, II, Q. 64, Art. 7.

56. For a classic historical study of the evolution of the doctrine, see J. Mangan, "An Historical Analysis of the Principle of Double Effect," *Theological Studies* 10 (1949): 41–61. See also P. Foot, "The Problem of Abortion and the Doctrine of Double Effect," in *Virtues and Vices*, ed. P. Foot (Oxford: Blackwell, 1978), 19–32.

57. J.D. Loeser and R.D. Treede, "The Kyoto Protocol of IASP Basic Pain Terminology," *Pain* 137.3 (2008): 473–477.

58. C. Sussman and B.M. Bates-Jensen, *Wound Care: A Collaborative Practice Manual for Health Professionals* (Philadelphia, PA: Lippincott Williams & Wilkins, 2006).

59. P.R. Wilkinson, "Neurophysiology of Pain Part I: Mechanisms of Pain in the Peripheral Nervous System," *CPD Anaesthesia* 3.3 (2001): 103–108.

60. K.J.S. Anand and P.R. Hickey, "Pain and Its Effects in the Human Neonate and Fetus," *The New England Journal of Medicine* 317.21 (1987): 1321–1329; T. Humphrey, "Some Correlation Between the Appearance of Human Fetal Reflexes and the Development of the Nervous System," *Progress in Brain Research* 4 (1964): 93–135.

61. Anand and Hickey, op. cit.; T. Humphrey, "Some Correlations between the Appearance of Human Fetal Reflexes and the Development of the Nervous System," *Prog Brain Res* 4 (1964): 93–135; H.B. Valnaan and J.F. Pearson, "What the Fetus Feels," *British Medical Journal* 280 (1980): 233–234.

62. See G.J. Annas, "A French Homonculus in a Tennessee Court," *Hastings Center Report* 19.6 (Nov/Dec 1989): 20–22.

63. R. v. Morgentaler [1988] 1 S.C.R. 30, at 3.

64. M.B. Mahowald, "Is There Life after Roe vs. Wade?" *Hastings Center Report* 19.4 (Jul/Aug 1989): 22–29, at 23.

65. See N.M. Simon, "Psychological and Emotional Indications for Therapeutic Abortion," in *Abortion*, ed. R.B. Sloane (New York: Grune and Stratton, 1971) 86 f, for a brief discussion of related issues.

66. For an explicit recognition of this (with the exception of the possibility of suicide), see *Criminal Code*, s. 287.

67. Compare Shaw and Doudera, *Defining Human Life,* ref note 3.

68. See *Re Eve*; *Re M,* etc.

69. Jewish law does not give a fetus the status of a person and in fact requires a 30-day postpartum viability to decide legal matters pertaining to the newborn. Compare F. Rosner, *Modern Medicine and Jewish Law* (New York: Yeshiva University, 1972), 66–69 ff. A version of this is also found in Thomson, op. cit.

70. A primary Canadian proponent of this is Christine Overall. See C. Overall, *Ethics and Human Reproduction: A Feminist Analysis* (Bristol: Allen and Unwin, 1987). See also M.A. Warren, *Moral Status: Obligations to Persons and Other Things* (Oxford: Clarendon Press, 1997).

71. This is known as the position of immediate animation. For a historical discussion, see J. Donceel, S.J., "Abortion: Mediate and Immediate Animation," *Continuum* 5 (1967): 167–171. See also E.-H. Kluge, *The Practice of Death* (New Haven, CT: Yale University Press, 1975), Chapter 1.

72. P. Ramsey, *The Patient as Person* (New Haven, CT: Yale University Press, 1970), 11–58.

73. For a statement of the thesis that life has intrinsic value, see R. Dworkin, *Life's Dominion: An Argument about Abortion, Euthanasia, and Individual Freedom* (New York: Random House, 1994). Dworkin concludes that a woman's autonomy permits abortion, because in a conflict between rights and values, values are trumped.

74. P.G. Ney and A.R. Wickett, "Mental Health and Abortion: Review and Analysis," *Psychiatric Journal of the University of Ottawa* 14.4 (Nov 1989): 506–516, at 506. See also B.K. Doane and B.G. Quigley, "Psychiatric Aspects of Therapeutic Abortions," *CMAJ* 125 (1981): 427–432.

75. Ney and Wickett (ref. note 74), 506. According to an older study, suicide is rare among pregnant women: M. Sim and R. Neisser, "Postabortive Psychosis: A Report from Two Centers," in *The Psychological Aspects of Abortion*, ed. D. Mall and F. Watts (Washington DC: University Publications of America, 1979), 1–13.

76. See S. Drower and E. Nash, "Therapeutic Abortion on Psychiatric Grounds," *South African Medical Journal* 54 (1978): 604–608, and 55: 643–647.

77. H.N. Babikian, "Abortion," in *Comprehensive Handbook of Psychiatry,* 2nd ed., ed. H.I. Kaplan and A.M. Freedman (Baltimore: Williams and Wilkins, 1975), 1496–1500, at 1498: "Women suffering from psychiatric illness before abortion showed no significant improvement after abortion and had more difficulties coping with the stress of abortion than psychologically more healthy women."

78. D.M. Ferguson, L.J. Harwood and J.M. Boden, "Abortion and Mental Health Disorders: Evidence from a 30 Year Longitudinal Study," *British Journal of Psychiatry* 193 (2008): 444–451.

79. A.C. Speckhard and V.M. Rue, "Postabortion Syndrome: An Emerging Public Health Concern," *Journal of Social Issues* 48.3 (2010): 95–119.

80. See *Humanae Vitae*, *supra*.

81. R. Hursthouse, *Beginning Lives* (Oxford: Basil Blackwell, 1987), and "Virtue Theory and Abortion," *Philosophy and Public Affairs* 20.3 (1991): 223–246.

82. D. Marquis, "Why Abortion Is Immoral," *Journal of Philosophy* 86 (Apr 1989): 183–202.

83. A.J. Wilcox et al., "Incidence of Early Loss of Pregnancy," *New England Journal of Medicine* 319.4 (28 Jul 1988): 189–194.

84. *Morgentaler*, p. 8.

85. Brachtenbach, *In the Matter of Colyer*, 660 P. (2d.) 738 (Sup. Ct. Wad. 1983).

1. Carol Ottridge, a forty-six-year-old successful middle executive with Baarnaard Corp. didn't intend to become pregnant and conscientiously practised birth control. However, as luck would have it, she did become pregnant—a statistic of the 1 percent expected failure rate of oral contraceptives. She did not want to have a child, because it would interfere with her career and her life plans. However, her long-time partner argued with her that they could very easily support a child on their combined salaries, and what with nannies, daycare and residential schools such as St. Michael's University School, the child would pose no hindrance to her career plans. After much soul searching, Carol agreed to continue with the pregnancy, but since she was at an elevated risk of a trisomy, she had an amniocentesis at 16 weeks in her pregnancy. She had been away on a business trip to Nepal that made it impossible to have the test earlier. The results came back a week and a half later and indicated that the fetus suffered from trisomy 18, which is associated with kidney and heart problems, esophageal atresia, mental retardation, developmental delays and muscle disorders. Moreover, the child would have at best a 50 percent chance of living to two months and an only 5 to 10 percent chance of surviving its first year of life. She therefore decided to have an abortion. The procedure—a dilation and evacuation (D&E) was performed ten days later.

2. Sadaf Yusuf was brought to the emergency room of the hospital with great difficulty breathing, an irregular heartbeat and dizziness that had lasted for several days. She was five months pregnant and had avoided seeing her family physician, because she was afraid that she would prescribe medications that would hurt her baby. The emergency room physician diagnosed her as in acute heart failure with heavy kidney insufficiency. The only way to save her life would be stabilize her, have a C-section and continue with follow-up treatment. Given the gestational age of the fetus, it was highly unlikely that the fetus would survive. Both Sadaf and her husband were also told that given her current medical profile, it was highly unlikely that Sadaf would survive if the C-section did not take place immediately. Sadaf and her husband were Coptic Christians who had emigrated from Egypt seven years ago and did not believe that an abortion—or what amounted to an abortion—was ethically defensible, because life was a gift from God. The medical team racked its brains trying to come up with some way to convince Sadaf and her husband that it was ethically acceptable to do the C-section to save her life.

Chapter 9

Health, Health Care and Social Justice

All other things being equal, people who are ill cannot compete on an equal footing with those who are not. They also have a lower quality of life than they would otherwise enjoy, and cannot fulfill their potentials as persons. To correct this, they require health care. This raises the question of whether health care is a right that society should provide, or whether it is a commodity that people should buy for themselves as and where they are able. This chapter looks at both of these options and at what they entail. However, it begins by first investigating the concepts of health and health care themselves, because without clarity on these notions, the whole discussion would be plagued by systemic ambiguities. It then analyzes the competing options and considers their implications. The chapter concludes with a brief look at the *Canada Health Act*, which provides the overall framework within which Canadian health care is delivered. It also takes a brief look at some of the suggestions that were made by the Royal Commission on the Future of Health Care on how to improve the Canadian medicare system.

Questions to Keep in Mind While Reading this Chapter:

1. What is health? Why is it sometimes claimed that the concept is value laden?

2. Is there a difference between a right to health and a right to health care?

3. What are some of the ethical implications of construing health care as a right? As a commodity? Which notion is ethically the most defensible—and why?

4. What are the fundamental principles of the *Canada Health Act*?

5. What is the relevance of the Romanow Report for health care in Canada?

INTRODUCTION

Most Canadians believe they have a right to health care irrespective of their medical condition or their financial resources.[1] They have not always felt this way. Until the 1930s they agreed with the citizens of many other countries that health care was a commodity that each individual should pay for, and that those who could not afford it simply did not have a right to it. The experiences of the 1930s fostered a change in this perspective, and by the 1940s the change was complete. First in Saskatchewan and then in other provinces, the now prevailing attitude began to dominate: Health care is a socially guaranteed right.

In 1944, this resulted in the establishment of universal health care and hospital insurance in Saskatchewan,[2] and the other provinces soon followed. It was reflected at the federal level in the Hall Report of 1964[3] and the Lalonde Report of 1974,[4] and ultimately resulted in the *Canada Health Act* of 1984.[5] Today, all Canadian provinces and territories have a universal health care system. It is sometimes referred to as medicare. Under this system, every "qualified resident" (the meaning of this phrase will be explained a little later) can access what is considered "medically necessary" health care (this phrase will also be explained later) as a publicly insured service. Physicians, hospitals, therapists and other health care providers supply these services according to province-wide schedules. Only certain services—including things such as cosmetic surgery and *in vitro* fertilization—have to be paid for by patients themselves.

As was said a moment ago, not all countries share the belief that health care is a socially guaranteed right; and even countries that share the belief do not necessarily share it to the same degree or, for that matter, agree on how this belief should be expressed in practical terms. For instance, the U.K.—which passed the *National Health Service Act* in 1946[6]—has the same general outlook as Canada. However, in contrast to Canada, it also allows a parallel private health care system that tends to provide speedier access to many services than the public system does, and that provides a wider variety of alternative and complementary treatments than the socially funded National Health Service, which is available to all.

The U.S., in turn, has a much more ambivalent attitude. On the one hand, it agrees that health care is a matter of right—as witness its Medicare and Medicaid programs. These programs provide free health care to U.S. residents who live below the poverty line (in the case of Medicaid)[7] or to people who are older than sixty-five years and who have paid federal income tax for ten years (in the case of Medicare).[8] On the other hand, the U.S. also believes that health care is a commodity like any other that can be bought and sold in the marketplace. Therefore, those who do not qualify for Medicare or Medicaid are responsible for financing their own health care. It is a matter of private responsibility. The U.S., therefore, does not have an overall public health care system as it exists in Canada or the U.K. but has what amounts to a two-tier health care system. As a result, more than 17 percent of the population (50.7 million people) have no access to health care at all. They do not meet Medicare or Medicaid requirements, but at the same time are too poor to afford private health care insurance premiums.[9] To put this into perspective, the average (2010) health insurance premium for a family of four in the U.S. was $13,770, whereby the employer paid $9,773 (if the employment benefits included health insurance) and the employee paid $3,997.[10] In 2007, 61 percent of all personal bankruptcies in the U.S. were health cost related. Most of those who went bankrupt for health-cost-related reasons were well educated, owned their own homes and had middle-class occupations, and three-quarters of them had health insurance. By contrast, medical bankruptcies in Canada and the U.K. are essentially non-existent. It is expected that the proportion of health-care-related bankruptcies in the U.S. will continue to rise unless a national health insurance system similar to that of either the U.K. or Canada is introduced.[11]

Of course, these are merely factual considerations. In and of themselves, they say nothing about the ethics of health care, nor do they say anything about whether health care is a right or a commodity. The inability to access health care may be unpleasant and even have tragic consequences; however, there are all sorts of facts that are unpleasant or have tragic consequences without, for all that, being unethical. For instance, it is tragic that everyone is going to die, but that does not make it unethical; likewise, it is tragic that it is currently impossible to entirely remove all HIV viruses from blood supplies,[12] but that it not unethical either. It is merely a fact of life.

Moreover, even if health care is a right, that says nothing about whether society should in fact institute a public health service. There are some rights where it does not really matter, in practical terms, whether that right is violated. For instance, in most cases it matters very little whether someone's right to scratch her right ear before scratching her left ear is violated, or whether putting on her left shoe before her right is prohibited. By contrast, there are some rights where it is extremely important whether they are violated or whether the corresponding duties are met. Failure to honour these rights may seriously affect people as persons. The right to legal representation is one of these, and so is education. The question, therefore, is not only whether health care is a right, but whether it is a right that matters.

So it is against this backdrop of facts and considerations that one has to ask whether health care is a right or a commodity—and if it is a right, how it is grounded. And if indeed it is a right, a series of other questions immediately arise: What is included under the right to health care? Are only life-saving or -sustaining services included, or are others included as well? Is this right—if it is a right—effective under all circumstances, or are there situations in which it loses its force? And finally, does it matter how the relevant care is provided? Is there a role for private enterprise? Or, if ethics is to be served, must all health care be provided by a public provider?

There is a wide variety of opinions on all of these issues. However, before addressing any of them, it is important to have some clarity on two even more fundamental issues: What is the nature of health? and Is there a right to *health* or a right to health *care*? Without clarity on these matters, any discussion of the right to health care will be plagued by fundamental ambiguities that have important practical implications, because, depending on how the notion of health is defined, different kinds of services will be included in the right to health care. And depending on whether one distinguishes the right to health from the right to health care, the orientation of health care services that are mandated will be different. Likewise, the whole debate about whether it would be appropriate to have a public-private parallel system (as in the U.K. and some other countries) will acquire a completely different perspective.

THE DEFINITION OF "HEALTH"[13]

To begin, then, with the notion of health. In a way, of course, the concept is intuitively obvious. To put it in terms that the World Health Organization (WHO) has made famous,[14]

> [h]ealth is a state of complete physical, mental and social well-being and not merely the absence of disease or infirmity.

This perspective tends to be in line with the notion of health as understood by First Nations, who define health in holistic terms and identify it as including "wellness of the body, mind, heart and spirit."[15]

However, as a whole series of authors have pointed out,[16] the WHO definition is extremely vague. For instance, what do "well-being" or "infirmity" mean? It is also circular because it defines "health" in terms of its correlative "disease." The notion of disease, however, can itself only be defined in terms of health, so this does not really help. Furthermore, the definition is far too inclusive. It would classify social and moral problems as health problems. While they are interrelated—the Assembly of First Nations definition above certainly acknowledges that fact—they are not the same. Nor does it help that the WHO tried to operationalize this definition in 1986, in the *Ottawa Charter for Health Promotion* when it said that[17]

> [h]ealth is, therefore, seen as a resource for everyday life, not the objective of living. Health is a positive concept emphasizing social and personal resources, as well as physical capacities.

Other definitions have been suggested to overcome these problems. For instance, health has been defined as a "proper working order of the human body,"[18] as a "mode of functioning [that] conforms to the natural design of that kind of organism" (with disease as a "deviation from the natural functional organization of the species"),[19] as "spiritual, moral or mental soundness or well-being,"[20] as the ability to function "in a given physical and social environment,"[21] as the "well-working of the organism as a whole . . . an activity of the living body in accordance with its specific excellence,"[22] or simply as "a state of physical well-being."[23]

Health and Values

But these definitions have also run into criticism. In fact, the very attempt to define health at all has been criticized. On a general level, the criticism has been that a proper definition is impossible, because concepts such as those of health and disease are inherently value laden.[24] They include not only descriptive components but also normative ones. The whole notion of health and disease is therefore ineluctably framed in terms of "state descriptions and normative claims"[25] because not only are they state relative—a point that will be addressed a little later—but they inevitably include value judgments. Tristam Englehardt, Jr. focuses on these normative components when he says that[26] discussion about what counts as health and disease involves considerations of what counts as the proper human state, and the latter is caught up with value judgements which are both explicit and implicit.

This critique is echoed by Joel Feinberg, who suggests an alternative definition in functional terms:[27]

> It may seem . . . that the ascription of functions to component parts or subsystems is a wholly factual matter consisting of, first, a description of a part's effect and, second a causal judgement that these effects are necessary conditions for the occurrence of some more comprehensive effects. But the illusion of value neutrality vanishes when we come to ascribe functions to the organism itself.

When the reasoning that underlies this perspective is taken to its conclusion, it leads to something like the position of Peter Sedgewick's claim that[28]

> illness and disease, health and treatment, (are) social constructions . . . Outside the significance that man voluntarily attaches to certain conditions, there are no illnesses or diseases in nature.

The position of Thomas Szaz is similar, although it is formulated more specifically with reference to mental illness. Szaz acknowledges that there is such a thing as organic brain disease, defined in terms of physiological dysfunction. However, he maintains that the concept of mental illness is a "myth." It is the legacy of a religious mythology and is heir to the notion of witchcraft, according to which "mastery of certain problems may be achieved by means of substitute symbolic-magical operations."[29] The value concept that Szaz sees buried in the notion of mental health is that of a smoothly functioning social order, where deviant behaviour of a divisive sort is eliminated under the guise of health care. More specifically, he characterizes the concept of mental illness as nothing more than an expression of society's current disapproval of certain ways in which individuals try to cope with the pressures of modern life. In support of this stance on mental health, which connects health and disease with values, one could point to the fact the former USSR incarcerated political dissidents in mental institutions as individuals who were mentally ill. Another example comes from North America, where the American Psychiatric Association (and the Canadian Psychiatric Association) considered homosexuality a disease and did not declassify it as such until 1973, after it had gained social acceptance as an alternative lifestyle.[30] Another—and more recent—example comes from India, where in 2011 the Minister of Health described homosexuality as an unnatural "disease" that resulted in socially aberrant behaviour.[31]

And finally, some have argued that the attempt to define "health" and its correlatives is really an open-ended task. The attempt to achieve "precision in defining health status always will entail a 'receding mirage,' but the further we go on the journey, the more accomplishments will be seen in the rearview mirror."[32]

What has just been sketched should give some idea of the range of positions on the very notion of health itself, and of the criticisms that have been levelled at any attempt to define it.[33] However, the issue is important. If one cannot give a value-free definition of health, then the question of what should be included under the rubric of health care remains irresolvable and is likely to be coloured by values that amount to political and cultural agendas.

Concepts and Values

The important question, therefore, is whether one can give a value-free definition of "health."

When all is said and done, the answer is probably "No." The reason lies in the relationship between concepts and language. One can define something only by using a language. Language, however, is cognitively meaningful only because the words of the language are associated with concepts. These concepts, in turn, are part of the overall conceptual framework that categorizes what is experienced and that structures the world-as-perceived. To borrow a metaphor from the philosopher Immanuel Kant, they are like a set of irremovable glasses.[34] It is these conceptual glasses that structure and impose significance on what would otherwise be completely meaningless sensory data.[35]

The metaphor of the irremovable glasses is fortunate, because it leads to the next point. How a pair of glasses is ground, and the colour and nature of the glass, condition what is seen through them. Therefore, the glasses may distort or colour what is seen, enlarge it or make smaller, etc. The parallel to concepts lies in the fact that the concepts that structure this conceptual framework are culture bound and even language related.[36] Therefore, any definition is necessarily bound to be a language-and-culture-bound definition. The further the language families (and hence the conceptual frameworks) are removed from each other, the greater the difference between these definitions. That is why—to use an example from Canadian health care—translators who facilitate communication between Inuit patients and non-Inuit health care providers have to be culturally sensitive and cannot simply reply on dictionary definitions.[37]

The concepts that form part of someone's conceptual framework therefore structure an individual's reality-as-perceived. However, languages and conceptual frameworks are not acquired in an isolated setting that is hermetically sealed from other influences. They are acquired as part of the lifestyle that defines the culture in which the individual is embedded, and because these embeddings differ, the concepts will inevitably be culture relative.[38] This means that the greater the overlap, the more similar the view of reality; and the less the overlap, the less similar the reality-as-perceived.

Moreover—and this becomes important when considering the question whether ill health is a mandate for treatment—the social context in which language is learned and concepts are acquired is characterized by social valuational gradients that condition individuals' reactions towards what they experience. These valuational gradients function like action-potentials. Negative values potentiate an unfavourable reaction to what is experience and, correspondingly, positive values potentiate a favourable reaction.[39] (See also Chapter 1.) This in turn influences the sorts of actions that persons find appropriate or inappropriate. The traditional way of putting this is to say that to learn concepts or to learn a language is to learn a way of life.[40] That is why to learn a language and acquire a conceptual framework is also to acquire a set of values that colour the concepts. To use a metaphor, they surround concepts like a halo. Whenever a concept comes into play, the values that surround it are called up as well.

The relevance of this to the issue of health lies in the fact that the socio-cultural context in which the concept of health is primarily acquired gives rise to what some have called a "normative" definition of health. However, the conceptual framework need not be socio-cultural in the usual sense of that term. It may be scientific in nature—and more specifically, it may be biological in orientation. The concept of health that then arises may be called a "naturalist" concept.[41] From such a perspective, the concept is geared towards functioning. Health is then the capability to exercise the biologically determined capacities within the environment in which the individual is embedded.[42] In other words, the definition of "health" from this perspective focuses on the functional ability of the individual to maintain itself in a homeostatic balance. This means that if the environment changes, a healthy individual will have to change as well. If the individual loses the capacity to maintain a homeostatic balance, the individual will be in ill health.

A naturalist concept of health is also surrounded by action-potentials. These are tied to the value of survival. Therefore, from a naturalist perspective, the judgment that someone is healthy does not activate the action-potential for treatment, whereas the judgment that someone is ill does, because it is grounded in the biological imperative of survival.

However, human beings are not merely animals but social animals. As such, the concept of a human being is not only the biological concept of a member of the species *homo sapiens* but the socio-cultural concept of a *person*—which is to say as a rational biological being who is embedded in a social context. That is why the concept of human health is not exhausted by the so-called naturalist parameters but includes the "normative" parameters mentioned a moment ago—the parameters that tie the functioning of individuals to the values of the society in question. Therefore, healthy *persons* are always individuals who are healthy relative to a conceptual framework. This means that they are persons who, in virtue of their constitution as embodied beings, have the capacity to take advantage of the opportunities that are presented by the social context in which they are embedded. If they cannot do so because of their constitution as embodied beings (as opposed to, say their embedding in terms of wealth, etc.), then they are in ill health. It follows that psycho-social considerations are important when talking about the health of human beings *as persons*.

This way of approaching the notion of human health not only explains why there is such a variety of definition, it also suggests several important conclusions. *First*, there is no objective and absolute way of telling whether someone is well or ill. It is all framework relative. Some frameworks are shared. For example, the scientific-biological framework is currently shared by most cultures. In that sense, and to that degree, they will at least partly share judgments about who is ill and who is not. However, even within this naturalist framework, the environmental context in which the judgment is made is very important, because the environmental embedding determines whether the individual can maintain homeostatic balance—or maintain it better, comparatively speaking. For instance, someone who carries a gene for sickle-cell anemia and is not homozygous for it will be healthier in a malaria-infested environment than someone who does not. However, that is not true in a geographic locale that does not include malaria.

Second, to say that someone is ill says nothing about the etiology of that condition. That has to be explored within the conceptual framework within which the judgment is made. It also says nothing objective and absolute about how the condition should be treated. That also is a function of the conceptual framework—and, of course, the traditions and the resources that are available.

Third, while the statement that someone is ill connotes a value judgment because of the action-potentials that are associated with the relevant concept, this does not necessarily entail that diagnosing someone as ill thereby constitutes a mandate for treatment. The decision to treat is a decision that is based on what is considered an appropriate reaction to a health status assessment, and the question of who should make that decision is again a function of the conceptual framework. These may differ from conceptual framework to conceptual framework. This is what grounds different approaches to health care decision-making in different cultures.

RIGHT TO HEALTH CARE

Right to Health versus Right to Health Care

Given this understanding of the concept of health, it now becomes meaningful to ask whether there is a right to health care—and it will be clear from the very start that because of the valuational components of the concept, the answer may well differ from socio-cultural framework to socio-cultural framework. However, it may be useful, before considering the question in more detail, to clarify a logical point; it is framework invariant (precisely because it is logical), but it is a point that is frequently overlooked when it comes to health care resource allocation and to deciding what should be included in the framework that operationalizes the notion of health care as a right. The point is simply this: One cannot have a right to something if the fulfillment of that right essentially lies outside the realm of what is possible. This follows from the Principle of Impossibility.[43] (See Chapter 1.)

That is to say, no one, no matter what they do, can guarantee that people will be healthy—any more than they can guarantee that they will be happy. The most that they can do is make every effort to ensure their happiness—or, as in the present context, to try to provide for their health. In other words, one can guarantee that one will make the attempt, and that one will do this to the best of one's ability—this would be in accordance with the Principle of Integrity (see Chapter 1.)—but that cannot and does not guarantee a successful outcome. For instance, one may be unable to do anything about a patient's genetic makeup, not even with the advent of contemporary germ and somatic cell line therapy. (For more on this, see Chapter 12.) And all other things being equal, one certainly cannot force people to take advantage of the health care opportunities that are offered to them and that must be used in order for them to have a successful outcome. People may insist on leading imprudent lifestyles by indulging in smoking, immoderate alcohol consumption, lack of exercise and so on. In these cases their health will suffer, no matter what the health care professional—or anyone else, for that matter—does. Furthermore, one cannot prevent all accidents. They are simply part of the human condition. Likewise, health care professionals cannot be expected to be perfect in what they do, any more than any other human being can. That is why all that one can expect from them is that they have appropriate skills, and exercise due diligence and care.[44] "Honest mistakes" and accidents happen. Finally, one cannot guarantee that there will be sufficient resources to provide all necessary health care services to the degree that may be necessary in each case.

Therefore, people do not have a right to health, no matter how health is defined. The best they can have is a right to health care. However, this immediately raises two questions: Is there such a right—and if there is, how would it be grounded? and, If there is a right to health care, what—if any—are its limits? The first question will form the subject of the next section; the second question will receive separate treatment in the next chapter.

Nature and Origin of the Right to Health Care

Legal versus Ethical Right to Health Care The first thing to do is to draw a distinction between a legal and an ethical right to health care. A legal right exists only if a duly empowered authority has declared that there is such a right. There is no legally recognized and universal right to health care in Canada—neither at the federal level nor at the provincial level. The reason there is no such right at the federal level lies in the Canadian constitution. It stipulates that health care, like education, is a matter of provincial jurisdiction. The only powers that the federal government has in this regard fall under controlling communicable diseases, licensing pharmaceuticals and similar matters. The *Canada Health Act*, therefore—which will be discussed later—does not deal with a right to health care but with the conditions under which the federal government will transfer health-care-related funds to the provinces.

Provincial legislation, in turn, does not guarantee a universal right to health care either. What it does is establish public, not-for-profit, provincial health insurance programs that provide access to certain specified health services *for the qualified residents of a given jurisdiction.*

Nor have Canadian courts affirmed a legal right. The closest they have come is in the *Chaoulli* case, in which the Supreme Court ruled that it was unconstitutional for Quebec to prohibit private health care insurance companies from offering their services in Quebec.[45] On the other hand, as several federal and provincial legislation make clear, and as has been affirmed by various Royal Commissions and federal reports, Canadians share a *belief* in the right to health care.[46] This is also what underlies the relevant legislation at both levels of government. However, that is not the same as a legal right.

Canadians, then, believe that there is an ethical right to health care. Can this belief be grounded in ethical principles, or is it merely a culture-relative matter of social value?

The right to health care has been defended in various ways. For example, it has been argued that health itself "is a primary good" and that it "generally helps people to carry out their life plans, whatever they may be."[47] It has also been suggested that health care "expresses and nurtures bonds of sympathy and compassion," and that therefore "a society's commitment to health care reflects some of its most basic attitudes about what it is to be a member of the human community."[48] In a similar vein, some authors have suggested that the right to health care is rooted in "a basic obligation of charity or beneficence to those in need."[49] Still others have suggested that access to health care is rooted in society's obligation to provide for equality of opportunity for its members.[50]

The sentiments expressed in some of these considerations are certainly laudable. Charity and beneficence are virtues that should be encouraged, and one could argue that providing health on a society-wide basis would certainly be an expression of care and concern. However, the fact that something is a virtue does not necessarily turn it into a duty, and the fact that something would be an expression of care and concern does not make its observance into an obligation. Therefore, these considerations may not be the most fortunate ones for establishing a universal and equal right to health care.

Beneficence and Non-Malfeasance There are three ethical principles, however, that do entail a social obligation to provide health care. They are Beneficence, non-Malfeasance, and Equality and Justice respectively. At first glance, Beneficence and non-Malfeasance seem to provide the strongest grounding. Clearly, health is generally considered a good. Therefore, providing services that maximize the probability of being in good health would be in keeping with the general duty to maximize the good for others. With due alteration of detail, the same thing is true of ill health and non-Malfeasance: Providing services that are likely to minimize the chance of ill health or that are likely to correct it would minimize harm.[51]

However—as Chapter 1 made clear—there is a difference between Beneficence and non-Malfeasance as construed from a utilitarian perspective and as construed from a deontological perspective. If they are construed from a utilitarian perspective then, arguably, they hold for any society, because they focus on the greatest good for the greatest number—and societies are more likely to flourish and survive if their members are in good health. This is well illustrated by the fate of West-Coast First Nations communities, which disappeared because of the ravages of untreated diseases such as smallpox and tuberculosis, and by the functional relationship between the depressed socioeconomic status of many First Nations and Inuit peoples and the ill health of their members.[52] This was also an integral part of the reasoning in the Heagerty Report of 1943,[53] which provided the impetus for federal politicians to consider instituting a national health insurance program, and was a central concept of the Hall Report of 1964 and the Lalonde Report of 1974. It also underlay the passing of the *Saskatchewan Health Services Act* and the *Saskatchewan Hospitalization Act,* and was one of the more prominent features of the

House of Commons debates that ultimately led to the passage of the *Canada Health Act*. Finally, it was also one of the sentiments that emerged in the Romanow Report.[54] Not only individuals but society itself will be advantaged if there is a social mandate to provide health care.

By contrast, if Beneficence and non-Malfeasance are construed deontologically, then the good to be promoted and the harm to be minimized are functionally dependent on the values of the individuals who would be the recipients of the relevant actions. This means that the duty to provide health care would not depend on whether good health would advantage society—not even if all members of the society shared that opinion. It would depend on the values of the individual person; and while it is reasonable to suppose that people would generally share a belief in the benefits of good health, any duty that would arise on the basis of individual values would be conditioned by the other values that are also held. So, for instance, if people considered free enterprise to be a fundamental right, then society would not necessarily have a duty to provide health services as a matter of social right, unless health care was considered more fundamental than free enterprise. At best, what would follow would be that society had a duty to control the expense of health services, so that they would be affordable for everyone who wanted it. This, however, would be perfectly compatible with a two-tier approach to health care. In other words, society would then have an obligation to control the cost that patients would have to pay for health, so that a minimum would be affordable for everyone; however, it would not rule out premium health services for those who could afford them. The only exception would be for those who could not afford the basic minimum. In their case, society would have to assist them.

Equality and Justice Beneficence and non-Malfeasance, therefore, give only a limited (and indeed somewhat ambiguous) answer to the question of whether there is a right to health care. By contrast, the Principle of Equality and Justice provides a clearer and more secure basis. Moreover, it would not allow for a two-tier health system. The reason lies in the nature of Equality and Justice itself. It will be recalled from Chapter 1 that the Principle is not satisfied when people are all treated the same; that is only a starting condition, subject to review. It goes on to say that people must be treated differentially if there are ethically relevant differences in their nature or condition. Therefore, if there are relevant differences between people, if these differences are not due to some inappropriate action on their part, then to ignore these differences is in effect to punish them for something over which they have no control. It is therefore to treat them unfairly. In that sense, justice consists not in rigidly applying the same rules equally and in the same way for all, but in applying them equitably. To use John Rawls's phrase, true justice is fairness.[55] This does not mean that the Principle of Equality and Justice allows for distinctions in how the quality of rights is understood or in the nature of the rights that it entails. If a right is entailed, then it is entailed for all, and then it belongs to everyone equally, simply because all people are the same as persons. The difference resides in their operationalization or, as it were, their metric.

As was pointed out before, the ability to take advantage of the opportunity that society offers to its members depends, to a considerable degree, on individual health status. Thus, people who suffer from malaria cannot take advantage of schooling to the same degree as people who do not suffer from malaria can, and people who suffer from cystic fibrosis, cancer or abscessed teeth are similarly disadvantaged. Therefore, a society that accepts Equality and Justice as a fundamental ethical principle, and that considers the principle as governing all social interactions including economic ones, must attempt to ensure equality of opportunity for all of its members. The only way to do that is to establish a health care system that covers the health care needs of all of its members, and that would maximize each individual's chances to compete on an even footing with everyone else.

It does not follow from this, however, that such a society cannot permit a two-tier health care system. It only follows that it cannot permit a two-tier system in which the lower tier does not provide all medically necessary services for levelling the playing field, whereas the higher tier does. Nor does it follow that the society has an obligation to provide all medically necessary services in the manner most convenient to its members, or even the medically most advanced and cutting-edge services. The point will be explored further when we consider the *Canada Health Act.*

Nor, finally, does it entail how society should provide the medically necessary services—i.e., whether it does so through a publicly owned and operated system or by using private health care providers. For instance, in 2000 Alberta passed its *Health Care Protection Act,*[56] which prohibits the establishment of private hospitals but allows private surgical facilities and the offering of services through private health care providers. The Act stipulates that if a private surgical facility offers a service that is an insured and publicly available service, then the private facility can charge no more for that service than the province itself pays to the public providers.[57] Moreover, it does not allow queue-jumping for patients who pay privately.[58] Therefore, this Act does not contravene the principle of a right to health care as grounded in the Principle of Equality and Justice. Nor does an Equality and Justice–based right entail that a public health care provider may not contract out health care services to a private health care corporation if that should turn out to be more cost-effective. If the services that are provided level the playing field, and if access to these services is equitably structured, then society has fulfilled its obligation.

Finally, Equality and Justice does not entail that, even if a particular service is identified as a medical necessity, it must be available everywhere. This can again be illustrated from the Canadian health care scene. The *Canada Health Act,* under section 5, stipulates "accessibility" as one of its fundamental provisions. This does not mean that the same level and type of service must be available everywhere, whether that be in Tuktoyaktuk or Montreal. It simply means that appropriate steps should be taken to facilitate reasonable access to health services without financial or other barriers. Individual differences in the ability to access health services because of the location of the services may therefore legitimately be dealt with by providing transportation services. This is particularly important in the Canadian setting, where the distance between patients and facilities can sometimes run into the hundreds of kilometres.

Health Care as Grounded in the Nature of Society Finally, the right to health care can also be grounded in the nature of society itself and in the presuppositions that condition membership in it. That is to say, in the words of Thomas Hobbes, life in a state of nature and outside the context of formalized social institutions is apt to be "solitary, poor, nasty, brutish, and short."[59] People form societies to ameliorate that condition. However, for societies to be possible, social interactions have to be integrated and rule governed. Therefore, there have to be some limits on unbridled and uncontrolled actions, lest the structure fly apart. It follows that members of society must necessarily limit their right of freedom of action—not entirely, perhaps, but sufficiently in order for society to be able to function. This does not amount to an abrogation of the Principle of Autonomy but is simply the application of its limiting clause (see Chapter 1) to a social context.

However, this limitation of freedom is conditional on the expectation that society will, to the best of its ability, provide for the fundamental needs of its members, and that it will do so by balancing the competing rights and the resources that are available. Finally, there is also the expectation that society will try to provide an opportunity for self-realization on the part of the individual person.

All of this has important implications. One of these, clearly, is that society undertakes to provide for the necessaries of life of its members. This involves two parameters. One is external, the other internal. The external parameter comes into play when an individual's life is threatened from the outside. Therefore, society has an obligation to provide against such things as aggression, natural disasters and so on. The internal parameter comes into play when the individual's life and welfare are threatened either by other members of society, by the conditions of the society itself or by the individual's ability to maintain him- or herself because of health conditions. Various social services are implicated here—and health care is one of them. In that sense, then, there is a right to health simply as a function of being a member of society. The right to health, therefore, flows primarily from the Principle of Equality and Justice but also can be grounded in Beneficence and non-Malfeasance and in the presuppositions that underlie membership in society itself.

Limits on the Right to Health Care

However, as was outlined in Chapter 1, a right is a justified claim that the right-holder may exercise claim if he or she so wishes but does not have to, and where there lies a corresponding duty on others to fulfill a corresponding obligation if the right-holder so wishes—or can reasonably be presumed to so wish, as, all other things being equal, is the case with incompetent persons. (See Chapter 5 on substitute decision-making.)

This means two things, which become important when considering the ethics of medicare in Canada. *First*, it means that all persons have the right to forego health care if they so wish, the only exception here being if foregoing that right puts others at serious risk. (See the limiting conditions of the right to autonomy discussed in Chapter 1.) Also, nothing that has been said so far entails that someone cannot decide to access health services outside of the public system that society is mandated to provide.

Second, a right is conditioned by the circumstances under which it arose, by the circumstances that obtain when the right is claimed and by the actions of the right-holder. The first condition entails that society does not have an obligation to provide medical services if these are not health care related and do not prevent individuals from taking equitable advantage of the opportunities that are otherwise available. The second condition entails that if society lacks the resources to provide certain kinds of health services, then society does not fail in its duties if it does not provide them. Therefore, the fact that some societies provide a more complete array of health services than others does not necessarily mean that the latter are unethical. The third condition entails that those who claim the right of health care must have made reasonable efforts not to need that care, insofar as this lies within their power.

The third condition is important, and will be explored more fully in the next chapter in relation to the distinction between auto- and hetero-induced needs. For now, the important point is that not taking appropriate care of one's health—insofar as that is possible under the circumstances that obtain—is to generate a preventable health care need. The satisfaction of a preventable health care need uses resources that would otherwise be available to meet the health care needs of other persons. When these resources are unavailable, the health care needs of these other persons cannot be met. This means that they will be harmed. People who do not take care of their health (insofar as that is possible under the circumstances that obtain) will therefore be responsible for preventable harm to others. It follows that although their actions will *prima facie* be justified in terms of Autonomy, they will in fact violate the Principle of Autonomy, because they do not take the equal and competing rights of others into account. Moreover they will have violated the Principle of non-Malfeasance.

Consequently, a socially guaranteed right to health care comes with the ethically grounded condition that people have an obligation to be prudent in their lifestyles and to take appropriate steps to minimize their demands on the health care system. As an aside, it is interesting to note that while these considerations have found acceptance in other areas of social endeavour under the rubric of contributory negligence, and while they are integral to private health care in that premiums are adjusted according to voluntary risk factors, they have found only limited reflection in socialized health care systems. The most obvious example in which they play a role is the fact the unreformed alcoholics are generally considered ineligible for liver transplants.

Allopathic Health Care versus Alternative Health Care

If there is a social duty to provide health care, then an issue that immediately arises is what would satisfy that duty, i.e., what would constitute legitimate health care? The question could also be expressed more contentiously by asking whether such practices as chiropractic, herbalism, homeopathy and naturopathy should be included; and whether culturally or ethnically grounded practices such as traditional First Nations medicine,[60] Chinese medicine or Ayurvedic medicine—to mention but three culturally based examples—should be included as well. Still another way of putting it would be to ask whether a publicly funded health care system is obliged to include only so-called allopathic or Western medicine or whether it should also include alternative health care practices.[61]

The answer is inherent in Equality and Justice. The reason for providing health care is to level the playing field for individuals who, for health-related reasons, cannot take advantage of the opportunities that are available to everyone else. This says nothing about how their health care needs should be met. The only condition is that they be met effectively—or as effectively as possible under the prevailing circumstances. Therefore, whether the health care is allopathic or alternative in nature is irrelevant. In fact, it may turn out that under certain circumstances non-allopathic medicine will provide better results than allopathic medicine, and that traditional First Nations medical practices or Ayurvedic or Chinese medicine are not merely more acceptable from a cultural perspective but are as good as or better than allopathic health care. An example here is acupuncture for chronic prostatitis/chronic pelvic pain syndromes.[62] Likewise, as has variously been reported in the literature, the placebo effect of many alternative health care practices may rival or even surpass the outcomes of allopathic medical treatment.[63] This, of course, does not mean that such practices should automatically be substituted for allopathic health care or, for that matter, that allopathic health care should automatically be provided rather than alternative medicine. The key is whether available data support a particular health care modality for a particular condition.

Moreover, the ability to provide health care is functionally dependent on the resources that are available and what, for want of a better term, may be called the level of sophistication of the society. A society that lacks the scientific tradition that vets health interventions by using the experimental protocols discussed in Chapter 6, and that relies on traditional knowledge and practices will arguably meet its obligation if it provides only traditional health care. However, it is an interesting (and potentially contentious) question whether, if that society now acquires access to scientifically validated allopathic health care that is more effective than the traditional care, the society may ethically refuse to embrace allopathic medicine.

What has been said so far suggests that it would be unethical to do so. However, this requires explanation. The key here lies in the ethical rationale for providing health care in the first place. A major part of the rationale, under Equality and Justice, is to facilitate equitable access to social opportunities—i.e., to level the playing field. However, the Principle of Integrity—which goes to whether a corresponding duty has been met—entails that if there lies a duty at all, the corresponding action should be performed in the best way possible. (See Chapter 1.) Therefore, if it turns out that allopathic medicine provides better results than traditional medicine, the society can satisfy the Principle only by adopting allopathic practices.

And here it would be inappropriate to reply that no one would be discriminated against if the society remained with traditional medicine, because no one would have access to allopathic medicine. Everyone would be treated the same. The point would be that remaining with the less effective model would be to institutionalize the health-related inequities by saying that adherence to traditional approaches trumped Equality and Justice. If no other type of health care was available, the matter would, of course, stand differently. Any health-based inequities that existed would be inherent in the situation, and not a matter of choice. The situation would be unfortunate, but not unethical, and the Principle of Impossibility would, so to speak, exonerate the community. However, once allopathic medicine was available, that would no longer be the case. The health-related inequities would now be a matter of social choice. Not using more effective allopathic treatments would be the result of a deliberate decision to confirm correctable inequalities. Of course, that does not mean that the society could not offer both types of care, so that its members would have a choice. However, that is another matter.

HEALTH CARE AS A RIGHT VERSUS HEALTH CARE AS A COMMODITY

Canada attempts to meet its obligation to provide health care through a public health care system that is governed by the *Canada Health Act*. However, before considering this Act and Canadian health care in more detail, there is one further issue that requires clarification. It is the ethical difference between a commodity- and a rights-based approach to health care.

The Commodity Approach

Under a commodity approach, health care is treated like any other article of commerce. As such, it is subject to the rules of the marketplace. Market forces determine the price of the services, and availability, access and distribution are a matter of a prospective purchaser's financial capability. Moreover, outcome measures are relevant only insofar as they affect the market position of the health care provider. If the market will support it, expenses incurred because of inefficiency can be passed on to the consumer. Health care providers can also engage in profit-oriented patient screening, and patients who will require expensive care that lowers profits will be refused service. This is sometimes referred to as "cream skimming."[64]

Moreover, because the service is purchased, patients become consumers, and the relationship between patients and health care providers becomes essentially a matter of contract. While that contract will have fiduciary aspects, these will be within the limits of the services contracted for, much as in the case of legal services contracted for with a lawyer. Therefore, the fiduciary obligations of the professional do not have the same flavour and do not extend as far as is entailed by a fiduciary model of the physician–patient relationship, as discussed in Chapter 3.

As well, health care resource allocation issues are self-solving. Market forces will determine the price of the service, and the ability to meet the price determines who has access—and to what. A possible exception is transplantation and blood transfusion, where the scarcity of available tissues, organs and blood may occasion allocation issues even though competing patients can all meet the price; and drug shortages when, for one reason or another, an insufficient number of doses has been produced. However, tissue, organ and blood availability are ethically problematic on a commodity approach in any case, as will be discussed in a moment.

Finally, issues that centre in professional matters such as salary, hours of service, etc., are resolved through professional and institutional bargaining. If the bargaining is unsatisfactory for the professionals they may go on strike, and if they are unsatisfactory for the institutions they may initiate a lockout.

The Rights Approach

By contrast, under a rights approach, availability, access and distribution of health care are a matter of social obligation. Allocation issues have to be solved within the context of a socially mandated right, and they become a matter of societal concern. Individual ability to pay does not enter the picture, and competing claims to scarce resources must be solved as a matter of balancing competing rights and obligations. There also is no limit to the number of times a given patient can access relevant services, because need and resource availability will be the only determinants. Physicians will practise on the basis of a Hippocratic fiduciary model, in keeping with the best interests of the patient, and irrespective of cost considerations.

Outcome and effectiveness measures, in turn, become centrally important, because costs cannot be passed on to the patients. That is why rights-oriented approaches to health care tend to be administratively more efficient than commodity-based approaches.[65] Moreover, health care providers cannot engage in cream skimming. They must provide health care solely on the basis of need and overall resource availability. As well, professional issues such as working hours and salaries cannot be settled by strikes or lockouts, because that would interfere with the social mandate to provide care. Instead, if no satisfactory solution can be found, they must be settled by binding arbitration. Emergency services must also be provided at all times.

Finally, since access to medically necessary services is guaranteed as a matter of right, geographic and other impediments to access must be resolved on a system-wide basis. This means that where services cannot be provided on site, transportation and transfer services must be provided. In countries such as Canada, this varies from ambulance services to medivac by air.

Discussion

The commodity approach is consistent with the position that there is no right to health care, and with a libertarian philosophical orientation that advocates a minimum of state interference in the lives of its citizens. Under this approach, citizens may, so to speak, contract with society to provide certain services including health care, but that would be a matter of choice, and both the nature and the extent of that care would be determined by the conditions of that contract. Therefore, although it might be unfortunate if a society did not provide health care as a matter of entitlement, and although this lack of provision might even reduce the ability of that society to function as effectively as possible (because its members would not be as healthy as they otherwise might be), that way of dealing with health care would not make the society unethical.

At first glance, this libertarian stance would seem inconsistent with John Rawls's suggestion that those social rules are just and fair that would be agreed on "behind a veil of ignorance" by individuals if they were in a position to set up a society. That is to say Rawls, borrowing the concept from John Harsanyi,[66] had argued that in an ideal world, where each person acted rationally, if people were to make choices about how to structure their society knowing nothing about their own abilities, tastes, and positions within the social order, they would decide on the following principles for the distribution of rights, positions and resources (and these would mark the society as just): *First*, each person in that society should have an equal right to the most extensive basic liberty compatible with a similar liberty for others;[67] *second*, social and economic inequalities in that society should be arranged in such a way that they would benefit the least advantaged; and *third*, the offices and positions in that society should be open to everyone under conditions of fair equality of opportunity.[68] However, Rawls himself had never applied this to health care. Norman Daniels, however, has argued[69]—much along the lines that were outlined in the discussion of health care as a right above—that equality of opportunity can exist only if the members of that society are healthy, because only then can they avail themselves of the opportunities that exist.

Of course, this has not gone unopposed. At the level of ethical theory and in opposition to Rawls, some philosophers—e.g., Robert Nozik—have argued that there are basic rights that are absolute, and that two of the most fundamental are the right to liberty and the right to property.[70] On that basis, so they continue, there is a right to dispose of the fruits of one's labour in any manner one pleases, as long as this does not lead to the dissolution of society itself. Those who adopt this perspective then argue that health care is a commodity, because it involves labour and the "fruits" of labour in that it uses devices and techniques, etc., that are the products of work. Therefore, while Beneficence may ground society's decision to develop a health care system, that decision is not a matter of duty, because it is always subject to the more basic Principle of Liberty or Autonomy.[71] This may mean that some unfortunate people will have no access to health care (or have only limited access), and that therefore they cannot compete on the same footing with those who either are healthier by nature or can dispose of more resources. However, not everything that is unfortunate is unethical—and this is one such instance.[72]

The rights approach, however, appears to be ethically more congenial to the physician–patient relationship than the commodity approach. More specifically, under the Hippocratic model of the physician–patient relationship—what was identified as the fiduciary model in Chapter 3—physicians have a duty to provide the best treatment for their patients, irrespective of financial considerations that may be occasioned by the cost of the care. By contrast, under a commodity approach to health care, if patients cannot pay for the services, there is no obligation to provide them. This becomes a matter of internal conflict for physicians who are acculturated into a Hippocratic model by their training but who, because they provide services within a commodity approach, must use a for-profit business model. Thus, under a commodity approach a physician has no duty to offer a transplant to a patient if the patient cannot pay for it or if it is not covered by the patient's insurance, nor does the physician have a duty to refer the patient to another health care provider except insofar as it is stipulated in the contractual arrangement. Hippocratic training therefore pulls physicians in one direction, whereas the business model under which they operate pulls them in another. That is why most (i.e., over 99 percent) of the Canadian physicians who left to practise in the U.S. between the years 2000 and 2009 returned to Canada.[73]

Moreover, under a rights approach, patient access to health care tends to be better than under a commodity approach, as illustrated by comparisons between the U.S. and Canada.[74] Outcomes also tend to be better for many interventions,[75] and costs tend to be lower.[76] Further, if a society that has adopted a commodity approach also provides a parallel system for those who cannot afford private health care (as is the case in the U.S.), the outcomes are less favourable for the uninsured patients than for the patients with private insurance, because care to the former is provided as a matter of charity rather than as a matter of obligation.[77] This suggests that a rights approach tends to have the edge on a commodity approach when it comes to satisfying the Principle of Integrity.

However, these advantages of a rights approach pale in comparison to two funda-mental ethical issues that beset a commodity approach. The may be called the *social-goods problem* and the *free-rider problem* respectively. The social-goods problem centres in access to and use of organs, blood and tissues. In most societies, there is no ownership in human organs and tissues. This means that these cannot (legally) be bought or sold. They can only be donated. While some societies do permit the sale of blood—Canada is one of them—blood is generally donated. In either case, however, when these biologicals are donated, they are not donated to enable a private third party to make money from their use. They are donated so that persons who need them as part of their health care will have access to them. This means that for all intents and purposes, organs, blood and tissues are social goods. Moreover, one cannot deal with burns, leukemia or perform major surgery, etc., without using blood, organs or tissues such as skin, bone marrow, etc. Therefore, a commodity approach effectively turns social goods into private goods without the consent—and probably against the intent—of the donors. *Prima facie*, at least, this is unethical.

As to the free-rider problem, it derives from the fact that under a commodity approach, those who cannot afford premium health care (or those who rely on charity or cannot afford premium service) tend to become the training ground for health care professionals. Moreover, the subject pool for Phase I trials—trials that are non-therapeutic in nature and set the stage for later therapeutic interventions—is generally drawn from the uninsured or underinsured.[78] Therefore, those who can afford health care benefit from the training that their health care providers receive while working on less fortunate patients, and they benefit from the experimental protocols that lead to the development of the therapy they receive without themselves having contributed.

THE *CANADA HEALTH ACT (CHA)*

Introduction

For reasons that have already been indicated, Canada has instituted a publicly funded health care system (medicare) that provides all medically necessary health care to qualified residents free of charge at point-of-service.

That is how Canadian medicare is generally understood by the public. Strictly speaking, however, this is not quite correct. It is not that the services are provided free of charge: They are paid for by taxes. Therefore, the only people who do not pay for them are those who do not pay taxes.

Moreover, the phrase *medically necessary* is somewhat misleading. It suggests that there is an objective way to determine what falls under this rubric, and it connotes that the same services are provided in all Canadian jurisdictions. Both of these impressions, however, are false. The services that are provided vary from jurisdiction to jurisdiction. The reason, as was mentioned before, is that constitutionally, health care falls under provincial and territorial (henceforth this phrase will be understood) jurisdiction. In each province, a medical services commission (or its equivalent) decides what is meant by that phrase. These commissions are usually composed equally of representatives of the government, the medical profession and the public. By considering such things as the incidence and prevalence of diseases or conditions, their severity, the available treatments and their effectiveness and cost, etc., they determine what is "medically necessary" and on that basis decide what should be an insured service.

Several further things are of note here. *First*, what is considered medically necessary changes over time as epidemiological patterns, cost and outcomes, etc., change. *Second*, even though oral health is important for health in general[79]—for instance, poor oral health can have serious cardiac implications[80]—routine dental health services that are provided outside of hospitals and that are not provided by physicians are not included in relevant health plans except for those who fall below the poverty line.[81] *Third*, experimental procedures are not covered under the relevant provincial legislation. *Fourth*, drugs are generally not included unless they are supplied in hospital. *Fifth*, if a particular service is not covered, coverage may be provided at the discretion of the relevant Minister of Health upon application. *Finally*, Aboriginal health services do not fall under the *CHA*. Originally provided by the Department of Indian Affairs, they were transferred to Health Canada in 1945.

The *CHA*

With this as background, we can now turn to the *Canada Health Act* (*CHA*). And it is important here to keep in mind that the *CHA* does not deal with health. It deals with the conditions under which the federal government will transfer moneys to a province for the health that the province provides.

The *CHA* contains five major clauses that govern, respectively, administration, comprehensiveness, universality, portability and access to the relevant health plans. Beginning with *administration*, the *CHA* stipulates that in order for a province to be eligible for an annual cash contribution from the federal government, the province must have a health insurance plan that is operated on a non-profit basis by a body that reports to the provincial government and that is subject to a public audit. This effectively means that if a province wishes to receive federal transfer funds for health care, it must treat health care as a right, not as a commodity.

Comprehensiveness, as the term has been interpreted, means that all medically necessary hospital and physicians' services (including dental surgery performed in hospitals) must be provided under the relevant plan, no matter what the medical condition of the individual may be or how many times the person has accessed the services. It will be recalled that the list of relevant services is decided by the provinces, not by anyone else.

Universality means that all qualified residents of a province, no matter where they live, what they do, how old they are, etc., must be treated the same way. This is expressed by the phrase *uniform terms and conditions*. A qualified resident is someone who fulfills the residency requirements for that province. Therefore, as soon as someone has established legal residency in a province, that person is covered. Since visitors to Canada are not residents, they will not be "insured persons." Hence, they will not be covered, and they will be billed for any services they receive, even emergency services.

Portability, in turn, means that if residents of a province require medical attention outside of their province, they are entitled to the relevant care in whichever province they find themselves *if* it is an insured service in their home province. Moreover, payment must be at the rate that is approved by the provincial insurer where the service is provided.[82] Also, if qualified residents require health care while outside of Canada (and have retained residency in their province of origin), they continue to be covered and their foreign expenses are paid—but only at the rate that is approved for the service in their province of residence. If residents move to another province, they will be covered by the health plan of their province of origin until they meet the residence requirement of their new jurisdiction. That time period, however, may not exceed three months.

Finally, *accessibility* means that there must be no impediment—and this is usually interpreted to mean financial impediment—for a qualified resident to access insured services. Therefore, *user fees* (charges that are levied for using the system) and *extra billing* (charges that are levied by professionals over and above the rate set by the relevant provincial health care commission) are prohibited. In fact, the federal government will deduct the amount charged in terms of user fees and extra billing from the amount that it transfers to a particular province.

However, accessibility does not mean that insured health services must be made available in every locality. Instead, appropriate transportation may be provided, such as ambulance services and medivac. Such transportation is not specifically identified as an insured service under the *CHA*; however, it is free in some provinces (e.g., Ontario) for residents if they have a valid provincial health insurance card and it is medically necessary. Where the service is not covered (e.g., B.C.), it is heavily subsidized.

The *CHA* and the Romanow Report

There are two important but logically distinct questions that may be asked about the medicare system that has arisen under the *CHA*. One is whether the *CHA* is consistent with the notion of health care as a right; the other is whether the medicare system as it is currently structured under the *CHA* is the most effective way of providing health care on a rights basis. The rationale for the first question is obvious; the rationale for the second question lies in the fact that how health care is provided may affect whether Equality and Justice are satisfied in real terms, the underlying philosophy notwithstanding.

At first glance, the answer to the first question is a resounding "Yes." However, that would be incorrect. As the Royal Commission on the Future of Health Care pointed out in its Report of 2002, the Act falls short in several areas. To begin with, First Nations, Métis and Inuit peoples are not covered by the Act. Their health care is provided by the federal government, and it falls appreciably below the health care that is provided for most non-Aboriginal peoples by provincial health care providers. This violates Equality and Justice (and also contravenes Beneficence and non-Malfeasance).[83]

Moreover, neither dental care nor prescription drugs are covered under the Act. Since both are integral parts of modern health care—the matter was already raised earlier—and since they are very expensive, this means that their absence from the list of insured services effectively constitutes a financial barrier to accessing health care on an equitable basis.[84]

One can therefore reply with only a qualified "Yes" to the first question. The underlying philosophy is indeed consistent with the notion of health care as a right, but the Act is too limited in scope as it stands. The Royal Commission therefore recommended that it should be changed to correct these shortcomings. In particular, it recommended that health care for Aboriginal peoples should be fundamentally restructured by integrating Aboriginal health services into provincial health care programs through Aboriginal health accords that respect their values, needs and traditions. It also recommended that dental care should be included as a publicly insured service for everyone (as had originally been envisioned in the Hall Report), and that prescription drugs be included as an insured service.[85]

On the question of whether medicare as it is currently structured under the *CHA* is the most effective way of providing health care on a rights basis, the answer is also only a qualified "Yes." In this connection, the work of the Royal Commission is again relevant. It found that the availability and quality of health care was seriously compromised by the fact that patient information is not always available in a timely manner—which, in turn, can have a negative effect on the ability of health care professionals to fulfill their fiduciary obligations and to provide care wherever and whenever it is needed. The Commission therefore recommended the introduction of electronic patient records that are universally available but uniquely linked to each patient.[86]

For similar reasons, the Commission recommended that health technology assessment be not only streamlined but also scientifically improved, so that it could provide reliable data on interventions, outcomes and costs.[87] It also recommended that there be an increase in the number of health care professionals at all levels; that primary care— which it considered the foundation of health care in general—be strengthened; that waiting times be more scientifically managed and reduced;[88] and that scientifically valid and standardized quality assurance measures be implemented.[89] The Commission's concern for equity also led it to recommend that rural and home care be improved by using new technologies such as telehealth and telemedicine.[90]

In a sense, however—and with the exception of Aboriginal health—this is to tinker with the *CHA*. There is a much more fundamental issue on the line: It is the question of whether it is possible to satisfy the concept of health care as a right *at all* under something like the *CHA*. The specific concern here is that waiting times become unacceptably high by having an only single-payer system; that the services that are available are unacceptably restricted—all because public funds are limited; and perhaps most importantly of all, that by prohibiting a parallel system of private health care, the Principle of Autonomy is violated.

The suggestion has therefore been made that the *CHA* should be abandoned, and that the whole approach to health care should be revamped and replaced by a two-track model. There would then be private as well as public providers, and people could access whichever system they preferred. Equity could be achieved by establishing medical service allowance (MSA), where each qualified resident would receive a yearly health care allowance based on a statistical model of average health care needs. People could use their allowance to "purchase" health care services, and if they had any funds left over at the end of the year, they could bank these for use in future years when their health care costs may be higher.[91] Not only would this reduce the load on the public system, it would also honour the Principle of Autonomy by allowing people to spend their resources in whatever way they wished.

The Royal Commission considered this suggestion—and rejected it. The major reason was that such a remodelling would be inherently incompatible with the underlying philosophy of health care as a right and with the principle of universal and equitable access. Instead of being merely a two-track and parallel system of health care, it would be a two-tier system, i.e., without the device of an MSA, the proposed system could not even begin to claim that health care as a right would be preserved. However, under an MSA approach, people whose health care needs exceeded the statistical norm would be penalized, and they would be thrown on their own resources—sometimes with catastrophic effect. By that very token, it would strike at the Principle of Equality and Justice, which is basic to the concept of health care as a right.[92] Staffing the parallel private system would also drain health care professionals away from the public system, thereby not only imperiling quality of care but also increasing wait times in the public system, contrary to what the proposal claims.[93]

CONCLUSION

It may be too facile to say that one can judge the ethics of a society by looking at the logic of its laws and institutional systems. However, there is some truth to this proposition. It certainly holds true with respect to its stance on health care. A just and equitable society will try to level the playing field for its members; and while it will respect autonomy and the right to self-determination, it will also accept that autonomy is not licence, and that the right to self-determination is limited by the equal and competing rights of others. Therefore, a just and equitable society will provide its members with a level of health care that is designed to minimize health-based differences; and while it will allow the purchase of health care on a private basis, it will ensure that such purchases do not introduce or confirm the very inequities that society is trying to eradicate.

That is why, in the case of *Chaoulli*, in which the Supreme Court of Canada had occasion to consider whether health care as structured under the *CHA* violated fundamental rights, the Court did not come up with such a ruling. The Court did find that section 7 of the Charter allowed Canadians to purchase private health care as a matter of security of the person; particularly if wait times were too long. However, the Court did not strike down the *CHA*. It upheld its legitimacy. It merely found that there are less restrictive ways of guaranteeing a universal right to health care than by ruling out entirely, by legal means, the ability to purchase private health care.

One can debate whether the *Chaoulli* ruling is consistent with empirical facts, and one can also accept that the Canadian health care system, as it is currently structured under the *CHA*, is not perfect. There are two points, however, that are important to keep in mind. *First*, the Supreme Court decision in *Chaoulli* is a matter of law, not ethics. If the analysis in this chapter is correct, then health care is a right, not a commodity. And even though the *Chaoulli* ruling is only a matter of law, the Supreme Court ruling did not put the issue of right into question. *Second*, how a particular right is implemented does not affect the nature of the right itself. Therefore, the fact that the *CHA* as it stands is not a perfect framework for guaranteeing a right to health care, and the fact that medicare as it is currently structured by the provinces has shortcomings, does not entail that the basic idea of health care as a right is incorrect. All it shows is that there is room for improvement.

Further Readings

Buchanan, A. "The Right to a Decent Minimum of Health Care" in *Securing Access to Health Care: A Report on the Ethical Implications of Differences in the Availability of Health Services,* President's Commission for the Study of Ethical Problems in Medicine and Biomedical and Behavioral Research (Washington DC: U.S. Govt. Printing Office, 1983).

Callahan, D. "The WHO Definition of Health." *Hastings Center Studies* 1.3 (1973): 77–87.

Canada Health Act

Daniels, N. *Just Health Care* (Cambridge and New York: Cambridge University Press, 1985).

Deber, R.B. *Delivering Health Care Services: Public, Not-for-Profit or Private?* Discussion Paper 17, Commission on the Future of Health Care in Canada (2002), available at www.teamgrant.ca/M-THAC%20Greatest%20Hits/Bonus%20Tracks/Delivering%20Health%20Care%20Services.pdf

Engelhardt, H.T., Jr. *The Foundations of Bioethics* (New York: Oxford University Press, 1986), Chapter 8.

Ereshefsky, M. "Defining 'Health' and 'Disease.'" *Stud Hist Philos Biol Biomed Sci* 40.3 (2009): 221–227.

Feinberg, J. "Disease and Values" in *Doing and Deserving: Essays in the Theory of Responsibility*, ed. J. Feinberg (Princeton, NJ: Princeton University Press, 1974), 253–255.

Freedman, B., and F. Baylis. "Purpose and Function in Government-Funded Health Coverage." *Journal of Health Politics, Policy and Law* 12.1 (1997): 97–122.

Kaufert, J.M., R.W. Putsch and M. Lavallée. "Experience of Aboriginal Health Interpreters in Mediation of Conflicting Values in End-of-Life Decision Making." *International Journal of Circumpolar Health* 57, Suppl 1 (1998): 43–48.

Nielson, K. "Autonomy, Equality, and a Just Health Care System." *International Journal of Applied Philosophy* 4.3 (1989): 39–44.

Veatch, R. "Just Social Institutions and the Right to Health Care." *Journal of Medicine and Philosophy* 4.2 (1979): 170–173.

World Health Organization. Preamble to the Constitution of the World Health Organization, available at www.who.int/about/definition/en/print.html

Endnotes

1. R.J. Romanow, *Building on Values: The Future of Health Care in Canada. Final Report* (Ottawa: Royal Commission on the Future of Health Care in Canada, 2002), 65 *et. pass.*

2. *Saskatchewan Hospitalization Act*, 1946, which followed the *Health Services Act* of 1945. The program outlined in this legislation did not become fully operative until an agreement was reached with the College of Physicians and Surgeons of Saskatchewan with the so-called Saskatoon Agreement of 1962. See also Mr. Justice Emmett Hall, *Report of the Royal Commission on Health Services* (Ottawa: Queen's Printer, 1964). For a discussion of the evolution of health services in Canada, see M.G. Taylor, *Health Insurance and Canadian Public Policy: The Seven Decisions That Created the Canadian Health Insurance System and Their Outcomes* (Kingston and Montreal: McGill-Queen's University Press, 1987).

3. The Hall Report, *supra.*

4. The Honourable Mr. M. Lalonde, *A New Perspective on the Health of Canadians* (Ottawa: Minister of Supply and Services, 1974).

5. *Canada Health Act*, R.S., 1985, c. C–6.

6. The *National Health Service Act* was passed in 1946 but came into effect in 1948. It did not include Scotland, which was included in the U.K.–wide system in 1947 through the *National Health Service (Scotland) Act.*

7. For eligibility criteria, see www.cms.gov/MedicaidEligibility/03_MandatoryEligibilityGroups.asp#TopOfPage

8. For eligibility details, see www.medicare.gov/MedicareEligibility/home.asp?dest=NAV|Home| Resources|EligibilityCalcQuestions|ResourcesOverview&version=default&browser=Firefox|5| WinXP&language=English

9. U.S. Census Bureau, *Income, Poverty, and Health Insurance Coverage in the United States: 2009*, 22–28, available at www.census.gov/prod/2010pubs/p60-238.pdf

10. Kaiser Family Foundation and Health Research & Educational Trust, *Employer Health Benefits: 2010 Summary of Findings*, available at http://ehbs.kff.org/pdf/2010/8086.pdf

11. D.U. Himmelstein et al., "Medical Bankruptcy in the United States, 2007: Results of a National Study," *The American Journal of Medicine* 10.10 (2009): 1–6.

12. The tests available for screening blood against HIV include ELISA, Western Blot and p24 Antigen testing. They do not guarantee a 100 percent specificity and validity.

13. For a useful discussion of the definition of "health," see M. Ereshefsky, "Defining 'Health' and ' Disease,'" *Studies in History and Philosophy of Science* 40.3 (2009): 221–227. See also J.S. Larson, "The Conceptualization of Health," *Medical Care Research and Review* 56.2 (1999): 123–136.

14. WHO, *The First Ten Years of the World Health Organization* (Geneva: World Health Organization, 1958).

15. Assembly of First Nations, *First Nations Public Health: A Framework for Improving the Health of Our People and Our Communities* (2006), available at http://fnpublichealth.ca/wp-content/uploads/ PDF/FNPB-IH.pdf; see also National Aboriginal Health Organization, *Environmental Scan of Cultural Competency/Safety in Health Curricula* (2006), available at http://fnpublichealth.ca/wp-content/ uploads/PDF/FNPB-IH.pdf

16. The best known is D. Callahan, "The WHO Definition of Health," *Hastings Center Studies* 1.3 (1973): 77–87. See also Ereshefsky, op. cit.

17. WHO/HPR/HEP/95.1 *Ottawa Charter for Health Promotion*, available at www.who.int/hpr/NPH/docs/ ottawa_charter_hp.pdf

18. J. Feinberg, "Disease and Values," in *Doing and Deserving: Essays in the Theory of Responsibility*, ed. J. Feinberg (Princeton: Princeton University Press, 1974), 253–255.

19. C. Boorse, "On the Distinction between Disease and Illness," in *Medicine and Moral Philosophy*, ed. M. Cohen, T. Nagel and T. Scanlon (Princeton, NJ: Princeton University Press, 1981): 49–68, at 57.

20. *Oxford English Dictionary*.

21. R. Dubos, "Health as Ability to Function," in *Contemporary Issues in Bioethics*, ed. T.L. Beauchamp and L. Walters (Belmont, CA: Dickenson Publ. Co., 1978), 99.

22. L. Kass, "Regarding the End of Medicine and the Pursuit of Health," in Beauchamp and Walters, op. cit., 108.

23. See Callahan, op. cit. A somewhat more theoretical and developed analysis is offered by E. Lidler, "Definition of Mental Health and Illness and Medical Sociology," *Social Science and Medicine A* 13 (1979): 723–731. She claims that these and other definitions are based on a Parsonian model of illness and disease: one that defines it as "an abstract, biomedical conception of pathological abnormality in people's bodies, where this is indicated by certain abnormal signs and symptoms which can be measured, recorded, classified and analyzed." To be quite correct, so she argues, the concept should be modified so that "subjective reality plays a role in determining whether an individual becomes ill in the first place."

24. See Ereshefsky, op. cit.

25. Ereshefsky, loc. cit.

26. H.T. Englehardt Jr., "Human Well-Being and Medicine: Some Basic Value Judgements in the Bio-medical Sciences," reprinted in *Biomedical Ethics*, ed. T.A. Mappes and J.S. Zembaty (New York: McGraw-Hill, 1981), 214.

27. See "Disease and Values," reprinted in *Biomedical Ethics*, ed. T.A. Mappes and J.S. Zembaty (New York: McGraw-Hill, 1981), 211.

28. P. Sedgewick, "What Is Illness?" *The Hastings Center Studies* 1.3 (1973), reprinted in Beauchamp and Walters, op. cit., 114.

29. T. Szaz, "The Myth of Mental Illness," in Mappes and Zembaty, op. cit., 227.

30. R. Bayer, *Homosexuality and American Psychiatry: The Politics of Diagnosis* (Princeton, NJ: Princeton University Press, 1987).

31. CBC News, accessed 21 Jul 2011 at www.cbc.ca/news/world/story/2011/07/05/india-gay-slur.html

32. Larson, op. cit., at 134.

33. For other attempts to define "health," see President's Commission for the Study of Ethical Problems in Medicine and Biomedical and Behavioral Research, *Securing Access to Health Care: A Report on the Ethical Implications of Differences in the Availability of Health Services*, 3 vols. (Washington, DC: U.S. Govt. Printing Office, 1983), Vols. 2 and 3.

34. Immanuel Kant, *Critique of Pure Reason* (Hartknoch: Jena, 1792).

35. See R. Chisholm, *Realism and the Background of Phenomenology* (New York: Glencoe, 1960); D.C. Dennett, *Content and Consciousness* (London: Routledge and Kegan Paul, 1969); J.M. Hinton, *Experiences* (Oxford: Clarendon Press, 1979).

36. See E.F.K. Koerner, "Towards a Full Pedigree of the Sapir–Whorf Hypothesis: From Locke to Lucy" in *Explorations in Linguistic Relativity*, ed. M. Pütz and M. Verspoor (Amsterdam: John Benjamins Publishing Company, 2000), 11–24. See also J.S. Bruner, J.S. Goodnow and G.A. Austin, *A Study of Thinking* (New York: Wiley, 1962); E. Sapir, *Culture, Language and Personality* (Berkeley: University of California Press, 1958) and B.L. Whorf, "Science and Linguistics," *Technology Review* 42.6 (1940): 229–231, 247–248.

37. See J.M. Kaufert, R.W. Putsch and M. Lavallée, "Experience of Aboriginal Health Interpreters in Mediation of Conflicting Values in End-of-Life Decision Making," *International Journal of Circumpolar Health* 57, Suppl 1 (1998): 43–48.

38. See L. Wittgenstein, *Philosophical Investigations* (Oxford: Basil Blackwell, 1958), #19.

39. See R.M. Gordon, *The Structure of Emotions: Investigations in Cognitive Philosophy* (New York: Cambridge University Press, 1987).

40. Wittgenstein, op. cit.

41. Cf. Ereshefsky, op. cit.

42. Compare Dubos, op. cit.

43. See also R. Veatch, "Just Social Institutions and the Right to Health Care," *Journal of Medicine and Philosophy* 4.2 (1979), and J.S. Millis, "Wisdom? Health? Can Society Guarantee Them?" *New England Journal of Medicine* 283 (30 Jul 1970): 260–261.

44. For more on this and related issues, see P.C. Hébert, A.V. Levin and G. Robertson, "Bioethics for Clinicians: 23. Disclosure of Medical Error." *CMAJ* 164.4 (20 Feb 2001): 509–513.

45. Chaoulli and Zeliotis v. Quebec (2005) SCC 35.

46. See *Building on Values*, loc. cit.

47. President's Commission for the Study of Ethical Problems in Medicine and Biomedical and Behavioral Research, *Securing Access to Health Care*, 3 vols., "The Ethical Implications of Differences in the Availability of Health Services," (Washington, DC: U.S. Govt. Printing Office, 1983), Vol. 1, 16.

48. See *Securing Access*, Vol. 1, 17.

49. A. Buchanan, "The Right to a Decent Minimum of Health Care," in *Securing Access*, Vol. 2, 232. See also D. Gauthier, "Unequal Need: A Problem of Equity in Access to Health Care," in *Securing Access* (ref. note 33), Vol. 2, 179–205.

50. N. Daniels, "Equity of Access to Health Care: Some Conceptual and Ethical Issues," *Milbank Memorial Fund Quarterly* 60.1 (1982), reprinted in *Securing Access* (ref. note 33), Vol. 2, especially 41–47; and D. Wikler, "Philosophical Perspectives on Access to Health Care: An Introduction," *Securing Access*, Vol. 2, especially 219 ff.

51. For a good economic analysis of the right to health care, see R.G. Evans, *Strained Mercy*, available at www.chspr.ubc.ca/files/publications/1997/Strained_Mercy/StrainedMercy_bookmarked.pdf

52. For a current perspective on the need for expanded health services for Aboriginal communities, see Health Council of Canada, *The Health Status of Canada's First Nations, Metis and Inuit Peoples* (2005), available at http://healthcouncilcanada.ca.c9.previewyoursite.com/docs/papers/2005/Bkgrd HealthyCdnsENG.pdf

53. J.J. Heagerty, *Report on Public Health in Canada* (Ottawa: King's Printer, 1943).

54. R.J. Romanow, *Building on Values: The Future of Health Care in Canada. Final Report* (Ottawa: Royal Commission on the Future of Health Care in Canada, 2002)

55. J. Rawls, *A Theory of Justice*, rev. ed. (Oxford: Oxford University Press, 1999), Chapter 1.

56. *Health Care Protection Act*, Revised Statutes of Alberta 2000, c. H-1, available at www.qp.alberta.ca/documents/Acts/H01.pdf

57. Ibid., s. 4.

58. Ibid., s. 3.

59. Thomas Hobbes, *Leviathan* I, 13. As J. Rawls, op. cit., has pointed out, this formalization need not be explicitly codified or even explicitly entered into in a formal way. It may merely exist *de facto.*

60. For a brief overview of First Nations medicine, see First Nations Health Society, *Environmental Scan: Traditional Models of Wellness* (2010), available at www.fnhc.ca/pdf/Traditional_Models_of_ Wellness_Report_FIN-_2010.pdf. For a First Nations Medicine Wheel (First Nations University), see www.firstnationsuniversity.ca/files/File/Science/Fidji/Medicine%20Wheel%20Booklet,%20reduced.pdf

61. For a brief overview of some alternative medicines, see Mayo Clinic Staff, "Complementary and Alternative Medicine: What Is It?," available at www.mayoclinic.com/print/alternative-medicine/PN00001/METHOD=print

62. S.H. Lee and B.C. Lee, "Use of Acupuncture as a Treatment Method for Chronic Prostatitis/Chronic Pelvic Pain Syndromes," *Current Urology Reports* 12.4 (Aug 2011): 288–296. For a somewhat more guarded conclusion for asthma, see T.Y Choi et al., "Moxibustion for Rheumatic Conditions: A Systematic Review and Meta-Analysis," *Clin Rheumatol* 30.7 (Jul 2011): 937–945; C.A. Smith et al., "Acupuncture or Acupressure for Pain Management in Labour," *Cochrane Database System Review* 7 (6 Jul 2011): CD009232.

63. F. Benedetti, I. Rainero and A. Pollo, "New Insights into Placebo Analgesia," *Curr Opin Anaesthesiol* 16.5 (2003): 515–519; M.E. Wechsler et al., "Active Albuterol or Placebo, Sham Acupuncture, or No Intervention in Asthma," *N Engl J Med* 365.2 (14 Jul 2011): 119–126.

64. P.P. Barros, "Cream-Skimming, Incentives for Efficiency and Payment System," *Journal of Health Economics* 22.3 (2003): 419–443; R.B. Deber, *Delivering Health Care Services: Public, Not-for-Profit or Private?* Discussion Paper 17, Commission on the Future of Health Care in Canada (2002), available at www.teamgrant.ca/M-THAC%20Greatest%20Hits/Bonus%20Tracks/Delivering %20Health%20Care%20Services.pdf

65. For a comparison of Canada and the U.S., see S. Woolhandler et al., "Health Care Administration in the United States and Canada: Micromanagement, Macro Costs," *Int J Health Serv* 34.1 (2004): 65–78.

66. J.C. Harsanyi, "Cardinal Welfare, Individualistic Ethics, and Interpersonal Comparison of Utility," *J. Polit. Economy* 63 (1955): 309–321.

67. Rawls, op. cit., 53.

68. Loc. cit., 47.

69. N. Daniels, *Just Health Care* (Cambridge: Cambridge University Press, 1985).

70. R. Nozick, *Anarchy, State and Utopia* (New York: Basic Books, 1974).

71. See H.T. Engelhardt Jr., *The Foundations of Bioethics* (New York: Oxford University Press, 1986), Chapter 8.

72. For a further critique of health as a right, see J.C. Moskop, "Rawlsian Justice and a Human Right to Health Care," *Journal of Medicine and Philosophy* 8.4 (Nov 1983): 329–338.

73. Canadian Institute for Health Information, *Supply, Distribution and Migration of Canadian Physicians, 2009,* available at http://secure.cihi.ca/cihiweb/products/SMDB_2009_EN.pdf

74. K.E. Lasser, D.U. Himmelstein and S. Woolhandler, "Access to Care, Health Status, and Health Disparities in the United States and Canada: Results of a Cross-National Population-Based Survey," *Am J Public Health* 96.7 (2006): 1300–1307.

75. Lasser et al., op. cit.

76. J. Antoniou et al., "In-Hospital Cost of Total Hip Arthroplasty in Canada and the United States," *Journal of Bone and Joint Surgery* 86.11 (2004): 2435–2439; M.J. Eisenberg et al., "Outcomes and Cost of Coronary Artery Bypass Graft Surgery in the United States and Canada," *Arch Intern Med* 165 (2005): 1506–1513; A.J. Pozen and D.M. Cutler, "Comparing Health of People with Heart Disease in the United States and Canada," *Forum for Health Economics & Policy* 12.2 (2009), electronic article.

77. F. Abdullah et al., "Analysis of 23 Million U.S. Hospitalizations: Uninsured Children Have Higher All-Cause In-Hospital Mortality," *Journal of Public Health* 32.3 (2010): 236–244.

78. There are exceptions. There are professional "lab rats" who earn their living as research subjects. However, these lab rats do not come from the well-to-do levels of society. For more, see www.msnbc.msn.com/id/23727874/ns/health-health_care/t/human-lab-rats-loan-bodies-science-cash/

79. P.E. Peterson, "The World Oral Health Report 2003: Continuous Improvement of Oral Health in the 21st Century—The Approach of the WHO Oral Health Programme," *Community Dental Oral Dental Epidemiology* 31, Suppl 1 (2003): 3–24.

80. R.A. Seymour, P.M. Preshaw and J.G. Steele, "Oral Health and Heart Disease," *Primary Dental Care* 9.4 (2002): 125–130; F. DeStefano et al., "Dental Disease and Risk of Coronary Heart Disease and Mortality," *British Medical Journal* 306 (13 Mar 1993): 688–691.

81. R.J. Romanow, *Building on Values: The Future of Health Care in Canada. Final Report* (Ottawa: Commission on the Future of Health Care in Canada, 2002), 5, 25, *et pass.*

82. Unless the relevant provinces have agreements that "apportion the costs differently." *CHA*, s. 11(1)(i).

83. Op. cit., 211–231.

84. Ibid., 189–210.

85. Ibid., 189–210.

86. Romanow, 76–82.

87. Ibid., 83–89.

88. Ibid., 128 ff.

89. Ibid., 150–153.

90. Ibid, 159–188.

91. Ibid., 28 f.

92. Ibid., 30 ff.

93. C.H. Tuohy, C.M. Flood and M. Stabile, "How Does Private Finance Affect Public Health Care Systems? Marshaling the Evidence from OECD Nations," *Journal of Health Politics, Policy and Law* 29.3 (2004): 359–396.

1. Marcia has been an IV drug user and sex trade worker since the age of 16. She was given up as a baby by her mother, who had left her reserve to live in Saskatoon. Marcia was disconnected from her Aboriginal heritage during her formative years, and, like her adoptive siblings, was mentally and physically abused as she grew older. She has recently been in contact with her extended biological family from her mother's reserve; they have suggested that she consult a native healer who has had great success in helping addicted First Nations people, and that she should petition the province for the necessary funds to detox and support herself without continuing her life as a sex trade worker. The province has refused her request, stating that Aboriginal people do not fall under the provincial health plan, and that in any case, native healing and Aboriginal health practices are not considered appropriate health care and are therefore not insured services.

2. R. is a convicted felon who is incarcerated in a maximum security prison for 25 years for aggravated sexual assault on a teenage boy. He had been using intravenous drugs and had contracted hepatitis C and is now in end-stage liver failure. He is evaluated by the prison medical team and found to be a suitable candidate for transplantation. He is listed with the transplant coordinator and awaits transplantation. J. is a primary caregiver of three young children but lives alone with them in subsidized housing, since he has no job. His end-stage liver failure is the result of hepatitis C, which he contracted through a blood transfusion after a car accident. He had to quit his job as a custodian in a local school on account of his illness. He has not been listed as a liver recipient because, aside from his ailing father, he has no support network, and without such a network, transplant recipients tend not to do well. This latter fact has led to the general policy that only people with support networks should receive transplants.

3. The health district of V. wants to build a state-of-the-art hospital. The planning committee for the health district decides that in order to pay for the building and the running of the hospital, they will have two VIP floors. These will be called "special service" wards to distinguish them from the "basic medical service" wards in the rest of the hospital. The VIP floors are not reserved for people with high social status but are open to all who are willing to pay an extra premium. These patients will receive amenities such as private rooms with private toilets, telephones, colour televisions, Internet access, refrigerators, better food, flowers, newspapers and other comforts that are not available to regular patients on the other floors. However, all patients, regardless of whether they are "basic service" patients or "special service" patients, will receive the same standard of medical care. The additional revenue the VIP floors bring in is added to the general hospital funds to cover, among other expenses, the cost of new equipment and extra staff that the hospital could not otherwise afford.

Chapter 10
Resource Allocation

This chapter deals with the right to health care when resources are limited. It distinguishes between macro-allocation (allocation at the policy level involving groups of individuals) and micro-allocation (allocation at the hands-on level of individual patients) and suggests some important considerations that are relevant when trying to resolve the conflicts that arise between competing claims.

Questions to Keep in Mind While Reading this Chapter:

1. Are there limits to society's obligation to provide health care? What would ground such a limit?

2. What is the difference between macro-allocation and micro-allocation in health care? What is vertical ethical conflict? Can it be avoided?

3. What are some ethically acceptable criteria for macro-allocation? For micro-allocation? What are some ethically dubious criteria? Why are they acceptable or dubious?

4. Are special considerations relevant when considering health care resource allocation to First Nation, Inuit and Métis peoples? To health care professionals? What about poverty?

5. What is the difference between hetero- and auto-induced health needs? Does the distinction have any relevance when it comes to allocating health care resources?

6. What is the phenomenon of the identified victim? What role (if any) should it play in resource allocation?

INTRODUCTION

As was indicated in the previous chapter, a just society has an obligation to provide some level of health care to its members. However, society also has an obligation to provide education, transportation and in general those services and infrastructures that underlie society's very existence and make its survival possible. All of these have to be funded from the same resource pool—and that resource pool is limited. Therefore, health care will always compete with other social services for these finite resources.

Resource limitation may not present much of a problem when health services are relatively cheap and the demands on them are not overwhelming. However, as the services become more expensive, the number of people who demand them increases and the types of services that are demanded goes up, society has to develop a rational decision matrix to decide how the available resources will be divided. In other words, society then has to develop a rational, and above all ethically consistent, way of dealing with the question of who shall have when not all can have. The issue becomes particularly pressing as the age demographic shifts towards the upper end, because health care for older people tends to be more expensive than health care for younger people.[1]

However, the problem is not simply one of demand and of demographics. The increasing technological sophistication of medicine and of health care itself is another driver. Thus, while the development of medical imaging technologies such as computerized axial tomography (CAT scans), magnetic resonance imaging (MRI)[2] and positron emission tomography (PET scans)[3] has improved the diagnostic abilities of physicians, their use comes with tremendous capital expenditure and operating costs. Similarly, the use of surgical procedures such as bypass surgery, mastectomies and prostatectomies, which nowadays have become almost routine, also have a cost attached to them that includes the material costs of the operations themselves, the patients' stays in hospital and the salaries for physicians, nurses, technicians, administrators, etc.

Moreover, the increased sophistication also has downstream costs. People who otherwise would have died now survive to acquire more illnesses and to require more treatments as they age. This applies to all health care interventions, whether one is looking at neonatal intensive care units, cancer treatment, treatment for chronic diseases or anything else. Increased sophistication brings increased survival—and everyone who survives becomes a downstream drain on the system.

It is easy to lose sight of this and focus only on the immediate benefits for individual patients. But when one loses sight of this, one forgets that with limited resources, what is given to one health care modality is unavailable for another, and what is given to one patient is taken away from the rest.

OVERALL HEALTH CARE BUDGETS WITHIN A SOCIALIZED CONTEXT

To back up a step, the socioeconomic capabilities of society set the overall limits within which any allocation of social resources must occur. Rational policy-making suggests that in order to establish the overall size of a health care budget—more accurately, perhaps, in order to determine how much money should be set aside for health care and how much money should go to other areas of social endeavour—society first needs some understanding of what the overall demands are for each area of social endeavour. This means that society has to develop a statistically valid average health profile for its members and combine this with numbers that describe the costs of current health conditions, the costs of conditions that are likely to develop, the cost of health-related capital expenditures, the salaries of health care professionals and so on. Society has to develop similar figures for all other areas of socially mandated services—i.e., for education, infrastructure, defence, etc. This then provides an overall framework that identifies the relative budgetary needs for all social service sectors and allows a calculation of the implications for each sector under different budgetary constraints.[4] However, these figures by themselves do not answer the question of how large the overall health care budget should be as opposed to, say, the education budget. The reason is that the figures themselves are decision-theoretically neutral and lack action gradients. (For values as action gradients, see Chapter 1, "Ethics as a Discipline.") What provides them with action gradients are the values that are placed on the various types of services. These values can come only from the people who look at the figures and who apply values to them.

The question, of course, is whose values should be used. Arguably, in a democratic society they should not be the values of political decision-makers—unless the latter have been elected precisely on the basis of their values. Instead, they should be the values of society itself. If this is correct, then the next step for a society that wants to have a rational approach to resource allocation is to identify the values that shape society and their relative weight. For example, is health a fundamental value? Security? Mobility? Education? What is the relative strength with which each of these is valued? This will then provide some understanding of what society as a whole is willing to give to one area as opposed to another.

However, ethically speaking, this is still insufficient. What has been outlined so far would allow a society to decide that it would prefer to devote the majority of its resources to aggressive warlike efforts rather than to things such as health care—which in turn would mean that people who needed health care to live decent lives or to have an equal opportunity to fulfill their life goals would be penalized for their ill health. That, however, would be unjust. Therefore, only social values that are congruent with the Universal Declaration of Human Rights would be ethically acceptable. When consistently applied, they would then lead to allocation decisions at the policy level that would provide an ethically defensible global health care budget.

MACRO-ALLOCATION

Once society has (ethically) determined the size of its overall health care budget, the fact that there are different types of health care services becomes important. In other words, the problem of *macro-allocation* now arises.

Macro-level of allocation, then, is concerned with competition between types of health care services—and the important question here is whether there is some ethically defensible mechanism for dealing with this issue. Various answers have been proposed. Some have suggested that cost/benefit considerations should be determinative, in other words, that only modalities that provide a positive economic benefit for society in return for its investment should be funded.[5] Others have focused on cost/effectiveness coefficients, arguing that only those modalities should be funded that can be shown to have the greatest level of positive outcome relative to other modalities.[6] Still others have suggested that quality-of-life years gained (QALYs)—which is to say modalities that predictably result in the best relative quality of life over the greatest number of years for their recipients—should be used.[7] A variant on this position is the suggestion that disability-adjusted life-years (DALYs) should be used—which is to say, a measure that compares modalities with respect to how much they reduce the disabilities of their recipients relative to each other. Et cetera.

So far, no clear favourite has emerged. There is a tendency on the part of health care funders (provincial governments, hospital districts and so on) to assume that efficiency and effectiveness are the primary determinants of just and fair allocation. However, this is not necessarily true. There may be no effective way of dealing with a particular health issue, simply because no appropriate treatment has been developed. Mental health problems in particular are here implicated, but so are congenital diseases such as Tay-Sachs, various metastasized cancers and others. Then there are the so-called orphan diseases. These are diseases that affect such a small number of people that pharmaceutical companies simply cannot afford to develop the relevant drugs, because the market would be too small to allow them to recoup their investment.[8] Given these various issues, it may be useful to take a closer look at some of the considerations that should play a role in ethically grounded macro-allocation.

Possible versus Impossible

One should perhaps start out with the fundamental ethical principle that one cannot have an obligation to do the impossible. (See the discussion of the Principle of Impossibility in Chapter 1.) Therefore, society cannot have an obligation to devote resources to treating conditions and illnesses that are incurable at the present time. Here, diseases such as Huntington's disease, Tay-Sachs and the various trisomies come to mind.[9] This does not mean that society should not fund research into these diseases. Nor does it mean that resources should not be allocated for symptomatic and ameliorative care. Since such care can be provided, it follows that by definition it is not impossible and therefore constitutes a legitimate area of allocation. However, it does mean that society does not have an obligation to fund experimental or non-validated treatments in the same way it funds treatments that are demonstrably possible and effective.[10]

At the same time, the mere fact that a particular treatment is possible and effective does not entail that it should therefore be funded. For example, liposuction is a possible and effective cosmetic treatment for fat deposits, as is Botox for wrinkles. However, these are not medically necessary treatments, and funding them would reduce the resources that are available for medically necessary treatments such as appendectomies or immunizations against mumps, measles and rubella.

In other words, the important thing to keep in mind is that macro-allocation should always occur within the context of the general right to health care. What ethically grounds the general right to health care is society's duty to maximize, to the best of its ability, equality of opportunity for all of its members. (See Chapter 9, "Health, Health Care and Social Justice.") To a considerable degree, the ability to take advantage of these opportunities depends on the health status of its members. People who suffer from malaria cannot take advantage of schooling to the same degree as other persons; people who suffer from cystic fibrosis, measles or abscessed teeth are similarly disadvantaged; and so on. This means that macro-allocation should always try to ensure that all members of society have access to what has been called a "decent minimum" of medically necessary health care.[11] Only in that way will it be possible to minimize health- or illness-grounded disadvantages.[12]

Threshold Effectiveness

Another important factor to be kept in mind is that not all levels of allocation are meaningful. That is to say, every area of health care has a certain basic funding level that must be reached before the service becomes effective. For instance, unless pediatric cardiac operations are funded at a sufficient level to allow the surgical teams to perform them a certain number of times in any given year, the success rate will deteriorate and cause a dramatic decline in positive outcomes.[13] Similarly, allocating funds to a cancer radiation treatment program or buying diagnostic equipment for case rooms but not providing sufficient funds for employing and training the necessary staff leaves the programs ineffective; and allocating only enough funds to cover immunization programs in urban centres without funding the same for rural areas threatens the effectiveness of the whole undertaking, because it assumes that rural and urban areas are isolated and independent of each other. In short, funding that does not permit threshold effectiveness is essentially wasted.

Vertical Ethical Conflict: Deontological versus Utilitarian Ethics

Also, and at an ethically much deeper level, there is the problem that while macro-allocation that satisfies the Principle of Fidelity involves using the best available statistical data and calculating budgets on that basis, this means that individual persons and their respective rights have to be treated as calculable quantities. However, individual patients are not statistical data, and rights are not calculable quantities.

It is at this point that the difference between deontological and utilitarian ethics becomes important. From a deontological perspective, persons cannot be treated in numerical terms, and the strength of a person's rights is not a function of the number of people who have the right or of the cost of providing the relevant service. Thus, from a deontological perspective, the fact that there are more people who need appendectomies than there are people who need HIV/AIDS treatment does not mean that the right of those who need HIV/AIDS treatment therefore weighs any less or merits less attention, even if HIV/AIDS treatment is more expensive than appendectomies. Rather, the effectiveness of a right is a function of the strength of the relevant claim itself, not of how many other people have a similar claim or what it costs to provide the service.

However—and this is a powerful argument in favour of using a utilitarian approach at the macro-level—it is simply impossible to develop a rational and, above all, consistent approach to health care policy-making without looking at outcomes and using numbers. In other words, the Principle of Impossibility seems to leave no alternative to using a calculative approach, because one cannot satisfy the Principle of Fidelity in any other way.

The upshot of this seems to be that the demand of rational macro-allocation makes *vertical ethical conflict* an inescapable feature of rational and ethically responsible health care itself. While at the macro- or planning level decision-making is governed by considerations of utility, at the micro-level of hands-on health care it is governed by deontological considerations. The difference between the two ethical approaches sets the stage for conflict—and this, of course, is what frequently happens.[14]

Non-Average Needs

Also, if macro-allocation were based solely on the statistically average medical profile of the population, it would violate the very duty that underpins the obligation to provide health services in the first place: the duty, namely, to maximize equality of opportunity for *everyone*. The reason here is that funding only statistically average health care needs would guarantee that persons whose health care needs fell outside the social norm—people who had statistically rare conditions[15] such as Huntington's disease,[16] Gaucher disease[17] or thalassemia[18]—would never have their health care needs addressed. The relevant funding would simply not be forthcoming.

For reasons that have already been indicated, the ethics of such a purely statistically based funding system is questionable. Genetic, environmental and socioeconomic factors produce inequalities that manifest themselves in different health status and health care needs. Social institutions that do not take this into account and treat everyone the same are egalitarian in nature, but by that very token they are unjust precisely because they treat everyone the same. In effect, they punish the disadvantaged for being the victims of bad luck, and reward the advantaged for their undeserved stroke of good fortune. While they treat everyone the same, they treat them unjustly.

That is to say, to treat people the same is to treat them as though there were no ethically relevant differences between them. In fact, of course, there are. That is why justice must be construed as equity.[19] Ethically defensible macro-allocation should therefore take into account the special needs of people who do not fit the statistically average health status profile of society; and a just society should adopt a macro-allocation approach that tries to reconcile the vertical conflict arising out of the need to use arithmetic calculations at the policy level while maintaining deontological considerations at the level of hands-on delivery.

Primary and Secondary Macro-Allocation

One way of achieving this without abandoning the undeniable need for calculations at the macro-level is to structure macro-allocation into two streams: one stream—what might be called *primary macro-allocation*—designed to provide the aforementioned "decent minimum" of health care by addressing the statistically average health care needs of society; and a second stream—what might be called *secondary macro-allocation*—intended to address the needs of individuals who are not served by primary allocation because their needs fall outside of the statistical norm.

However, to structure this second stream solely on the basis of need would be unworkable, because it would undermine the very possibility of health care itself. Need is like a bottomless pit. It can swallow up a whole health care budget—sometimes even without reasonable expectation of positive results. Funding for HIV/AIDS is a good example. If HIV/AIDS were funded solely on the basis of need, where need was identified as the need for a cure, the amount of money needed to achieve this would be staggering. Likewise for Ebola, Creutzfeldt-Jakob disease, diabetes and fatal familial insomnia. Justice therefore demands that both primary and secondary macro-allocation involve some limitation and some balancing. Considerations based on Justice, Beneficence and Fidelity suggest the following:

> 1. The condition that falls outside of the societal norm must result in a lower than statistically average health status.

The underlying reason here is that an unusual condition should not trigger special funding if it does not affect the ability of the affected persons to take advantage, on an equal basis, of the opportunities that are available to everyone else. For instance—and this is merely an example for illustrative purposes—the fact that some people suffer from baldness does not mean that special funds should be set aside for the treatment of baldness. It may be that baldness is a health condition. That does not, however, mean that it results in a lower-than-average health status and prevents the affected persons from participating on an equitable basis in social interactions.

> 2. The average health status of society (as achieved by primary macro-allocation) should not be adversely affected by the special, secondary macro-allocation.

That is to say, it is not as though those whose health care needs do not fit the societal norm do not also have needs that are shared by the rest of society. To continue with the previous examples, the people who get Ebola, Creutzfeldt-Jakob disease or suffer from fatal familial insomnia also get the flu, mumps, measles and have heart attacks—and these are precisely what would be funded under primary macro-allocation. It is just that they have special needs that exceed the statistical norm, and it is these special needs that are to be addressed by the secondary macro-allocation.

> 3. The projected (reasonably-to-be-expected) health status of the recipients of preferential (secondary) macro-allocation must be at least as good as the one that existed

prior to the allocation, where the improvement/retention of the status must be trace-able to the secondary allocation.

This condition derives from the Principle of Fidelity. That is to say, there is an old saying that it is silly to throw good money after bad. In health care, it is not merely silly but unethical. The fact that resources are limited means that what is not used effectively is misused. Therefore, while it may be necessary to provide a greater-than-average alloca-tion for a particular disadvantaged group, that allocation must be effective. Otherwise, it wastes resources that could be used to raise the overall health status of every member of society. Therefore, if neither the improvement in the health status of this group nor even the retention of its current health status is traceable to secondary allocation, then the special allocation violates the Principle of Fidelity. This means that both primary and secondary macro-allocation should involve only scientifically valid modalities. Every-thing else should fall under the rubric of research and experimentation—which falls under a separate rubric of health care resource allocation.

More could be said about primary and secondary macro-allocation. The preceding comments are merely intended to give some idea of the mix of ethical and pragmatic variables that go into developing an ethically defensible macro-allocation policy. How-ever, three points are perhaps worth separate mention. *First*, the threshold-level effect that was mentioned in the discussion of primary macro-allocation also applies in the case of secondary macro-allocation. This may entail that even with secondary macro-allocation there will be health care needs that will not be met.

Second, the preceding discussion is based on the assumption that there is no absolute and universally valid pattern of health care macro-allocation that holds for all societies. This seems valid, because the general health profile of a given society is a function of its population makeup, the total socioeconomic environment in which it is embedded and related factors. All of these play an important role in determining what the society can afford and what it is ethically obligated to provide in terms of health care.

Third, while it is ethically appropriate to recognize the legitimacy of special needs, adjustments to meet these needs cannot be open-ended. Ethical health care macro-allocation should distinguish between what is possible and what can reasonably and fairly be expected.

SPECIAL NON-MEDICALLY DEFINED GROUPS

First Nations

The discussion so far has focused on parameters that find their basis in purely medical conditions and has assumed that society is socially more or less homogeneous. However, that is not necessarily true—particularly in the Canadian context. First Nations, Métis and Inuit peoples are here implicated. It is therefore important to ask whether this makes an ethically relevant difference with regard to macro-allocation.

To answer this question, and to put the matter into perspective, some background may be useful. As was mentioned in the preceding chapter, First Nations, Métis and Inuit peoples are not covered by the *Canada Health Act*. In fact, in 1974, the Minister of National Health and Welfare stated in Parliament that the Government of Canada had no statutory or treaty obligations to provide health services to Canada's Aboriginal peoples, although he did go on to say that Government would make every attempt to ensure "the availability of services by providing it directly where normal provincial services [were] not available, and giving financial assistance to indigent Indians to pay for necessary services when the assistance [was] not otherwise provided."[20] It was on this basis that the federal government moved to provide First Nations, Métis and Inuit peoples with health services through its Medical Services Branch either directly, by providing nursing and medical care, or indirectly, by funding private health care practitioners to provide such services on reserves and in First Nation communities.[21]

However, as the Royal Commission on Aboriginal Peoples stated in 1996,[22] the health services that were made available under this rubric were entirely inadequate and did not meet their health care needs nor, quality-wise, were they on a par with what was available to all other qualified Canadian residents. The Recommendations of the Royal Commission therefore included the proposal that there be a progressive transfer of control over health care to First Nations and Inuit communities through a Health Transfer Policy, whereby this transfer should be formalized through transfer agreements between the federal government and the various communities of Aboriginal peoples.

Irrespective of how successful this policy development has been—and if current health status indicators are anything to go by, it has not been very great[23]—the whole issue raises the question that was intimated in the preceding chapter and that was the point of departure of this digression: Is it ethically appropriate, from the perspective of health care allocation policy, for a society to distinguish between different groups, not on the basis of medical need but on the basis of ethnic or cultural background, and to have distinct approaches to resource allocation depending on the socio-cultural or ethnic status of the groups in question?

It is at this juncture that the difference between ethical and legal considerations becomes important. Legally, neither Canada's constitution[24] nor any applicable treaties oblige the Canadian government to provide health services to its Aboriginal citizens. Ethically, however, the situation is different.[25]

To see why, let us return for a moment to the relationship between a society and its members. All members of a society are equal as persons. Therefore, ethically speaking, all have the same entitlements and are subject to (and are the beneficiaries of) the same ethical considerations. Anything else constitutes discrimination. Hence, it follows that, ethically speaking, if society has a duty to provide health care to its members, then that duty extends to *all* of its members. Of course, how that duty is met may differ from situation to situation. In fact, differences in individual situations may require appropriate adjustments in order to preserve equity. The important point is that the treatment accorded to the individuals and groups in question must be equitable and fair.

Moreover, Canadian society has an obligation to ensure that the resources available to an administrative health care unit are sufficient to ensure the same decent minimum of health care that is available to the constituents of all other administrative units. In the case of First Nations and other Aboriginal communities, this means that (subject to a consideration that will be raised in a moment) the same level of funding should be available to them as is available to all provincial jurisdictions under the *Canada Health Act*, so that their macro-allocation policies can be developed and implemented in an equitable manner.

From a purely administrative perspective, therefore, this means that the allocation policies that govern the delivery of health care should be shaped by the very same ethically grounded macro-allocation considerations, and that differences between the administrative structures that provide that care, irrespective of whether they are provincial, federal or Aboriginal in nature, should not make any difference—as neither should the source of funding. In other words, while the identity of a particular administrative health unit may be variable—and constitutional factors here play a legitimate role—the ethics of the administration should be uniform, because all members of society, no matter what their identity or origin, are equal as persons.

This, however, is only a partial answer. Aboriginal communities tend to be characterized by a lower socioeconomic profile than non-Aboriginal communities. Arguably, this disadvantaged position is the result of historical injustices. Moreover, a lower socioeconomic status tends to translate into a lower health status. In light of the above, this entails that as a matter of equity, First Nations, Inuit and Métis communities have a right to special macro-allocation considerations in order to compensate for and, if possible, overcome these disadvantages, so that the members of these communities will truly be on an equal footing with the rest of Canadian society. Historical injustices, therefore, seem to entail special consideration.

Further discussion of the topic of historical social injustices towards Aboriginal peoples (and of what this entails in terms of compensation and redress) transcends the scope of the present discussion. With respect to the ethics of macro-allocation in health care, however, at least this much seems clear: The federal government has an ethical duty, under its Health Transfer Policy, to provide its First Nations, Inuit and Métis communities with funding which, although independent of standard transfer arrangements between federal and provincial levels of government, nevertheless is sufficient to allow these communities to provide the same kind and level of health care, subject to the same macro-allocation considerations, as the health care that is provided to all other Canadians. This may mean that the proportion of health care funding for these communities should be larger than that for other communities, no matter what statutes or treaties are in place. The important point here is that statutes and treaties are legal in nature. They do not determine the ethics. Legal rights and obligations are a matter of contract; ethical rights and obligations are a matter of the interrelationship between persons as persons.

Poverty

It is a short step from asking whether historically grounded differences in social embedding mandate ethically distinct treatment, to the question of whether economically grounded differences in social embedding mandate ethically distinct treatment. In both cases, after all, one is dealing with groups of people who are identified not on the basis of health status but on the basis of social considerations. The question assumes particular importance because poverty tends to be correlated with poor health status.

The short answer is that the two are not on a par. Logically, the position of peoples whose very identity as peoples gave rise to distinct and discriminatory social treatment and socioeconomic conditions is different from the position of peoples whose socioeconomic position is not grounded in their identity as peoples. To treat them the same is to say that the causes of a particular state of affairs have no bearing on the ethical considerations, just so long as the situation itself is the same. That is to confuse a cause with an effect.

Moreover, one has to distinguish between the causal factors that lead to health issues and the health issues themselves. The determinants of health are multifactorial. Poverty is certainly one of them—but so are education, housing, nutrition, sanitation and even transportation.[26] The function of health care is not to deal with health and health-related determinants in this global sense. If it were, then, directly or indirectly, health care would include all social services. In fact, health care would be the only rubric of social obligation.[27] Instead, the function of health care is to deal with health-related issues insofar as these directly and clinically involve physical and mental well-being. (See the discussion of the nature of health in Chapter 9.)

If certain health conditions are preferentially associated with or even caused by certain socioeconomic factors, then these factors will be addressed under a properly structured overall social macro-allocation policy, i.e., the non-clinical causal factors giving rise to health conditions are properly dealt with as a matter of general social policy, because a rationally structured social policy will want to take health determinants into account. To deal with these determinants is not a matter of health care itself. Consequently the federal government's Health Transfer Policy for First Nations, Inuit and Métis peoples should not properly be seen as a matter of health care but as an attempt to deal with historically grounded social injustices that express themselves in health care terms.

Age

There are other approaches to macro-allocation. Age, for instance, has increasingly emerged as a possible criterion.[28] The argumentation here takes various forms. One version—the so-called "fair innings" argument[29]—maintains that the elderly have already lived and have had their opportunity to access health care resources, whereas the younger people have not yet had their turn. Equity therefore demands that younger patients be given priority over older ones. Another version focuses on the fact that in most instances—and in particular for acute care—interventions on older patients are less likely to have a positive outcome than on younger patients. Since the whole point of allocation is to make the best use possible of what is available, it is only reasonable to use those resources where they will do the most good. A still different argument says that the benefits of health care, both for society and for patients, decrease with advancing age. Therefore, to provide the elderly with health care when the benefits are seriously reduced is to be guilty of mismanagement—and thus violate the Principle of Fidelity.

The problem with age-based rationing in general is that it covertly defines the right to health care in terms of effectiveness of treatment and cost.[30] If the issue really is one of effectiveness and cost—and this will be discussed further in a moment—then it does not necessarily single out the elderly as being less worthy of treatment. It applies to anyone whose treatment is less effective than anyone else's, irrespective of age. In particular, those who suffer from chronic conditions or are incurably disabled will be particularly implicated.

Furthermore, the notion of being elderly is a moving target. It changes as the demographics of society change and with advances in medical science, pharmacology and social services such as housing, nutrition and sanitation[31]—as well as with reproductive patterns. Consequently it will not yield an objective criterion that is stable over time—which means that it will lead to discrimination even within the very same population.

As to the fair innings version of the argument, while it may be true that some older people have already had the opportunity to access health care, this is not true of all older people. Those in outlying and underserviced communities would certainly not fall into that category, as neither would First Nations, Inuit and Métis peoples who, as was already pointed out, have not had access to properly structured health care services in the first place.

Moreover, the elderly may have reached old age not because they used the health care system in their younger years but because they have led responsible lives by exercising, eating a proper diet, minimizing stress, etc., and generally have taken care of themselves. It is now, because of the very nature of the aging process (which inevitably entails that the human body will deteriorate at the cellular level and organ systems will start to fail)[32] that they require treatment. To deny such people access to health care because of their age would be to punish them for having been responsible.

MICRO-ALLOCATION

The fact that a particular area of health care has been funded does not guarantee that everyone who needs that type of health care will get it—or will get it right away. Frequently, what happens is that more patients need the relevant care than the caregivers can provide for. Consider, for example, the following case:

> Mark is a seventy-five-year-old carpenter who has been a smoker for sixty years and continues to be a moderate smoker (one pack a day). Among other things, he now suffers from emphysema and has been told by his primary care physician and his respirologist that his life expectancy is extremely limited unless he gets a new lung. However, there are fifteen other patients on the transplant waiting list. One of them is

a nurse whose lungs were severely damaged by an infection contracted from a patient; another is a police officer whose lungs were burned when a meth lab she was taking down blew up. There also are several teenagers and young adults who suffer from cystic fibrosis, and so on. Should Mark be put on the waiting list? And should the fact that his smoking demonstrably contributed to his lung disease be taken into account?

This case presents a classic problem of micro-allocation: The claim of one individual stands against the competing claims of others.

In a way, micro-allocation is emotionally more difficult than macro-allocation. The reason is simple: At this level one is not dealing with abstract entities, such as groups and subgroups of people, which one can do at a distance. Instead, one is dealing directly with the individuals who make up these groups, and one is dealing with them on a one-on-one footing. Here, the impact of a particular decision is as immediate as it is apparent. Such immediacy involves great psychological pressure.[33]

Another reason is that unlike the impacts of allocations involving groups, the impacts of micro-allocation decisions cannot be lessened by shifting them to another area. There is no slack, no subchoices that could spread the negative effect over a larger base. What is given to Mark will not be available to the nurse or the police officer. It is as simple as that.

Is It Possible to Avoid Micro-Allocation?

At this juncture, it is tempting to suggest that if macro-allocation decisions were made better, there would be no micro-allocation problem, or that the whole issue would disappear if the health care system were structured differently—perhaps by allowing a two-track system in which those who could afford it would be able to buy their care without having to wait. Not only would this make it unnecessary to triage, it would also take the pressure off the publicly funded health care system.

Let us take these suggestions in turn. As to the claim that better macro-allocation would do away with micro-allocation problems, it ignores reality. The reason for macro-allocation is that health care resources are finite. There is nothing anyone can do about that. There are only a certain number of health care professionals who can be trained and who can be available at any one time. The same thing is true of buildings, surgical and infectious disease facilities, medications and so on. Therefore, when demand exceeds supply—as sooner or later it invariably does—micro-allocation decisions have to be made. This is true no matter how efficient the macro-allocation protocols may be.

Second, society cannot simply set aside a certain amount of resources such as beds or drugs—or, for that matter, train and employ a sufficient number of health care professionals—so that each person who is a potential health care consumer would have the relevant resources ready and waiting when the need for these resources materializes. That would require virtually infinite resources. No society is in that position. It would turn health care into a bottomless pit that would swallow not only all available resources but also all of the resources that a society might ever develop. Other areas of legitimate social endeavour also have to be funded, because these other things—education, infrastructure, transportation, research, etc.—are what make society itself (as well as health care) possible. The only thing a society can do is make macro-allocation decisions that are based on the best data available. That is why Canada has established the Canadian Institutes of Health Research. Their role is to provide the relevant data—and these data are statistical in nature.

However, macro-allocation protocols based on statistical models may be flawed, as happened in a recent flu outbreak when the statistical forecast for a particular type of vaccine was simply inaccurate and insufficient doses of the right vaccine were ready for use. Or it may happen that all potential health care users *including the staff and personnel who run the health care services* will need the services simultaneously—as happened during the Spanish flu epidemic in 1918. Therefore, selective allocation at the level of individual persons is an inescapable result of the finitude of society itself. This does not mean that the right to health care at the individual level is a sham. It merely means that allocation criteria at the micro-level must dovetail with the allocation ethics of the macro-level.

As to the suggestion that micro-allocation problems would not exist or would be less severe if Canada adopted a two-track approach to health care, this ignores several important facts. *First*, the private provider track also needs health care professionals. Society can train only a limited number of health care professionals.[34] This means that the private track would compete with the public track and reduce the number of professionals available to the latter. Therefore, rather than this alleviating the pressure on the public system and minimizing micro-allocation problems, it would worsen the problems for the public system.[35]

Second, it would ignore the fact that by their very nature, certain health care resources are in limited supply. The case of Mark above illustrates this rather well. The fact that there are limited numbers of lungs has nothing to do with how well or ill a macro-allocation policy works or whether the health care system is wholly public or allows a private track. Only a limited number of people donate their organs; and given the fact that the number of people who need transplants exceeds the supply of available organs, the issue of micro-allocation remains, no matter what the system.

Third, a private track cannot function (except in a very limited way) unless it has access to public goods. To illustrate the point, let us return to the example of Mark. Mark needs a lung. If he were to go to a private health care provider, that provider would have to acquire a lung to do the transplant. Where would that lung come from? The private provider could not buy the lung because, to put it in legal terms, in Canada there is no ownership in human bodies. That includes organs. These are not sold but donated. Therefore, the private provider would have to compete with the public track for the organs— and not only for organs because, in Canada, blood is also implicated, as are gametes and other human tissues. However, blood, organs and other tissues are not donated with the expectation or the intention that they be used by private for-profit health care providers so that they can make money by selling their services to people who can afford to opt out of the public health system in order to receive quicker care. They are donated with the expectation and intention that people who need them will have an equitable chance of getting them. Allowing the private provider access to these resources and to provide Mark with a better and quicker chance at a transplant therefore assumes that someone can increase their right to health care simply by paying a private provider to take the relevant resources away from the public system. This is in clear contravention of the assumption on the basis of which the relevant resources were made available in the first place.

With due alteration of detail, similar remarks apply to the development of pharmaceuticals, medical and diagnostic equipment, etc. Their development requires research with human subjects and experimentation. Research with human subjects and experimentation relies on volunteers, none of whom volunteer with the expectation or intention of making private health care providers rich or allowing rich patients to receive better care than poor patients. The intent of non-therapeutic experiments is to help others; in the case of therapeutic experiments, it is to help themselves. While volunteers for non-therapeutic experiments may be rewarded, the reward may not be sufficient to overcome the humanitarian element and constitute undue enticement. (For more on this, see Chapter 6 "Research Using Human Subjects.")

Therefore, the whole suggestion that a two-track approach to health care would alleviate the micro-allocation problem is not only factually false but also ethically objectionable.

Ethically Questionable Micro-Allocation Criteria

The question therefore becomes "What criteria are ethically appropriate for making micro-allocation decisions?" There are various candidates, not all of which are ethically defensible. In particular, merit, legal status, "first-come, first-served" and the ability to pay fall into this category, as do economic considerations such as QALYs and DALYs.

Merit The merit criterion suggests that access to scarce resources should be on the basis of whatever contribution a particular patient has made to society. Whoever has made the most substantial contribution to the welfare of society should be first in line.

If this were the deciding criterion, then Mark in the case above would probably lose against the nurse and the police officer. Even though he made important social contributions as a carpenter, the social contributions of carpenters are generally not perceived as being on a par with those of nurses or police officers.[36]

However, this highlights one of the shortcomings of the merit criterion. Merit is a function of social perception, which may have nothing to do with what is actually the case. What is perceived to have merit may simply be the "flavour of the day." Thus, neither police officers nor nurses could function in a society where there were no carpenters to build and maintain the requisite facilities. In what sense, then, do carpenters have "less merit"? Moreover, the criterion would virtually guarantee that certain members of society would always lose in the competition for scarce resources. For example, it would entail that the teenagers and young adults on the transplant list would be even worse off than Mark (even if the lungs were size matches) because they have contributed comparatively little.

In other words, this approach makes two important assumptions: *First*, it assumes that everyone who needs a resource has had the same opportunity as everybody else to contribute to society or to acquire "merit." That is simply not true. *Second*, it assumes that merit is an objectively definable concept and therefore provides an objective ranking scale. That is also not the case.

Legal Status   A related but equally dubious criterion is legal status. It contends that criminals or social miscreants should always go to the bottom of the list. This stance underlies the claim that "to assume that there was little to choose between Alexander Fleming and Adolf Hitler [for access to scarce resources] . . . would be nonsense,"[37] and is in perfect alignment with the opinion that criminals should not have the right to vote,[38] that they should not receive pensions[39] and so on.

The legal-status criterion actually has two parts: that we are responsible for our actions, and that if we do something criminal our ethical status is diminished and we should suffer the consequences.[40] As to the claim that we are responsible for our actions, this claim is ethically defensible and is as old as Plato and Aristotle. However, it is precipitous to equate ethical status with legal status, nor would doing so alleviate the allocation problem. *First* of all, it would not resolve micro-allocation conflicts between people who have the same legal status. The vast majority of people who require access to scarce resources do not differ in this regard. Using the legal-status criterion would therefore provide no way of deciding the allocation problem in the case above.

Second, the criterion would run the risk of producing irremediable harm for people who are wrongfully convicted. Miscarriages of justice do occur. The wrongful convictions of David Milgaard,[41] Donald Marshall, Jr.[42] and Guy Paul Morin[43] are cases in point. In fact, if access to health care were governed by legal standing, Mahatma Gandhi would have had no right to health care because he had been convicted of what was then a criminal act.[44]

Third, the criterion assumes that what is illegal is unethical. This is not necessarily the case. Suicide was a criminal act until 1972; the conduct of commercial enterprises on Sunday was prohibited by the *Lord's Day Act* until 1985[45]; and the buying and selling of alcohol was illegal until the repeal of Prohibition. That did not make these activities unethical.

Finally, and perhaps most importantly, this criterion would turn health care into an instrument of the legal system. This is a fundamental error. The two have different rationales. While, as the United Nations has firmly recognized, access to health care should be equitable and just, that does not mean it should be part of the justice system.[46]

First Come, First Served   Another dubious criterion is first-come, first-served. It would allocate scarce resources in the order in which people accessed the health care system.[47]

The fact that this is a workable criterion does not make it ethically defensible. In the first place, it assumes that everyone has the same chance of accessing the health care system and, so to speak, of getting into line. That is not correct.[48] Geographic location importantly influences one's ability to access the system and to queue up, as does the ability to free oneself from other obligations or to afford appropriate transportation.

Moreover, there are other variables that influence how and in what order one can access the system: things such as the ability to communicate[49] or the bias that a particular medical professional may have in identifying someone as an appropriate candidate for the relevant service and therefore slotting the person into the queue. There even is evidence that mental disability,[50] gender[51] and ethnic extraction may play a role in this regard.[52] All in all, therefore, the first-come, first-served criterion is seriously flawed. It assumes equality of opportunity where none exists.

Age, QALYs, DALYs and Other Considerations

Age has also been suggested as a micro-allocation criterion. Arguments here focus on lower QALYs and DALYs for the elderly, their reduced life expectancy even with treatment,[53] the lower likelihood of successful intervention,[54] the cost-effectiveness and cost-benefit of having access to the intervention,[55] and so on.

The problem with all of these criteria is that they tacitly assume that greater life expectancy and better quality of life—however that may be defined (and there is no agreement on that score)—confer a greater right. Not only is that ethically questionable,[56] it would also mean that if this principle were applied consistently to all patients, it would apply not only to the elderly, but also to all persons who suffer from serious and debilitating diseases or conditions *no matter what their age*. Therefore, as an age-based criterion it would fail.

As to the QALY- and DALY-based arguments specifically, the reasoning here is similar to the age-based argument for macro-allocation. The QALY-based argument begins with the premise that allocation should proceed in a rational and above all objective manner. This, so it contends, is possible only if the allocation criteria are numerically quantifiable. It therefore assigns numerical values to the quality of life that patients would have with the intervention and combines this with the number of years that the patients are likely to survive if they receive the service. The result is a numerical quotient that allows an objective decision as to who should go to the top of the list and who should move further down, simply by ordering access on the basis of the QALY numbers.[57] The DALY-based argument is similar except that it focuses on disability. By combining mortality and disability into a single common metric it yields single quotients that allow objective comparisons.[58]

Quite aside from all else—and defining what counts as a low quality of life or as a disability is problematic in itself—both the QALY and DALY approach tacitly assume that all treatments are equally effective. However, that assumption is questionable. The effectiveness of a particular treatment is largely a function of how much money is invested in developing the treatment and in perfecting it—which, in turn, is functionally related to the number of people who suffer from the relevant condition and the likelihood of economic return for pharmaceutical companies and health care providers who have to develop the treatment modality.[59]

Ethically Possible Criteria

The fact that these criteria are ethically dubious raises the question of whether there are any that are any better. And of course there are.

Need   Need is definitely one of them. All things being equal—the reason for this qualifier will become clear in a moment—the right of patients who need a particular intervention takes priority over the right of patients for whom this is an elective procedure. The reason is simple: Patients whose request for a particular intervention is not need driven are able to wait a little longer without detriment, whereas need-driven patients are not in that position.

However, the notion of need has to be handled carefully. A demand is need driven in an ethically relevant sense only if failure to respond to the demand will lead to an irreparable deterioration of the health status of the individual. For instance, someone with tuberculosis or having a heart attack would suffer serious and irreparable harm if not treated right away, and might even die. By contrast, having a stiff elbow joint cleaned out or a foot defect surgically corrected can wait.

Life Saving versus Quality Enhancing   At the same time, not all need-driven claims are the same. Thus, one can distinguish between a need that is life preserving and one that is quality enhancing. The point is one of logic. The right to a certain quality of life presupposes the right to life as an enabling condition. Therefore, if the two right claims conflict, the one whose claim is for a life-saving intervention takes priority over the one whose claim is for a qualitative intervention. That is why the right to have a facial scar repaired has lower priority than the right to have surgery to remove a cancerous tumour.

Outcome   Another acceptable criterion is outcome. Thus, if an intervention is likely to have a positive outcome for a given patient, then it is ethically appropriate to slot the patient into the queue for the resource; if it is unlikely to be successful, entering the patient into the queue is inappropriate. The scarce resource would simply be wasted—which would violate the Principle of Fidelity.[60]

To illustrate the point, consider two patients: one is dying of metastasized bone cancer and needs a bypass, and another, who is obese, also needs a bypass. It is virtually certain that the cancer patient would not survive the surgery, whereas this is not true of the obese patient. The right of the cancer patient is therefore less strong than the right of the obese patient.

However—and there is always a "however"—one has to be careful here not to understand the notion of positive outcome too narrowly. It refers only to the expected and intended result of the particular intervention in question. While the cancer patient's right to cardiac surgery would be lower than the obese patient's, the cancer patient would still have a right to symptomatic and to palliative care. Likewise, an intervention should be considered successful if it slowed the deterioration in health status of a given individual or allowed that person to retain his or her current level of health.

Origin: Auto- versus Hetero-Induced   Moreover, one can sometimes distinguish between needs that are auto-induced—which is to say, needs that are completely or to a large degree the result of people's own voluntary actions—and hetero-induced needs—which is to say, needs that cannot reasonably be traced to such acts. For example, lung cancer and heart disease are often traceable to smoking and to an immoderate lifestyle, and severe lacerations, fractures and contusions are often the result of not wearing appropriate safety devices when in an automobile. On the other hand, genetically-based diseases such as Huntington's disease or cystic fibrosis lie outside the patient's control, and infectious diseases such as rubella, HIV/AIDS[61] and malaria can be contracted accidentally and despite appropriate precautions. This suggests that the difference between auto- and hetero-induced conditions can be used as a way of prioritizing competing right claims.[62]

That is to say arguably, and as a matter of justice, no one should deliberately interfere with the legitimate rights of others or bring about conditions that will endanger the exercise of their legitimate rights. Auto-induced conditions, however, do just that. They bring about preventable needs which, if met, reduce the amount of resources available and thereby create a scarcity that imperils other people's right to health care. Consequently, all other things being equal, auto-induced needs should have a lower priority than hetero-induced needs.

In other words, one could reasonably argue that distinguishing between the moral ranking of auto- versus hetero-induced needs is merely saying that being responsible and being irresponsible are not ethically on a par. To honour the right claims of irresponsible people to the same degree as those of responsible people would mean that those who lived responsibly and did not decrease the amount of resources available by their actions would have no better access to those resources than those who lived irresponsibly and without concern for others. However, this would mean that responsible people would effectively be punished for being responsible, and irresponsible people would be rewarded. This would violate the Principle of Equality and Justice.

At the same time, it may be difficult to determine whether a health care need is in fact auto-induced. The case of alcoholics and liver transplants illustrates this rather well. There is beginning to be evidence that susceptibility to alcoholism is partly genetically determined.[63] It is unclear of how many other diseases this could be true. It is also unclear what weight one should attach to a genetic predisposition in terms of being responsible for the actualization of that predisposition. Certainly, a predisposition is not a determination, and many people who have a predisposition to alcoholism do not succumb to it. Nevertheless, it seems only reasonable to suggest that while this criterion is appropriate in principle, it requires extreme caution in application.

On a related note, there are professions, such as mining and farming, which have statistically higher accident rates and higher rates for certain diseases than is normal in the population. No one is forced to become a miner or a farmer. One could therefore argue that the health care needs of such workers are auto-induced and therefore fall under this criterion. However, that would be inappropriate. These are socially approved and indeed necessary professions. Without mining, modern medicine would not be possible (metals are necessary for surgical and diagnostic instruments, etc.), and without farming there would be no food. Consequently it seems appropriate to say that if a health care need is associated with a socially approved lifestyle or profession or is necessary for the survival of society as we know it, then it should not fall under the rubric of auto-induced needs.[64]

Lots The criteria that have been sketched so far will not resolve all micro-allocation conflicts. Sometimes all things are equal. A good example would be a case in which two children have both been in the same accident, both require immediate attention and there is no way to tell which one is a better risk. In situations like this, the only option is to draw lots. Lots assign an equal chance to everyone. That is why they are inappropriate when all other things are not equal. In that case, they discriminate against those who are disadvantaged in some way. However, when all other things are equal, the fact that they assign the same chance to everyone is appropriate. They allow for discrimination while retaining the equality of those concerned.

TWO FINAL NOTES ON ALLOCATION

Health Care Professionals and Pandemics

The discussion so far has assumed that all people are equal as people and therefore should have equitable access to health care. In principle, this is certainly correct. However, one cannot provide health care without properly trained professionals. This means that any allocation schema, whether at the macro- or the micro-level, must ensure that a sufficiently large number of properly trained health care providers are available to keep the health care system functioning. And this, in turn, means that under certain circumstances—for instance, during pandemics—a sufficient number of properly trained health care professionals must be given access to the scarce resources, such as vaccines, independently of any ranking or prioritization schema. Of course, this does not mean that every health care professional should have priority over everyone else. The precise number (and identity) would depend on such things as the nature of the pandemic, the number of vaccine dosages available, the size of the potential patient pool and so on. However, *that* such a prioritization should occur is simply a matter of logic. The fulfillment of the right to health care presupposes that there is someone who can provide that care. If only health care professionals fit that category, then a sufficient number of them must be kept alive and functioning. Otherwise the right will fail.

Sidestepping Allocation Protocols: The Phenomenon of the Identified Victim

Finally, no matter what happens in allocation, someone is going to lose. It then may happen that the loser (or somebody on his or her behalf) turns to the media with an appeal for a special allocation that sidesteps the allocation process entirely.[65] This is frequently successful—which is not surprising. It is psychologically easier to refuse resources to a person we don't know than to someone we know. This is what grounds the *phenomenon of the identified victim.*[66] Presenting the identified victim to the public and appealing for help makes it very difficult for the public to refuse access to the needed resources, because now the individual is anonymous no longer. The anonymous group with whom this person stands in competition tugs much less strongly at our heartstrings.

However, as has been argued elsewhere, this approach is seriously flawed.[67] It is to say that the particular individual on whose behalf the appeal is launched somehow should not be subject to the ranking procedures that determine access to the resources. However, to do so would be to exempt this person from these criteria by definition. Ethically, such an approach cannot be defended. The fact that allocation may have a tragic outcome for those who lose does not mean that therefore the allocation process is unethical. Not everything that is tragic is unethical. It would be unethical only if the criteria themselves were unethical or were applied in an unethical manner.

CONCLUSION

Canadian society assumes that just and equitable access to an appropriate level of health care is a matter of right. However, all rights have limits. Health care is no exception, and its limits are inherent in the finite nature of social resources. Given the fact of limitation, there has to be some way to allocate the health care resources in a just and equitable fashion. Moreover, any allocation will advantage some and disadvantage others. That, however, is not really the issue. The issue is whether the fact of comparative disadvantage amounts to unethical discrimination. It is all too easy to lose sight of that fact that what is experienced as a disadvantage, either at first-hand or by considering the plight of others, may be strongly coloured by the psychology of our experience. The phenomenon of the identified victim is a powerful force in the politics of health resource allocation. However, it would ultimately be to everyone's disadvantage if a perception that has its roots in the psychology of experience were to govern a process that should really be determined by considerations of ethics.

Further Readings

Boyle, J. "Limiting Access to Health Care: A Traditional Roman Catholic Analysis," in *Allocating Scare Medical Resources: Roman Catholic Perspectives*, ed. H.T. Engelhardt Jr. and M.J. Cherry (Washington DC: Georgetown University Press, 2002), 77–95.

Callahan, D. "Rationing, Equity, and Affordable Health Care." *Health Progress* 81.4 (2000): 38–41.

Churchill, L.R. "Age-Rationing in Health Care: Flawed Policy, Personal Virtue." *Health Care Analysis* 13.2 (Jun 2005): 137–146.

Cookson, R., and P. Dolan. "Principles of Justice in Health Care Rationing." *Journal of Medical Ethics* 26.5 (2000): 323–329.

Denier, Y. "On Personal Responsibility and the Human Right to Healthcare." *Cambridge Quarterly of Healthcare Ethics* 14.2 (2005): 224–234.

Fleck, L.M. "Just Caring: In Defense of Limited Age-Based Healthcare Rationing." *Cambridge Quarterly of Healthcare Ethics* 19.1 (2010): 27–37.

Hirose, I. "Should We Select People Randomly?" *Bioethics* 24.1 (2010): 45–46.

Kaposy, C. "Accounting for Vulnerability to Illness and Social Disadvantage in Pandemic Critical Care Triage."*Journal of Clinical Ethics* 21.1 (2010): 23–29.

Kerstein, S.J., and G. Bognar. "Complete Lives in the Balance." *American Journal of Bioethics* 10.4 (Apr 2010): 37–45.

Kluge, E.-H. "Resource Allocation in Healthcare: Implications of Models of Medicine as a Profession." *MedGenMed* 9.1 (2007): 57.

Persad, G., A. Wertheimer and E. Ezekiel. "Principles for Allocation of Scarce Medical Interventions." *The Lancet* 373.9661 (2009): 423–431.

Rachels, J. "Who Shall Live When Not All Can Live?" *Soundings: An Interdisciplinary Journal* 53 (1970): 339–355.

Rescher, N. "The Allocation of Exotic Medical Lifesaving Therapy." *Ethics* 79 (1969): 173–180.

Scheunemann, L.P,. and D.B. White. "The Ethics and Reality of Rationing in Medicine." *Chest* 140.6 (2011): 1625–1632.

Tsuchiya, A., and A. Williams. "A 'Fair Innings' between the Sexes: Are Men Being Treated Inequitably?" *Soc Sci Med* 60.2 (Jan 2005): 277–286.

Williams, A. "The Rationing Debate: Rationing Health Care by Age: The Case for." *British Medical Journal* 314 (1997): 820.

Endnotes

1. See M.S. Marzouk, "Aging, Age-Specific Health Care Costs and the Future Health Care Burden in Canada" *Canadian Public Policy* 17.4 (1991): 490–506; J.J. Polder et al., "Age-Specific Increases in Health Care Costs," *European Journal of Public Health* 12.1 (2002): 57–62.

2. This is a computer-assisted technique for visualizing cellular structures in the body by exposing them to alternating magnetic fields. It does not involve X-rays or similar radiation.

3. A PET scan is a nuclear diagnostic tool that involves the injection of a slightly radioactive compound which, when taken up by cells in the body, allows visualization of body functions such as blood flow, oxygen use and sugar (glucose) metabolism, and thus assists in determining how well organs and tissues are functioning.

4. As an aside, it should be noted that while such data have been more or less available for other social sectors, this has not been the case for health care and was identified as a serious shortcoming in the Romanow Report, *Building on Values: The Future of Health Care in Canada. Final Report* (Ottawa: Royal Commission on the Future of Health Care in Canada, 2002), available at www.cbc.ca/healthcare/final_report.pdf. As a result, the federal government established the Canadian Institutes of Health Research (CIHR; www.cihr-irsc.gc.ca). Their mandate is to provide just such data. These data are used by the federal and the provincial governments to rationalize their health budgets.

5. Cost/benefit analysis assigns numerical coefficients to the costs for a given treatment modality and to the financial benefits to society of the outcomes, and then compares the different modalities relative to each other. For a good discussion, see M. Drummond, "Guidelines for Health Technology Assessment: Economic Evaluation," in *Health Care Technology: Effectiveness, Efficiency and Public Policy*, ed. D. Feeny, G. Guyatt and P. Tugwell (Montreal: Institute for Research on Public Policy, 1986).

6. Cost/effectiveness analysis compares numerical coefficients assigned to costs as opposed to the amounts of resources (money) saved for comparable forms of treatment. For several good

discussions, see M.F. Drummond, *Principles of Economic Appraisal in Health Care* (Oxford: Oxford Medical Publications, 1980); R. Sugden and A. Williams, *The Principles of Practical Cost-Benefit Analysis* (Oxford: Oxford University Press, 1978); H.E. Klarman, J.O. Francis and G.D. Rosenthal, "Cost-Effectiveness and Analysis Applied to the Treatment of Chronic Renal Disease," *Medical Care* 6 (1968): 48–54; and N. Daniels, *Just Health Care* (Cambridge and London: Cambridge University Press, 1985).

7. QALYs (Quality Adjusted Life Years) calculations assign numerical coefficients to quality-of-life evaluations and compare them to the cost involved in bringing about the extended lifespan.

8. It is estimated that it costs between $800 million and $1.5 billion to develop a new drug and bring it to market. Given a small number of affected persons, no pharmaceutical company can afford to invest in such development unless its development costs are subsidized. That is why the U.S. has put in place the *Orphan Drug Act* (January 1983). The European Union has similar legislation (Regulation EC 141/2000). Canada does not.

9. Compare N. Rescher, "The Allocation of Exotic Medical Lifesaving Therapy," *Ethics* 79.3 (Apr 1969): 174–186. Although somewhat dated, this is a classic discussion.

10. The issue is considered more fully under the rubric of experimentation and the right to experimental treatment.

11. A. Buchanan, "The Right to a Decent Minimum of Health Care," in *Securing Access to Health Care*, 3 vols., President's Commission for the Study of Ethical Problems in Medicine and Biomedical and Behavioral Research (Washington, DC: U.S. Govt. Printing Office, 1983), Vol. 2, 179–205.

12. Of course, this does not mean that providing a basic level of health care will, in and of itself, maximize equality of opportunity. However, it is a necessary component of maximization. In other words, it is a necessary, albeit not sufficient, condition.

13. See Associate Chief Judge Murray Sinclair, *The Report of the Manitoba Pediatric Cardiac Surgery Inquest: An Inquiry into Twelve Deaths at the Winnipeg Health Sciences Centre*, accessed 4 Jan 2011 at www.pediatriccardiacinquest.mb.ca/index.html

14. E.-H.W. Kluge and K. Tomasson, "Health Care Resource Allocation: Complicating Ethical Factors at the Macro-Allocation Level," *Health Care Analysis* 10.2 (2002): 209–220.

15. In the U.S., a rare (or orphan) disease is generally considered to have a prevalence of fewer than 200,000 affected individuals.

16. An inherited progressive disease of the central nervous system, characterized by progressive spastic involuntary and convulsive movements, dementia, disturbed speech and reduced life expectancy. Death usually occurs within twenty years after the patient has become symptomatic. It is incurable, and its onset is usually in adult life.

17. Gaucher disease is an inherited metabolic disorder. Type 1 Gaucher disease results in low blood platelets and fatigue due to anemia, enlarged liver and spleen, skeletal disorders and, in some instances, lung and kidney impairment. There is brain involvement. In type 2, there is liver and spleen enlargement and extensive and progressive brain damage. Death usually occurs before the age of two years. In type 3, liver and spleen enlargement, skeletal irregularities, eye movement disorders and blood disorders are present, and there may be brain involvement. There is no treatment for brain damage occurring in types 2 and 3.

18. Thalassemia is an autosomal recessive blood disease that results in a reduced rate of synthesis (or of no synthesis at all) of one of the globin chains that make up hemoglobin, leading to the formation of abnormal hemoglobin molecules and causing anemia. The estimated incidence of thalassemia in Canada is 119 per year. See www.cureresearch.com/t/thalassemia/stats-country_printer.htm

19. J. Rawls, *A Theory of Justice* (Harvard University Press, 1971; rev. ed. 1999).

20. Health Canada, "History of Providing Health Services to First Nations People and Inuit," accessed 22 Dec 2010 at www.hc-sc.gc.ca/ahc-asc/branch-dirgen/fnihb-dgspni/services-eng.php. See also Romanow Report, 212.

21. See Romanow Report, 213.

22. Royal Commission on Aboriginal Peoples, *Report of the Royal Commission on Aboriginal Peoples* (Ottawa: Canada Communications Group, 1996).

23. See Romanow Report, 218 f.

24. *Constitution Act*, 1982, available at www.solon.org/Constitutions/Canada/English/ca_1982.html

25. See Romanow Report, *pass*.

26. T. McKeown, *The Origin of Human Disease* (Oxford: Basil Blackwell, 1988). See also B. Harris, "Public Health, Nutrition, and the Decline of Mortality: The McKeown Thesis Revisited," *Social History of Medicine* 17.3 (2004): 379–407.

27. See D. Callahan, "The WHO Definition of Health." *Hastings Center Report* 1.3 (1973).

28. D. Callahan, *Setting Limits: Medical Goals in an Aging Society* (New York: Simon & Schuster, 1987); L.M. Fleck, "Just Caring: In Defence of Limited Age-Based Healthcare Rationing," *Cambridge Quarterly of Healthcare Ethics* 19.1 (Winter 2010): 27–37; A. Williams, "The Rationing Debate: Rationing Health Care by Age: The Case For," *British Medical Journal* 314 (1997): 820; and G. Persad, A. Wertheimer and E. Ezekiel, "Principles for Allocation of Scarce Medical Interventions," *The Lancet* 373.9661 (2009): 423–431. For a contrary position, see L.R. Churchill, "Age-Rationing in Health Care: Flawed Policy, Personal Virtue," *Health Care Analysis* 13.2 (Jun 2005): 137–146; and S.J. Kerstein and G. Bognar, "Complete Lives in the Balance," *American Journal of Bioethics* 10.4 (2010): 37–45.

29. See Williams, op. cit.

30. I. Dey and N. Fraser, "Age-Based Rationing in the Allocation of Health Care," *Journal of Aging and Health* 12.4 (2000): 511–537.

31. See T. McKeown, R.G. Record and R.D. Turner, "An Interpretation of the Decline of Mortality in England and Wales During the Twentieth Century," *Population Studies* 29 (November 1975): 391–422.

32. T. De Meyer et al., "Studying Telomeres in a Longitudinal Population Based Study," *Frontiers in Bioscience* 13 (2008): 2960–2970.

33. T. Kogut and I. Ritov, "The 'Identified Victim' Effect: An Identified Group, or Just a Single Individual?" *Journal of Behavioral Decision Making* 18 (2005): 157–167.

34. This raises the question of whether it is ethically appropriate for a society to meet its needs for health care professionals by importing them from other countries. Currently, Canada's immigration policy gives preferential status to physicians and nurses. Is that ethical, given that this will reduce the number of such professionals available in countries such as Ghana, Zaire or Peru?

35. C.H. Tuohy, C.M. Flood and M. Stabile, "How Does Private Finance Affect Public Health Care Systems? Marshaling the Evidence from OECD Nations," *Journal of Health Politics, Policy and Law* 29.3 (2004): 359–396; S.J. Duckett, "Private Care and Public Waiting," *Aust Health Rev* 29.1 (2005): 87–93.

36. See Gallup poll, 24 Nov 2008, accessed 29 Dec 2010 at www.gallup.com/poll/112264/nurses-shine-while-bankers-slump-ethics-ratings.aspx

37. See F.M. Parsons, "Selection of Patients for Haemodialysis," *British Medical Journal* (11 Mar 1967): 622–624. Rescher (see note 9, *supra*) seems to accept something like this in what he calls the "retrospective service" factor.

38. For a discussion of the history of prisoners' right to vote in Canada, see A. Schaefer, "Ballots Behind Bars: The Struggle for Prisoners' Right to Vote," special to *The Globe and Mail*, accessed 2 Jan 2011 at www.umanitoba.ca/faculties/arts/departments/philosophy/ethics/media/Ballots_Behind_Bars.pdf

39. Cf. Speech by Mark Warawa (MP for Langley, B.C.) in Parliament, 8 Jun 2010, accessed 2 Jan 2011 at www.markwarawa.com/EN/mark_in_the_news/no_cash_for_cons:_elderly_inmates_shouldn%E2%80%99t_get_pension,_says_mp/

40. For a critical discussion of some of these issues, see B. Clark, "The Hidden Costs of a Cruel and Unusual Prison Health Care System," *Bioethics Forum* 18 Sep 2006, accessed 30 Dec 2010 at www.thehastingscenter.org/Bioethicsforum/Post.aspx?id=276

41. Reference re Milgaard (Can.), [1992] 1 S.C.R. 866.

42. www.danielnpaul.com/DonaldMarshallJr.-1971.html

43. *Report of the Kaufman Commission on Proceedings Involving Guy Paul Morin*, accessed 30 Dec 2010 at www.attorneygeneral.jus.gov.on.ca/english/about/pubs/morin/

44. For a popular account of Gandhi's trial and sentence in 1922, see "Trial of Mahatma Gandhi-1922," accessed 2 Jan 2011 at http://bombayhighcourt.nic.in/libweb/historicalcases/cases/TRIAL_OF__MAHATMA_GANDHI-1922.html

45. R. v. Big M Drug Mart Ltd., [1985] 1 S.C.R. 295.

46. *Standard Minimum Rules for the Treatment of Prisoners,* adopted by the First United Nations Congress on the Prevention of Crime and the Treatment of Offenders, held at Geneva in 1955, and approved by the United Nations Economic and Social Council by its resolutions 663 C (XXIV) of 31 July 1957, and 2076 (LXII) of 13 May 1977, accessed 2 Jan 2011 at www.unhcr.org/refworld/docid/3ae6b36e8.html

47. See E. Anscombe, "Who Is Wronged?" *The Oxford Review* 5 (1967): 16–17.

48. See N. Daniels, *Just Health Care* (Cambridge and London: Cambridge University Press, 1985).

49. Those who have a language barrier will not be able to access the queue easily. This is particularly important in the multicultural context of Canadian society.

50. See D. Crane, *The Sanctity of Social Life: Physicians' Treatment of Critically Ill Patients* (New York: Russell Sage Foundation, 1975), Part I, Chapters 3 to 5, with respect to treatment options considered appropriate for the mentally handicapped.

51. A.R. Sehgal, "The Net Transfer of Transplant Organs across Race, Sex, Age, and Income," *Am J Med* 117.9 (1 Nov 2004): 670–675; L.K. Kayler et al., "Gender Imbalance in Living Donor Renal Transplantation," *Transplantation* 73.2 (27 Jan 2002): 248–252; F. Carlsen and O.M. Kaarboe, "Norwegian Priority Guidelines: Estimating the Distributional Implications across Age, Gender and SES," *Health Policy* 95.2–3 (May 2010): 264–270.

52. B. Vissandjée et al., "Sex, Gender, Ethnicity, and Access to Health Care Services: Research and Policy Challenges for Immigrant Women in Canada," *Journal of International Migration and Integration* 2.1 (2001): 55–75.

53. N. Rescher, "The Allocation of Exotic Medical Lifesaving Therapy," *Ethics* 79.3 (Apr 1969): 173–180.

54. Op. cit.

55. H. Hemingway et al., "The Effectiveness and Cost-Effectiveness of Biomarkers for the Prioritization of Patients Awaiting Coronary Revascularisation: A Systematic Review and Decision Model," *Health Technology Assessment* 14.9 (Feb 2010): 1–15. See also D. Feeny, G. Guyatt and P. Tugwell (eds.), *Health Care Technology: Effectiveness, Efficiency and Public Policy* (Montreal: Institute for Research on Public Policy, 1986); and R. Young, "Some Criteria for Making Decisions Concerning the Distribution of Scarce Medical Resources," *Theory and Decision* 6 (1975): 439–455.

56. See J. Boyle, "Limiting Access to Health Care: A Traditional Roman Catholic Analysis," in *Allocating Scare Medical Resources: Roman Catholic Perspectives*, ed. H.T. Engelhardt, Jr. and M.J. Cherry. (Washington, DC: Georgetown University Press, 2002), 77–95.

57. P.P. Reese et al., "How Should We Use Age to Ration Health Care? Lessons from the Case of Kidney Transplantation," *J Am Geriatr Soc* 58.10 (Oct 2010): 1980–1986.

58. See WHO, "Metrics: Disability-Adjusted Life Year (DALY)," accessed 31 Dec 2010 at www.who.int/healthinfo/global_burden_disease/metrics_daly/en/index.html. For a discussion of DALYs and related measures, see P. Zweifel, F. Breyer and M. Kifman, *Health Economics,* 2nd ed. (London and New York: Oxford University Press, 1997), Chapter 2, "Economic Evaluation of Life and Health." See also Feeney, Guyatt and Tugwell, op. cit.

59. It is estimated that it costs approximately $802 million U.S. (2000) to bring a new drug to market. See J.A. DiMasi, R.W. Hansen and H.G. Grabowski, "The Price of Innovation: New Estimates of Drug Development Costs," *Journal of Health Economics* 22 (2003): 151–185. In 2011 dollars, that would amount to approximately $1.1 billion U.S.

60. M.E. McKneally et al., "Ethics for Clinicians: Resource Allocation," *Canadian Medical Association Journal* 157.2 (1997): 163–167.

61. HIV/AIDS has been contracted through tainted blood. In fact, it is impossible to prevent nosocomial HIV/AIDS infections through blood transfusions, because Western Blot and ELISA are neither 100 percent specific nor 100 percent sensitive.

62. K. Sharkey and L. Gillam, "Should Patients with Self-Inflicted Illness Receive Lower Priority in Access to Healthcare Resources? Mapping Out the Debate," *Journal of Medical Ethics* 36.11 (2010): 661–665; A.H. Moss and M. Siegler, "Should Alcoholics Compete Equally for Liver Transplantation?" *Journal of the American Medical Association* 265 (1991): 1295–1298. For discussion, see D. Brudney, "Are Alcoholics Less Deserving of Liver Transplants?" *Hastings Center Report* 37.1 (2007): 41–47.

63. D.M. Dick et al., "Evidence for Genes on Chromosome 2 Contributing to Alcohol Dependence with Conduct Disorder and Suicide Attempts," *American Journal of Medical Genetics Part B: Neuropsychiatric Genetics* 153B.6 (Sep 2010): 1179–1188.

64. For a classic discussion of this criterion, see President's Commission for the Study of Ethical Problems in Medicine and Biomedical and Behavioral Research, *Securing Access to Health Care*, 3 vols. (Washington, DC: U.S. Government Printing Office, 1983), Vol. 1, Chapters 1 and 2.

65. "Be my HERO! I need a new KIDNEY!," accessed 29 Dec 2010 at www.youtube.com/watch?v=oa0A6PC5CUo&feature=related; "Vanessa, Mother of 2 little kids URGENTLY needs a kidney! Save her life! Contact Chaya Lipschutz," accessed 29 Dec 2010 at www.youtube.com/watch?v=6MdN4t8MAac&feature=related

66. K.E. Jenni and G. Loewenstein, "Explaining the 'Identifiable Victim Effect,'" *Journal of Risk and Uncertainty* 14 (1997): 235–257; T. Kogut and I. Ritov, "The 'Identified Victim' Effect: An Identified Group, or Just a Single Individual?" *Journal of Behavioral Decision Making* 18 (2005): 157–167.

67. See E.-H.W. Kluge, "Designated Organ Donation: Private Choice in Social Context," *Hastings Center Report* (Sep/Oct 1989): 10–15, for similar considerations.

68. Based on a case in which the author acted as ethics consultant.

69. Based on Auton (Guardian ad litem of) v. British Columbia (Attorney General), [2004] 3 S.C.R. 657, 2004 SCC 78.

SAMPLE CASES

1. S.P. is a woman in her thirties who has been a severe insulin-dependent diabetic for fifteen years. She has followed her dietary regimen only sporadically and when it suited her momentary lifestyle. She has also quite often taken her medication inappropriately and therefore has been in and out of hospital on many occasions—often several times a year. She is now in hospital for severe ketoacidosis. Ulcerations have developed on her legs during her last alcoholic episode, and they are not healing. She is going into renal failure. Dialysis resources are stretched to the limit and there are other candidates waiting for dialysis, but they cannot be dialyzed because there

simply are not enough machines. A resident says, "We really ought to reduce the burden on our end-stage renal dialysis program, particularly given the current budgetary restrictions. It's only reasonable to ration under these circumstances. We ought to start here." Some of the staff agree. What considerations are relevant when it comes to deciding this case?[68]

2. The parents of an autistic child brought an action against the Province of British Columbia, because it refused to fund ABA/IBI (Applied Behaviour Analysis/Intensive Behaviour Intervention) therapy for autistic children between the ages of three and six on the grounds of existing financial constraints and the experimental and controversial nature of this therapy. The parents alleged that the failure to fund the therapy violated section 15(1) of the Canadian Charter of Rights and Freedoms and the *Canada Health Act*. The British Columbia Ministry of Health has funded a number of programs for autistic children, but not ABA/IBI therapy. The trial judge found that the failure to fund ABA/IBI therapy violated the petitioners' equality rights, directed the province to fund early ABA/IBI therapy for children with autism and awarded $20,000 in damages to each of the parents. The Court of Appeal upheld the judgment. The Province appealed the decision to the Supreme Court of Canada, which overturned the judgment of the lower courts. Is the Supreme Court's decision ethically appropriate? Why or why not?[69]

Chapter 11
Reproductive Ethics and the Right to Have Children

Is there a right to have children? Is sex selection ethically defensible? Is surrogate motherhood? Like most questions in biomedical ethics, these cannot be answered in isolation and on the basis of pure theory. Since they deal with matters in the world, they can be answered only by taking into account relevant facts. Relevant material facts are that the capacity for procreation is inherent in human beings as biological organisms; that survival of the human species depends on the exercise of this capacity; that some human beings carry genes which, if expressed in their offspring, will result in agonizing, irremediable and incurable conditions that are unlikely to contribute to the survival of the species from an evolutionary perspective; and that the world is a finite place with limited resources. There also are certain ethical facts that are relevant. They include the fact that all persons, insofar as they are persons, have the right to self-determination, subject only to the equal and competing rights of others; that children are persons; that all persons insofar as they are persons are equal; and that there lies a general duty to be responsible in one's decision-making and to avoid doing harm to others.

The question whether there is a right to have children, whether surrogate motherhood is ethically defensible or whether sex selection should be prohibited can be answered only against this constellation of facts. The discussion that follows explains why and how this is the case, and what this means in actual practice. It will also look at some of the legal considerations that define the Canadian context, since this is the setting in which Canadians would exercise their right to have children.

Questions to Keep in Mind While Reading this Chapter:

1. What are some of the arguments in favour of the right to have children? What are some arguments against asserting such a right? Is there any particular argument that is more convincing than others? Why?

2. Does the state have a role in controlling the reproductive practices of its citizens?

3. Is sex selection ethically defensible?

4. Is surrogate motherhood ethically defensible?

INTRODUCTION

Resolution 217A(iii) of the *Universal Declaration of Human Rights* reads as follows:[1]

> Men and women of full age, without any limitation to race, nationality or religion, have the right to marry and found a family.

It was drafted in the aftermath of the eugenics[2] program that had become an integral part of the population policies of Nazi Germany. The *Declaration* was adopted by the United Nations General Assembly on December 10, 1948. Twenty years later, on May 13, 1968, the United Nations reiterated its position in the *Proclamation of Teheran* in the following statement:[3]

> Parents have a basic right to determine freely and responsibly the number and spacing of their children.

This stance was reaffirmed in 1974 at the International Population Conference in Bucharest when 137 members of the United Nations World Population adopted the *World Population Plan of Action:*[4]

> Individual reproductive behaviour and the needs and aspirations of society should be reconciled . . . All couples and individuals have the basic right to decide freely and responsibly the number and spacing of their children and to have the information, education and means to do so; the responsibility of couples and individuals in the exercise of this right takes into account the needs of their living and future children, and their responsibilities towards the community.

This was again restated, in essentially the same words, ten years later at the International Population Conference in Mexico City.

It is easy to see that a shift had occurred from the time of the *Universal Declaration of Human Rights* to the *World Population Plan of Action* of Bucharest and Mexico City. Rather than talking only about rights, the conferences and the resolutions stated that the right to have children also implies certain responsibilities, and that a balance must be struck between the two. More specifically, they stipulated that a balance must be struck between people's reproductive freedom and their obligation to "take into consideration their own situation, as well as the implications of their decisions or the balanced development of their children and of the community and society in which they live."[5]

These considerations also appear to underlie the People's Republic of China's *White Paper on Family Planning*,[6] which states that because China cannot sustain an uncontrolled population growth, and because the Chinese state, as formal representative of the Chinese people, is obligated to put into place rules and regulations that are designed to promote the general welfare of its citizens, it has the duty to institute laws which, all other things being equal, restrict each family to one child.[7]

However, these documents and resolutions are essentially a matter of politics and merely stipulate. They do not provide any ethically grounded reasoning as to why one should accept them. Therefore, it is not untoward to ask whether there are any ethically valid reasons for saying that there is a right to have children. And if such a right can be ethically grounded, it becomes important to consider whether it is inalienable and unconditioned or merely a *prima facie* right subject to limitations and conditions; and finally, it becomes appropriate to ask whether society—that is to say, the state—has an ethically legitimate role in monitoring or enforcing adherence to these limitations and conditions, as is averred by the People's Republic of China.[8]

These questions have more than merely theoretical significance. If there is an inalienable and unconditioned right to have children, society would have no mandate to interfere with the reproductive rights of its citizens—which, in turn, would mean that it could not (as it has done in the past) sterilize people on the basis of mental disability[9] or for having criminal personalities,[10] nor could it engage in non-consensual birth control.[11] This would also mean that society would have a positive duty to assist persons whose attempts to become biological parents have failed. And this, in turn, would entail an obligation to provide services such as artificial insemination (AI), *in vitro* fertilization (IVF) and so on. Further still, Equality and Justice would entail that society would have a duty to provide sperm for women who do not have access to male partners, and surrogate mothers for those men who might be unable to convince a woman to become pregnant by them and carry their child to term.

On the other hand, if the more limited interpretation is correct, then society might indeed have both a right and a duty to interfere in the reproductive activities of its members if there were ethically appropriate reasons for doing so. Specifically, society would have a duty to interfere in circumstances where the reproductive practices were "irresponsible"—for instance, if people did not take into account "the needs of their living and future children, and their responsibilities towards the community." While it might require interpretation as to precisely what this last clause amounts to, this understanding of the general thesis would nevertheless legitimate the principle of state interference.

It is therefore important to know which interpretation is correct, because it has tremendous personal and social consequences. The discussion that follows will identify some of the more important considerations that are relevant when trying to find an answer.

SOME LEGAL AND HISTORICAL CONSIDERATIONS

To get some background on the whole issue, and to situate it in the Canadian context, it may be useful to begin with some historical and legal facts.

The first thing to note is that Canada's acceptance of the *Universal Declaration of Human Rights* and of the *Proclamation of Teheran*, etc., does not mean that Canada is legally bound by these declarations, proclamations and resolutions. They become Canadian law only when the relevant provisions have been passed by Parliament and have been proclaimed by the Governor General.

In fact, there is only one piece of Canadian legislation that deals specifically with human reproduction. It is the *Assisted Human Reproduction Act*.[12] However, that Act says nothing about the right to have children. It deals only with reproductive technologies. In other words, it deals only with certain *methods* of producing children and leaves the issue of whether there is a right completely alone.

There is Canadian case law that deals with the right to have children, but it deals with it only tangentially. The most important cases are those of *E. (Mrs.) v. Eve*[13] and *Muir v. The Queen*.[14] The *Eve* case dealt with a woman who was mentally severely disabled and was not a medical candidate for birth control medication; if she had children, they would become a burden to Eve's mother (who was already of advanced age) and ultimately the state. Eve's mother had brought an application to allow her daughter to be sterilized. While a lower court had given permission, the Supreme Court struck it down June 29, 2011, with the following words:

> [A] court can [not] deprive a woman of that privilege [of bearing children] for purely social or other non-therapeutic purposes without her consent. The fact that others may suffer inconvenience or hardship from failure to do so cannot be taken into account.

The *Muir* case—which was decided after *Eve*—applied the reasoning in *Eve* in what essentially was a retrospective look at the Alberta legislation under which Ms. Muir had been non-consensually sterilized. Ms. Muir had been sterilized at age fourteen because she had been diagnosed as a "mental defective moron" incapable of taking care of children. Even though this sterilization was conducted in accordance with the sterilization statute that was then in force,[15] the Supreme Court held that her rights had been infringed and awarded damages.[16]

If we assume that Canadian judgments reflect public standards, then Canadian values have undergone a fundamental change since the 1930s, when the Alberta statute (and the corresponding British Columbia and Saskatchewan statutes) was enacted: Canadian society has come to accept that there is a fundamental right to have children, and that this right may not be subverted, even by the state. In other words, the judgment suggests that Canadian society has come to accept that there is an absolute and unconditioned right to have children.

However, such an interpretation of the judgments would be premature. In neither case did the Supreme Court go so far as to recognize a right to have children.[17] In the *Eve* case, it asserted that there was a *fundamental privilege*; and in the *Muir* case it used similar language. One can only speculate why the Courts used such language, but the logic of rights and privileges may well hold a clue. As we saw in Chapter 1, rights are justified claims, and in that sense are entitlements whereby, all other things being equal, someone has a corresponding duty. Privileges, however, are not entitlements. They are special advantages that the privilege-holder enjoys over other persons. Therefore, if the Court had recognized that there was a right to have children, that right could not belong only to women, because that would constitute discrimination on the basis of sex—which is specifically ruled out by section 15 of the Charter. It would also have to be a right for men.

The Court was also justifiably reluctant to recognize such a right for another reason. It would have removed reproduction from the domain of health care, where it traditionally belonged, into the domain of fundamental rights, and thereby would have taken it out of provincial jurisdiction and placed it into the realm of federal powers. This would have meant that the federal government not only could regulate reproductive services in all of their aspects, but also would have a duty to enact legislation criminalizing any impediment to the provision of these services.

This, in turn, would have had a curious consequence. Logically, the right to have children is not synonymous with the right to become pregnant. It is synonymous with the right to have (biological) offspring. Men also have the capacity to have biological offspring. Therefore, if the Court had recognized a right to have children, it would have recognized, by implication, a social duty to remove any impediment to a woman's access to sperm if she wanted to become pregnant and, correspondingly, to remove any impediment that might interfere with a man's access to female reproductive services. This would have had serious consequences not only for the legality of commercial surrogate motherhood but also for the ability of Parliament to pass the *Assisted Human Reproduction Act*, which criminalizes commercial surrogacy and prohibits reproductive practices whose sole purpose is to facilitate having children. Not surprisingly, therefore, the Court recognized only a "fundamental privilege" of becoming pregnant and bearing children.

SOME PRELIMINARY ETHICAL CONSIDERATIONS

Canada, therefore, does not recognize a fundamental and absolute legal right to have children. However, that is a matter of history and law, not a matter of ethics. It therefore becomes important to inquire into the ethics of the matter. Is there an *ethical* right to have children? How would such a right be grounded? Are there limits to the right—supposing for the moment there is such a right? And how would such limits—if there are limits—be enforced?

The Ambiguity of the "Right to Have Children"

With this, however, one is immediately brought face to face with another question—one which so far has received little attention in either the literature or public debate: What exactly does the claim of a right to have children amount to? Does it mean that one has the right to biological offspring of one's own? Or does it mean that one has the right to be a parent? Or does it mean a combination of these?

Depending on how one answers these questions, different consequences follow. If the right to have children is understood as the right to be a parent, then in principle nothing would bar society from interfering in the reproductive capacities of its citizens as long as people were provided with children to parent. Their right to have children would be fulfilled by making adoptions possible for everyone who wanted to parent a child (and was capable of doing so). Moreover, it would not rule out involuntary sterilization for reasons unrelated to the health of the individual person. Furthermore, as long as society provided anyone who wanted it with the opportunity to parent, society would have no obligation to investigate and correct the causes of infertility.

On the other hand, if the right to have children is understood as the right to have biological offspring of one's own, then society would have an obligation to try to prevent or cure infertility. Research efforts and relevant health services would be mandated. However, it would then not follow that biological parents had a right to keep any of their own biological offspring. This consequence would assume particular significance in the contemporary context, in which surrogate motherhood has become a reality. It would mean that surrogate contracts could become legally enforceable.[18]

Finally, if the right to have children included both the right to have biological offspring as well as the right to be a parent, the picture would shift once again. Not only would society have an obligation to fund research aimed at eradicating or curing infertility, it would also have an obligation to assist people who had difficulties functioning as parents by providing ancillary services. This would have important implications in the case of mentally or otherwise disabled persons.

Given these distinct consequences, it is important to become clear on which of the three interpretations (if indeed any) is correct. What follows is an attempt to give at least a partial answer. It begins by looking at some of the ethically based arguments in favour of the right to have biological offspring of one's own.

SOME ARGUMENTS AND THEIR ANALYSIS

Argument from Biology

One of the more traditional arguments for the right to have children is based on the biological nature of the human species. It is surprisingly simple. It centres in the fact that unless human beings reproduce, the species *homo sapiens* will disappear. It follows, so the argument contends, that there is a right to have children because this is grounded in the biological nature of humanity itself.

However, even though it has a factual basis, the argument is logically flawed. First of all, the fact that the human species will disappear unless it does something (whatever that might be) does not entail either the right or the duty to engage in the actions that are necessary to ensure its survival. For that to follow, another premise is necessary: specifically, that it would be unethical to allow the species to disappear. That premise, however, cannot simply be assumed. It has to be established on its own terms.

In this connection it seems relevant to note that, like all other species, the species *homo sapiens* is subject to evolutionary processes. The species itself appeared only about 500,000 years ago,[19] and has undergone evolutionary changes since then. For instance, evolutionary processes have produced changes in the ability to metabolize alcohol,[20] the ability to synthesize vitamin D[21] and the ability to live in a rarified oxygen environment such as Tibet and the high Andes.[22] Similarly, blue eyes and blond hair appeared only about 10,000 to 25,000 years ago as a result of mutations,[23] and the presence of HIV resistance is another example.[24] This means that, all other things being equal and given sufficient time, the species itself will alter dramatically and ultimately evolve out of existence. If allowing the human species to disappear would constitute moral negligence, then there would be a duty to take all appropriate measures to prevent this from happening. In other words, there would be a duty not only to have children but also to prevent genetic evolutionary changes which, cumulatively, would lead to the demise of humanity as a species. It is not at all clear how one could argue for such a position aside from assuming that allowing the species to disappear is unethical—which of course would be to beg the question.

The argument also fails for another reason. Even if one accepted the thesis that there is a duty to preserve the species and that, therefore, there is a corresponding right to have children, this would not entail that every member of the species—that is to say, every person—would have that right. In fact, the very opposite would follow. What would follow would be that all and only those people who could reasonably be expected to contribute to the survival of the species would have that right. That would certainly not include everyone; e.g., it would exclude all those who carry genes that reasonably could be described as not contributing to the evolutionary fitness. Clearly, this would be incompatible with the claim that there is a universal right to have children.

Argument from Desire

Another argument for the right to have children begins with the claim that most people want to have children.[25] From this, the argument concludes that therefore there is a *prima facie* right to have children. The argument admits that this right may be overruled on certain occasions, but insists that there must always be a reason—an ethically valid reason—for doing so. It cannot simply be a matter of social whim.

It takes little reflection to see that this argument is also problematic. Logically, the conclusion would follow only if one assumed the general premise that the existence of a desire was sufficient to ground a *prima facie* right. That assumption, however, is questionable at best. If it were true, anyone who really wanted something would have a *prima facie* right to it. Arguably, then, psychotic killers would have a *prima facie* right to murder their victims, kleptomaniacs would have a *prima facie* right to steal and sex maniacs would have a *prima facie* right to satisfy their sexual urges.

Nor would this argument be saved by saying that only "natural" or instinctive desires are implicated, and by interpreting these in terms of Maslow's theory of needs.[26] According to that theory, only natural needs are genuine needs, and people have natural needs that can be arranged hierarchically: Physiological needs take priority over safety needs, which take priority over social needs, which in turn take priority over esteem needs which, finally, take priority over self-realization needs. In the first place, it is not at all clear under which heading the need to have children—if indeed there is such a need, rather than there merely being a need for sexual gratification (which is an entirely different matter)—would fall. In the second place, even if the theory of needs were correct (which some have doubted),[27] this does not show that the existence of a need establishes a right to fulfill that need. That would require the additional premise that a "natural" need automatically establishes a right. However, that amounts to begging the question, because it is the very point at issue.

Argument from the Realization of Personal Potential

Closely related to the argument from desire in its Maslowian form is the argument from personal potential. It starts from the premise that human beings have the potential to grow as persons in the context of their own families: as nurturers and as providers of security, comfort and education to their children. It then goes on to say that without children, this potential will never be fulfilled. It concludes by saying that because there is an inherent need to develop one's potential, and because interference with this development constitutes malfeasance, it follows that people have a right to have children.[28]

One of the problems with this argument is that—like many arguments that are based on a potential—it begs the question. To be valid, it has to assume that the mere existence of a potential establishes the right for realizing that potential—and that is the very point at issue.

Another problem is that if the premise were granted, it would lead to all sorts of otherwise questionable consequences. For instance, it would entail that potential Nobel Prize winners would have the right to laboratory space so that they could do Nobel Prize–winning work; potential Olympic swimmers would have the right to be trained to enter the Olympics; and potential axe murderers would have the right to have their psychotic tendencies developed so that they could actually murder someone. All of these involve personal potentials. All of them involve the development of capacities inherent in individuals.

A third problem is that this argument would establish such a right if, and only if, there were such a potential. Fertility issues aside, not everyone has the relevant potential which, after all, centres in the potential for personal growth that can be realized through the birth and raising of a child.[29]

The Manitoba court case of *B. (B.) v. Child and Family Services*[30] is interesting in this regard. It concerned mentally disabled parents whose child was to be taken away from them because the parents were alleged to lack the capability for parenting: to put it in terms of the present discussion, because they allegedly lacked the relevant potential. The lawyer for the parents brought a section 15 Charter argument—that is to say, an argument based on the equality section of the Charter of Rights and Freedoms. He argued that taking a child from parents with mental disability is "justified only if the parents are unable to provide appropriate care despite the provision of supportive services." The child was ultimately returned to the parents, because the lawyer was able to persuade the

Court that the Manitoba provincial *Human Rights Code* requires reasonable accommodation provisions. "All of the relevant evidence points to the capability of the parents to care for their child, and the parents are willing to accept reasonable conditions as to monitoring and supervision."[31]

The point of mentioning this case is twofold: *First*, it shows that even in the legal context, the argument from personal potential is considered successful only if in fact there is the relevant potential. This means that the argument could not be used to establish a right to have children for people who are mentally so severely disabled that they cannot "provide appropriate care" to their children even with assistance. By that very token, it shows that even if it were granted that the existence of a potential to have children confers a right, this does not mean that the right would be absolute.[32]

Second, it suggests that the notion of the right to have children cannot be considered merely in the context of the individuals themselves. It has to be considered within the overall social context, which includes the capacity of society to provide relevant and appropriate supportive services. (This agrees with the more limited interpretation of the *Proclamation of Teheran* mentioned above, as well as with the position staked out in the *White Paper* of the People's Republic of China.)

Third, it allows us to see that the whole question of whether there is a right to have children cannot be settled simply in terms of the perspective of the right-holder. The fact is that the fulfillment for such a right—if indeed there is one—would involve *children*. However, children are not objects. They are persons. Therefore, any argument for the right to have children must be careful not to deteriorate into an argument for the claim that it is ethically acceptable to use persons as a means for realizing one's own potential. The issue will be discussed further when considering the question of whether having children might be unethical because it produces harm.

Argument from Social Expectation

The argument from social expectation maintains that there is a universal and unconditioned right to have children, because having children is something that is normally expected of members of society.

However, as it stands, the conclusion it draws is too strong, and the inference does not follow. One could easily admit that there is a general and socially sanctioned presumption that people in society will normally have children. One could even admit that this presumption is built into the very nature of social existence, so that the mere fact of being a member of society would license this expectation as a matter of right. However, none of this would establish the existence of a right that was absolute and unconditioned. What it would establish is something much more limited: namely, a right that was subject to parameters that derive from the nature of society itself.

In other words, if one understands the right to have children as a socially guaranteed right based on social expectation, then the conditions that normally surround the expectation are relevant. However, even though people may be aware that there is a statistical chance that their children may not fit that profile, the usual expectation is that the children will be healthy and at least statistically average in their mental and physical endowments. Therefore, the expectation comes with the built-in limiting conditions of the societal norms in terms of the standard social expectations about infant health. This means that if someone's children are not likely to fall within that expected norm, then by that very token, the argument from social expectation would entail that such a right does not exist in their particular case.

One should, of course, be careful not to misunderstand this. The norm is not a unique and precise set of characteristics that is fixed and endures forever—something like the specific weight of a given material. Nor is it something that a particular society decides in an explicit and formal manner. It is a range of characteristics that are usually encountered in children in the context of a particular society: the sorts of health conditions or functional characteristics that one could normally expect of or for them. This means that the range of normal expectations may not be the same for all communities. But it would still follow, on this interpretation, that if people have reasonable grounds to believe that their children would probably fall outside this norm-range—whatever that range might be—then they could not claim a right to have children. In their case, the operant condition of this right would not be met.[33] Therefore, if one is going to argue for a right to have children on this basis, the argument can establish only that there is a limited right at best.

Another aspect of the argument from social expectation is that any right that was based on it would be conditioned by the equal and competing rights of others. Therefore, even if there were a right to have children, it would be a *prima facie* right only. There would be no guarantee that it would be an effective right in a given setting.

For instance, suppose that a society was so impoverished as to food, water, medical resources, etc., that adding another member into the community and supplying that person's needs would imperil the very existence of the people who were already on the scene. If one took the argument from social expectation seriously, one would also have to accept that members of society have a social expectation not to have their very existence threatened by the actions of fellow members. In fact, one could combine this with the claim that their right to life was more fundamental than other people's right to procreate—which is essentially a matter of quality of life—because the right to life is more fundamental than (and therefore takes priority over) the right to a certain quality of life. (See Chapter 1 for the ranking of rights. See also Chapter 10.) One could then go on to say that ignoring their existential needs would not only usurp this logical relationship between different kinds of rights, it would also contravene their expectation not to have their very existence threatened. Therefore, having a child would not only be pragmatically unwise in such an impoverished context but would be ethically objectionable, because it would violate, in its resource implications, the more fundamental right to life of other persons.

The preceding also suggests a set of quality-based considerations. Suppose that a society's resources are so strapped that it can barely support its present members. The members of that society might not necessarily expect an improvement in their lot (although they might have that hope), but they would certainly expect that the quality of their lives would not be threatened by society permitting actions that would threaten the current ability of society to meet their needs. However, the advent of more children would have that effect, because these children would also have needs that would have to be met. The advent of more children would therefore entail an increased drain on already stretched resources, and would predictably lead to chronic malnutrition, health levels would drop seriously, life-expectancy would be lowered and so on. A society that accepted the fact of social expectations as the basis of the right to have children would therefore have to balance the right to have children with the right to a certain quality of life. In some respects, this analysis mirrors the position staked out in the People's Republic of China's *White Paper*.

Argument from the Right to Personal Integrity

But what about the claim that the right to have children has nothing to do with the social context? That what is really important is an individual's right to the integrity of their person? That any interference with a woman's ability to carry a pregnancy to term would constitute a violation of her integrity as a person?

The Supreme Court's decision in *Eve* may be considered relevant in this connection:[34]

> The importance of maintaining the physical integrity of a human being ranks high in our scale of values, particularly as it affects the privilege of giving life. I cannot agree that a court can deprive a woman of that privilege for purely social or other non-therapeutic purposes without her consent.

However, an argument along these lines would also not establish a right to have children (and the appeal to the Supreme Court's judgment in *Eve* would fail), because it is based on a logical confusion. Specifically, it is based on a confusion between the right to have a capacity and the right to exercise that capacity. To draw an analogy, the right to the integrity of the person entails the right not to have one's vocal chords removed. However, the right not to have one's vocal chords removed does not entail the right to yell ethnic slurs at people or to shout "Fire!" in a crowded theatre when there is no fire. Therefore, while the right to personal integrity includes the right not to have one's reproductive capacity interfered with, this is logically distinct from the right to use one's intact body and its capacity to produce biological offspring.

IS THERE A RIGHT TO HAVE CHILDREN?

Introduction

If the preceding analysis is correct, then the right to have children would have to be established on other grounds. Are there such grounds?

To answer that question, it may be useful to go back to basics and begin with the fact that human beings are members of a biological species that maintains itself through reproduction, and that humans therefore have a reproductive capacity as part of their natural biological makeup. Of course, as was pointed out a moment ago, having the biological capacity to have children is not the same as having the right to exercise that capacity. It merely ties the capacity to reproduce to the nature of human beings.

However, that capacity, as well as the fact that human beings are *rational beings* who can exercise their capacity on the basis of volition, may just be successful in establishing such a right—by identifying it as inherent in the autonomy of human beings as volitional and rational biological agents.

That is to say, human beings are rational animals possessed of will and understanding. Some of their capacities as rational biological beings—in particular, their capacity for reproduction—are not automatically exercised in the same way as the breathing reflex in response to high CO_2 concentration in the blood, or the patellar reflex in response to mechanical cues to the patellar tendon. Instead, their reproductive capacity lies under their conscious control.[35] In other words, human reproductive behaviour is not like that of lower animals who respond instinctively to pheromonal cues. It is a matter of volition. This places the ethics of reproduction on the same footing as the ethics of any other voluntary human activity.

If one frames the argument in this way, then the right to have children is seen as inherent in the autonomy of human beings as biologically embodied rational agents. The right is then no more special than the right to run, the right to speak or the right to think, and its exercise is then subject to the same ethical considerations that apply to the exercise of any other volitional act. This also means that the right belongs to everyone who has that nature—that is to say, to all human beings as embodied rational agents. However, it also means that like all other rights, this is a *prima facie* right only, and is subject to the conditions that obtain and the equal and competing rights of others.

The implications of this can be clarified by distinguishing between acts that have no implications for anyone other than the individual who performs them, and acts that have implications for others. An act—that is to say, the exercise of a capacity—that has no implications for anyone other than the actor is not subject to ethical limitations that are grounded in anyone other than the actor him- or herself, whereas an act that has such external implications is always subject to the equal and competing rights of others. This is inherent in the Principle of Autonomy, which governs voluntary actions. (See Chapter 1.) It therefore follows that if there is a *prima facie* right to have children—more specifically, if there is a *prima facie* right to exercise one's reproductive capacity—it is subject to the equal and competing rights of others. That, in turn, takes the analysis back to the beginning of this chapter. It shows why the *Universal Declaration of Human Rights* should be interpreted in a limited fashion, and why the *Proclamation of Teheran* is correct in stating that there are limits on the general right to reproduce and have children.

However, another important fact conditions the right to have children: To procreate is to bring children into existence. Of course, this is a tautology, and therefore trivially true. However, what is not so trivial is that children are not objects. They are persons. Therefore, the ethical fabric in which the right to have children is situated is not confined to people who are already on the scene. It also includes the children who will be produced. In other words, the right to have children has to be evaluated not only with respect to the equal and competing rights of current people but must also take into account the children who will come into existence. This, again, would be in keeping with the *World Population Plan of Action,*[36] which says that people should take into account the rights of their present and future children.

As opposed to this, it could be argued that this conclusion about future children—and indeed the underlying logic of the *Proclamation of Teheran* and of the *World Population Plan of Action*—is on very tenuous grounds, precisely because it deals with the rights of *future* children. Future children do not exist. However, logically speaking, rights are relational properties. Non-existent things cannot have properties, relational or otherwise, precisely because they do not exist. This means that, unless one is willing to say that future children who do not exist in fact do have some sort of existence, future children cannot have any rights. The best one can say is that *if* the children came into existence, then they *would* have rights. However, that is entirely different from saying that they have rights *here and now*, and it does not yield the conclusion that their rights should in any way figure in one's current, rights-based deliberations.

In other words, the counter-argument would be that to make sense of the claim that the rights of future children should be taken into account, one would have to accept the thesis that beings who do not exist do in fact exist in some way or other. That is either nonsense or constitutes a commitment to a very strange metaphysic—specifically, to a metaphysics that would recognize the real existence of possible objects (future children, after all, are merely possible objects here and now) as well as the real existence of merely possible objects that will never exist. After all, not all possible future children will be born, because some future pregnancies will result in miscarriages. Absent any otherwise valid reason for accepting such an arcane ontology, one could reasonably argue that future children have no existential standing. Consequently—so the argument would continue—it is hard to see why their rights should be taken into account at this point in time.

The matter of future children will be discussed further in Chapter 12, which deals with biotechnology, gene modification and related issues. However, one can avoid framing the issue in terms of the metaphysical status of future generations by framing it as an issue about the ethical status of the act of procreation itself.

The argument here begins with the fact that to act is to set into motion a chain of events that will lead to a certain outcome. That outcome may occur within a short period of time, as when someone produces an explosion by lighting a match in a gas-filled environment; or it may have a delayed outcome, as when someone shoots an arrow and the arrow takes a few seconds to travel to the human target and kill that person; or it may be temporally delayed even more, as when someone buries a mine in a road where others will foreseeably travel. The shooting of the arrow is part of the temporally somewhat extended act of killing the victim, and the burying of the mine is part of the temporally even more extended act of killing the person who steps on the mine. In each case, the act is complete only when the result of initiating the causal chain comes to fruition. If one considers only the initiating action and not the total chain, then shooting the arrow or planting the mine are ethically neutral, whereas when one considers the overall chain, they are morally reprehensible.

If one applies this to reproduction, one can argue that reproduction is a temporally extended act that includes gestation and ultimately the birth of a child, i.e., that the act of reproduction becomes complete only when the child is removed from the mother. The child, however, is a person. Therefore, an ethical evaluation of reproduction as an act has to take into account not simply the effect on present persons but also on the child that is produced, because the child is integral to the complete act itself.

To illustrate how this may have a conditioning effect on the exercise of the right to have children, consider a case in which procreation will predictably lead to the birth of a child that will be born with cystic fibrosis. By engaging in intercourse and reproducing, the parents set in motion a chain of events that will be complete when the child is born and, moreover, one in which the child will suffer harm at the same time it is born.[37] Being born and being harmed are, so to speak, contemporaneous. To engage in acts that harm other persons is to violate the Principle of non-Malfeasance—which is unethical. Therefore, to reproduce—that is to say, to have children—when the children who will be born will foreseeably suffer is to do something unethical, because that is inherent in the nature of the act.[38]

This way of looking at the matter avoids any ontological commitment to future beings while at the same time showing why the welfare of the children who will be born is a relevant factor when evaluating the right to have children in a given case.[39] All one has to do is look at the nature of the chain of causal events initiated by the reproductive act itself. This way of approaching the issue also shows what is meant by saying that the right to have children is a *prima facie* right only, and why saying that there may be cases where it is overruled by the harm that will befall the children who will be born does not entail an arcane ontology.

At the same time, this overruling is not an absolute matter. In a society that has the means to deal with severe health problems or severe disabilities—i.e., with health problems which, absent appropriate intervention, would be experienced as agonizing, incurable and irremediable—the Principle of non-Malfeasance would not be engaged. By contrast, in a society that lacks the resources and cannot mobilize them without seriously interfering with the welfare of its members, the reverse would be true. Therefore, what would constitute harm is always context relative, and whether the right to have children is effective depends on the facts of the case. However, this should not be surprising. All rights are context dependent—not in their nature, but with respect to whether they remain merely *prima facie* or become actual.

The Control of Reproduction

This, in turn, raises the question of how to translate the notion of limits and conditions into actual practice.

Voluntary Control Voluntarily adhering to relevant limiting conditions seems to present no ethical problems. People constantly refrain from exercising *prima facie* rights because they see that their *prima facie* rights are overruled by the equal and competing rights of others. One could, of course, argue that the method that people use to voluntarily control their reproductive activity is ethically important. Specifically, one could argue that methods that do not permanently alter their bodily makeup and do not destroy their capacity to reproduce are ethically acceptable (birth control pills, abstention, mechanical devices and so on), whereas methods that involve destruction of the capacity (sterilization, for example) are not, because they would constitute self-mutilation, and thus would violate what Kant called self-regarding duties, that is to say, the duties people have towards themselves simply because they are persons.[40]

However, this reasoning would ignore the fact that people are not identical with their bodies, and that what makes them persons is not their capacities as biological entities but their capacities as rational and volitional beings. Therefore, voluntary body modification—in this case, sterilization—would be unethical only if it did away with, diminished or interfered with the capacities that are characteristic of individuals as persons. Reproductive capacity, however, is not essential in this regard. If it were, women who suffered from Turner syndrome, men with advanced Klinefelter's syndrome or people who had been rendered sterile by accident, medical misadventure or any other means would not be persons. Therefore, not only is voluntary birth control using only temporary means ethically acceptable, so is using permanent means such as sterilization.

It follows that if the notion of limits and conditions is translated into practice by individuals exercising voluntary control over their reproductive behaviour, there is nothing inherently unethical about it, and that the method used—whether temporary or permanent in nature—is ethically irrelevant as long as it does not violate the Principle of Autonomy and Respect for Persons.[41]

Non-Voluntary Control At the same time, not everyone always acts ethically. It is generally assumed that if people insist on not doing so—and if the matter is important—society has a duty to take appropriate steps to curtail their unethical behaviour. The criminal law is based on this assumption. The difficult question, therefore, is whether society can ethically enforce reproductive limits when people do not voluntarily control their reproductive behaviour when, ethically speaking, they should.[42]

Bioethicists have generally shied away from this question, and those who have addressed it have usually focused on women's issues, tending to characterize externally imposed reproductive control as patriarchal and oppressive. Unfortunately, this is not much help, because it simply avoids the issue of what to do when limitation is mandated but people refuse to act responsibly. The only discussion that is specific to the issue is found in China's *White Paper*.[43] However, it expresses itself only in generalities. While it insists that society has a duty to ensure that individual procreation does not infringe on the rights of others, it presents no suggestions as to how this may be ethically enforced.

In the absence of any considered treatment, therefore, it may be appropriate to confine the discussion to indicating a few relevant considerations. *First*, even if society has a right or duty to intervene in the reproductive freedom of individual persons, this intervention must always respect the individual as person. Interventions or policies that ignore this and treat individuals as mere counters are ethically unacceptable.

Second, any interference with individual procreative rights must always be subject to what has sometimes been called the *Principle of the Least Restrictive Alternative*. This principle stipulates that an ethically justified interference with someone's right is limited to using only those means that interfere with the individual's rights to the least degree that is necessary under the circumstances that obtain.[44] Therefore, if the right to have children is conditioned by the equal and competing rights of others, and if society has a duty to ensure that individuals do not ignore this limitation, then society may use only the least restrictive means at its disposal. In the words of the Law Reform Commission of Canada,[45]

> [t]he application of this principle would require that coercive regulations could be applied only when non-coercive methods would not achieve the same goals . . . In practice, this would mean that it would have to be demonstrated that an individual either could not be taught to use . . . other forms of birth control, or was not responsible enough to use them even if capable.

Whether this mandates interference with the sexual activities or capacities of the individuals in question or whether it mandates abortion is unclear and warrants further investigation. However, it would seem reasonable to suggest that *if* interference is mandated, and *if* society has to step in to ensure that ethically appropriate reproductive behaviour is followed, *then* the least restrictive alternative would entail that whoever would be subject to such interference should be given the choice of the method to be applied. That would respect individual autonomy to the greatest degree possible while being consistent with the mandate of interference itself.

The Mentally Disabled and the Right to Have Children

This leaves the issue of what to do with persons who are incapable of exercising voluntary control because they are mentally severely disabled—which in turn opens up the general question of whether the mentally severely disabled have the right to have children.

As to the general question, ethically the answer is very simple: If the right to have children is limited only by the equal and competing rights of others, then—contrary to what it has done in the past[46]—society has no mandate to interfere with the procreative activities of the mentally disabled solely on the grounds of their mental disability. Mental disability might, barely, constitute an ethically acceptable reason if the mental disability was severe, produced harm, was genetically grounded, would be passed on to progeny and could not be accommodated by supportive social services. But even here, it would have to be shown that the children who would be born would suffer severe harm and, moreover, that society could not take appropriate steps to deal with the disability once it manifested itself and to mitigate the harm by providing appropriate assistance.

Moreover, in this connection it is worth noting that, as the Law Reform Commission of Canada put it, "there is nothing inherent in mental handicap that determines whether or not a person is competent to raise children,"[47] and that[48]

> [w]ithout some proof (beyond simple mental handicap) that a person is unable to care for children, the justification for state intervention in the procreative ability, that is the state's interest in protecting those unable to protect themselves, does not appear adequately established.

Furthermore, as the Supreme Court put it in *Eve*,[49]

> [t]he argument relating to fitness as a parent involves many value-loaded questions. Studies conclude that mentally incompetent parents show as much fondness and concern for their children as other people; . . . Many, it is true, may have difficulty in coping, particularly with the financial burdens involved. But this issue does not relate to the benefit of the incompetent; it is a social problem, and one, moreover, that is not limited to incompetents.

In other words, severe mental disability constitutes a ground for limiting the *prima facie* right to have children if, and only if, society does not have the means to compensate for the disability or when compensating for the disability would predictably interfere with society's duty to provide the necessaries of life for its members, or would make it impossible for society to provide a minimally acceptable level of socially mandated services either to the disabled themselves or to their progeny. But this limiting condition is the same for all persons, irrespective of the existence or level of any disability, and would not target mentally disabled persons in any specific way.[50]

By the same token, it follows that if a mentally severely disabled person needed a substitute decision-maker to decide whether to have a child, or whether to have his or her reproductive capacity limited in some way or other, the choices open to the duly empowered substitute decision-maker should be the same as those open to any objective reasonable person faced with a similar decision on his or her own behalf. Not to allow this latitude of options—including that of sterilization—is to limit the options open to the disabled, simply because they are disabled. Unfortunately, that is precisely what the Supreme Court did in *Eve*. Ironically, contrary to what the Court intended, that constituted discrimination on the basis of disability.[51]

COMMERCIAL SURROGATE MOTHERHOOD AND RELATED ISSUES

The preceding has dealt with *limitation* of the (*prima facie*) right to have children. But what about the converse of this question? What about persons whose *prima facie* right is not overruled but who cannot have children because they are infertile, are sterile or carry a serious genetic load? Arguably, these are health issues, and as was pointed out in Chapter 9, the right to health care is a matter of equality and justice. This suggests that society has a *prima facie* duty to provide reproductive health services for people in this position.

However, as was also made clear in Chapter 9, the duty to provide health services has to be seen in the context of limited resources. That is why treatments for conditions that cause no pain, do not affect an individual's ability to function or for which the available treatments are not very successful generally tend not to be covered by provincial health insurance plans. Relative to the present context, this explains why the provincial plans tend to cover such things as surgery to repair scarred or blocked fallopian tubes or to deal with such conditions as endometriosis, but tend not to cover IVF.[52] IVF is expensive—each cycle costs approximately $6,000 (in 2011)[53]—and it has a comparatively low success rate for a live take-home baby—somewhere in the neighbourhood of 21.3 to 33 percent per cycle[54] at best, with several cycles being required. That is why, in Canada, reproductive services are essentially a privately funded matter.

However, as soon as a service becomes a matter of private funding, it opens up the possibility of exploring various options for providing that service. Moreover, some people who need reproductive assistance cannot be helped by medical means because their problem is medically incurable. For instance, a woman who has no uterus cannot be helped by medical means because she cannot have her uterus replaced; a man who is fertile but who has difficulty finding someone who will carry his child cannot be helped by medical means either. Moreover, there are situations in which it would be possible for a woman to have a child, but to do so would put her at a tremendous disadvantage because it would mean interrupting her career and seriously (and negatively) affect her life plans. That is where ectogenesis and surrogate motherhood enter the picture. Ectogenesis and related technologies will be considered in the next chapter under the rubric of biotechnologies. Surrogate motherhood, however, is appropriately discussed in this chapter because, in contrast to the inherently technical solutions, it raises issues that focus in the reproductive capacities of human beings themselves.

In surrogate motherhood, a woman becomes pregnant (usually by means of an assisted reproduction procedure) and bears a child on the understanding that she will give the child up for adoption to an antecedently specified person or persons. The child's genetic origin may be ova and sperm retrieved from the couple who will adopt the child, ova from the female partner and donated sperm, ova from the surrogate mother and sperm from the male partner, ova from the surrogate mother and donated sperm, or any other combination of these. Of course, surrogacy need not involve a heterosexual couple or even a couple at all but may involve a single person. However, this is irrelevant to the issue of surrogacy itself.

There are two types of surrogate motherhood. In commercial surrogate motherhood, the woman enters into a contractual arrangement with those who will adopt the child and is paid a fee for her services; in altruistic surrogacy, no money changes hands. Altruistic surrogacy is legal in most countries; commercial surrogacy is illegal in many jurisdictions, including Canada. Thus, the *Assisted Human Reproduction Act* stipulates that[55]

> 6. (1) No person shall pay consideration to a female person to be a surrogate mother, offer to pay such consideration or advertise that it will be paid.
>
> (2) No person shall accept consideration for arranging for the services of a surrogate mother, offer to make such an arrangement for consideration or advertise the arranging of such services.

It is, however, legal in countries such as India[56] and the Ukraine.[57] The issue, of course, is not one of law—one can always change the law—but one of ethics. Is commercial surrogacy ethical?

Arguments Contra

The objection to commercial surrogacy centres in four claims: that surrogacy is exploitative of and degrading to the surrogate mother;[58] that it amounts to baby selling;[59] that it harms the children who are born, as well as the children of the surrogate mother;[60] and that it harms society.[61]

The argument that commercial surrogacy is exploitative focuses on the fact that women who enter into commercial surrogacy arrangements generally do so because they have a financial need. Also, most surrogate mothers come from lower socioeconomic backgrounds. Therefore, so the argument contends, commercial surrogacy takes advantage of these women. Furthermore, in so doing, it also fosters a negative stereotype of women as nothing more than baby makers.[62]

The argument that commercial surrogacy is a covert form of baby selling is rather straightforward. While surrogacy involves giving up the baby that is born for adoption to those who hire the surrogate mother, the adoption takes place only if the surrogate mother is paid. To exchange something for a financial consideration is to sell. Therefore, commercial surrogacy constitutes baby selling. This violates the Principle of Autonomy and Respect for Persons, because it treats the children as commodities,

The argument that it harms both the children who are born as well as the children of the surrogate mother is somewhat more complex. The reason it is said to harm the children who are born is that when the children of surrogate mothers find out that they have been handed over by their gestational mothers to their non-biological parent(s) for a fee, they will come to see themselves as commodities. Moreover, they will see themselves as not having "been created . . . as ends in themselves but to serve the needs of another."[63] The children will experience this as demeaning, and possibly believe they have been found unworthy of being kept by the mothers who gave them life. The argument that it harms the surrogate's children (if she has children) is that when they become aware that their sibling has been handed over to a third party for money, they may come "to wonder whether they too will be relinquished by their parents" for money.[64]

The argument from social harm centres in the claim that commercial surrogacy alters the understanding of parenthood, of the nature of a family, and of both women and children. It turns the concept of a family from that of an organic and nurturing environment into that of a commercially based unit; it changes the concept of parenthood from that of a loving and responsible interrelationship involving children as ends in themselves into a relationship based on a commercial contract; and it fosters the perception of women and children as beings whose value can be measured in financial terms.

It is not at all clear, however, that these arguments are cogent. For instance, with due alteration of detail, the claim that commercial surrogacy arrangements are exploitative because the women who enter into them need money could be made about almost all persons who are paid for their physical labour. However, performing physical labour for money is not seen as inherently exploitative. It is considered exploitative only when the working conditions are dangerous or demeaning or when the wages that are paid are inappropriately low. Whether this may apply to commercial surrogacy, however, cannot be stated *a priori*. It can be determined only by looking at the fee structure for individual surrogacy services. In this regard, the 2011 fees for surrogate mothers range from $12,000 to $35,000 plus a monthly nutrition allowance, a clothing allowance and health insurance fees if applicable.[65] Moreover, surrogate mothers have their own legal representatives when negotiating their contracts, and are screened to ensure that they are capable of giving free and informed consent. Finally, surrogates are paid an agreed-upon fee even if the pregnancy fails to result in a live take-home baby.

As to the claim that surrogacy fosters a stereotype of women as mere baby makers, this assumes that surrogate motherhood will be seen as representative of womanhood. That, however, assumes that the activities of an exceedingly small subset of the total number of women (which numbers into the billions) will be considered representative of the whole set of women. Absent any data to support such a contention, it must remain speculative at best. Similarly, the suggestion that surrogacy would result in the social stratification of women into those who bear babies and those who raise them is based on the assumption that surrogacy would become a widespread practice. Given the fee structures involved and current patterns of child-bearing, that appears highly unlikely.

Of course, the contention that commercial surrogacy amounts to turning the baby into an object and constitutes baby selling would be true if the fee were for the child. Arguably, however, the fee is not for the baby but for the gestational services. Specifically, the fee is for supplying an environment in which the self-extracting blueprint that is the baby's genetic code can go to work (i.e., the uterus) and for the raw materials with which the baby is able to do so (i.e., the blood supply). This is corroborated by the fact that the surrogate is paid even if she miscarries. The fact that she is paid a higher fee if she actually delivers a baby does not alter the picture. Successful completion of a task generally entails a higher fee than its partial completion.

It is, of course, possible to argue that things are different when the ovum involved in the pregnancy is that of the surrogate mother herself. In this case the surrogate would not merely be the gestational parent but the biological parent as well.

However, to see whether this really changes the situation, it may be useful to consider what actually goes on in surrogate pregnancy. To make this clear, an analogy may be of use: Suppose someone supplies raw materials and a place of work to an automated self-directing assembly line that builds itself according to a complete set of internal instructions. Suppose further that the basic unit from which this self-directing assembly line starts is the product of an interaction between the supplier and a third party, whereby the supplier and the third party each contribute half the instructions for the assembly code and half the material for the basic unit that begins the work of assembly. It does not follow from this that—if the supplier is paid for half the starting unit, the space, the raw materials and half the instruction—the supplier is being paid for the final product.

The point of the analogy is that the zygote is a self-directing assembly line that works according to its internal code (DNA). By providing the blood supply that the zygote uses, the surrogate is like the supplier of raw materials, and the uterus in which the zygote grows is like the work space. This makes it clear that the surrogate is paid for the use of her uterus and her blood supply, not for the child. The situation does not change even if she is paid for her ovum, because even if the ovum is included in the total original supplies for which she is paid, this does not amount to a child.

In this connection, it is perhaps also worth pointing out that if altruistic surrogacy is considered ethically acceptable, then it becomes puzzling why commercial surrogacy should be considered unethical. In both cases, a child is gestated by a woman who will not be its social mother. The only difference is that in the one case the gestating mother is paid, whereas in the other she is not. However, since in both cases a child is handed over, then if handing the child over for money is to turn the child into a purchased object, then handing the child over free of charge is to turn the child into a gift—which is also an object. In other words, the difference between the two types of surrogacy has nothing to do with what is done to the child—it is handed over in both cases—but what happens to the woman and her work.

Regarding the claim that commercial surrogacy would result in harm to the child, there is no logical link between paying someone to do the work of bearing a child and a negative effect on the quality of the relationship between the child that is born and the contracting parents, nor are there any data that would support such a contention. In fact, it may be more reasonable to assume that people who engage a surrogate mother would be more likely to be nurturing and caring parents, given that they have gone to the trouble and expense of hiring someone just to have a child. As to the possibility that the child itself would feel that it has been created simply to serve the needs of another, that holds true for any child, be it in a surrogacy context or in the context of a traditional family. Whether the child feels that way depends on the nature of the parent–child relationship.

As to the claim that the surrogate's children might fear that they too would be sold, this is hypothetical. Commercial surrogacy has been practised for years in India and the Ukraine (and in certain states of the U.S.), and there are no data that would substantiate the claim that this has ever happened. And even if one were to accept this hypothetical, such a fear could only arise at a point when the children would have attained self-awareness and a relatively sophisticated understanding of the parent–child relationship. By that very token, however, parents could easily counteract such a fear by having a nurturing and loving relationship with their children and by pointing out to them that they have long passed the newborn baby stage and therefore no longer meet the criteria for surrogacy arrangements.

Arguments Pro

The arguments against commercial surrogacy, therefore, are either based on mistaken assumptions or do not establish their point. However, absence of proof is not proof of absence—that is to say, showing that an argument does not establish a particular position is not the same as establishing its opposite. It is therefore appropriate to ask whether there are arguments in favour of commercial surrogacy, and if so, whether they fare any better.

There are two such arguments: One is based in autonomy, the other on the right to have children. The argument based on autonomy begins with the premise that women have the right to decide what shall happen to their bodies. This means that, all other things being equal, they have the right to decide whether to become pregnant and under what circumstances. Furthermore, they have the right to be paid for the work they do. Therefore, if there are no ethically valid reasons for being paid to be pregnant—and the preceding discussion has shown they are paid for being pregnant, not for selling children—then to prohibit women from entering into surrogacy contracts is an unwarranted interference with their liberty as persons.

As to the argument from the right to have children, it is fairly simple: If there is a right to have children, and if this right can be met only if someone else bears the child, then this may legitimately be prohibited only if there is something unethical about the other person doing so. The preceding analysis has shown that there is nothing inherently unethical about such a practice. Consequently, surrogacy itself is not unethical. The only question then becomes whether payment makes an ethically relevant difference to the status of the child; and as was pointed out a moment ago, that is in fact not the case.[66] After all, it is not the child that is being paid for but the service.

With these considerations in mind, it may be appropriate to reconsider the *Assisted Human Reproduction Act*. It allows altruistic surrogacy but prohibits commercial surrogacy on pain of criminal sanction. The question to ask, therefore, is whether the Act has an ethical basis or merely reflects political values.

SEX SELECTION[67]

One of the more difficult questions that arises in the context of reproductive ethics is, whether it is ethically defensible to ensure that the child that will be born is of a specific sex. This is generally referred to as the issue of sex selection.

There are several reasons why people may want to embark on sex selection: one is medical, another is valuational, and a third is preference based. Medical sex selection consists in employing techniques to prevent the birth of a child that will suffer from a serious sex-linked disease; value-based sex selection consists in preventing the birth of a child of a particular sex because people of that particular sex are not valued; and preference-based sex selection is sex selection that prevents the birth of children of a sex that does not meet the preferences of their parents.

Medically-Grounded Sex Selection

Canada permits medically grounded selection under section 6 (2) of the *Assisted Human Reproduction Act* which specifically states that no person may knowingly,

> (e) for the purpose of creating a human being, perform any procedure or provide, prescribe or administer any thing that would ensure or increase the probability that an embryo will be of a particular sex, or that would identify the sex of an *in vitro* embryo, *except to prevent, diagnose or treat a sex-linked disorder or disease.* [Emphasis added]

Of course, that is only the law, and does not by itself establish that medically grounded sex selection is ethically defensible—and there are arguments on both sides.

Arguments Pro

Medically grounded arguments in favour of sex selection usually find their ethical roots in the Principle of non-Malfeasance. They begin with the fact that some seriously debilitating health conditions are sex specific, and they cite hemophilia, Lesch-Nyhan syndrome, Graves' disease and Alport syndrome as examples.[68] They then point out that available treatment for these conditions is only symptomatic and tends to be so limited that the affected persons will never enjoy a normal quality of life. Moreover, in many cases the affected persons die relatively young and under agonizing circumstances. Therefore, preventing the birth of someone who would have such a sex-linked disease is to prevent harm and, conversely, that not to do so is to become a passive co-agent of the resulting harm.[69] Hence, in these cases sex selection is ethically obligatory.[70] Medically based sex selection—so the argument concludes—is not sex-directed but disease-directed, and therefore is ethically defensible as a type of preventive medicine.

Arguments Contra

This reasoning has been criticized on three grounds: It is an unwarranted interference in human reproduction, it promotes discrimination on the basis of disability and it involves sex discrimination.

The first type of criticism usually has a religious basis and tends to be part of a general position that rejects all (scientific) interference with reproduction as a violation of fundamental moral principles that find their root in the will of the Supreme Deity. This stance is particularly well illustrated by *Donum Vitae* and *Humanae Vitae*, two encyclicals promulgated by the Roman Catholic Church.[71] However, this kind of critique is trenchant only if there is proof that the belief on which it is based is correct. Absent such proof, it is compelling only within the framework of the religious belief that underlies it.

The second type of argument is based on the claim that medically based sex selection treats severely disabled people as not worthy of inclusion in the human community[72] and not only rejects the "radical moral equality of all human beings"[73] but also subverts the development of moral virtues such as kindness and compassion towards the disabled—virtues that can fully emerge, and be fostered and strengthened only when witnessing pain and suffering.[74]

This line of reasoning is emotionally very powerful because it appeals to our fundamental conviction that all persons, insofar as they are persons, have equal worth. It is therefore easy to miss the fact that it involves a fundamental logical error. It confuses a claim about the condition from which an individual suffers with a claim about the individual him- or herself.

That is to say, because of their disabilities, some persons endure lives of irremediable, incurable and extreme suffering. Not only is the quality of their lives demonstrably different from those who do not suffer from such handicaps, it is essentially not worth living.[75] This does not mean—as it did in Nazi Germany—that these persons should be killed. It merely means that if one were to give reasonable persons the choice, behind a Rawlsian veil of ignorance[76], between being born into such a life or not being born at all, they would choose not to be born.[77] Therefore, the claim that the quality of their lives is not worth living is to make a claim about the qualitative nature of their way of living, not about the persons themselves.

By way of illustration, consider the case of Huntington's disease. Some people who carry the gene for the disease choose not to have children, because they do not want to run the risk of their children experiencing their own terrible fate. People who make this choice do not make it because they believe that whoever has the disease (or carries the gene) does not merit inclusion in the human community. They make it from a desire to prevent harm.

Therefore, to say that the quality of someone's life makes it not worth living is perfectly compatible with the claim that the people who lead such lives have the same worth as anyone else. It is precisely because the two are logically compatible that one can go on to say that the persons who lead such lives deserve sympathy, compassion and even admiration—and that one should do everything in one's power to help them.

It is also worth pointing out that medically based sex selection is not sexually discriminatory. It is disease based because it treats female- and male-linked diseases the same. The sex merely happens to be a characteristic of the relevant disease. Absent the disease, medically based selection would not occur. Consequently, it can be appropriately characterized as a kind of preventive medicine.[78]

Non-Medical Sex Selection

Preference versus Values   Sex selection on personal grounds differs fundamentally in that its aim is not to prevent harm but to ensure that the child will be of a specific sex.

It is generally assumed that sex selection on such a basis is ethically unacceptable, because it is based on sexist values that rank one sex as having more worth than the other. However, that is not necessarily the case. One can distinguish between personal grounds that are based in preferences, and personal grounds that are grounded in values; and one can then argue that while sex selection based on sexist values is ethically objectionable, sex selection that is based on personal preferences is not.

To see why this is so, it may be useful to examine the relationship between ethical principles, personal values and personal preferences a little more closely. Values are logically distinct from preferences. Values judge the worth of a person;[79] preferences are concerned with the feelings that people have—that is to say, with their likes or dislikes.[80] For instance, one may prefer the company of women to that of men without believing that men have less worth than women; one may prefer the company of the auditorily disabled (deaf) to those who can hear, because one is deaf oneself,[81] without thereby making a value judgment about those who can hear; and one may prefer to associate with adults rather than children without thinking that children have lower value as persons. Of course, a preference may be rooted in values. However, this is not necessarily the case. It may simply be grounded in emotions and feelings. That is how we choose our friends and preferentially associate with them. This does not mean that we consider our friends to have greater moral worth. We simply *like* them more than others. They are *simpatico*.[82]

Arguably, therefore, preference-based selection is no more ethically discriminatory than the preference-based selection of one's friends. The situation would be different if preference-based sex selection involved killing a person. For instance, it would be different if preference-based sex selection involved the abortion of a fetus that had passed the stage when it would be considered a person. (See Chapter 8 for a discussion of fetal personhood.) However, that would be unethical irrespective of sex selection.

These considerations, of course, leave untouched the fear that people might in fact predominantly choose to have children of a specific sex. However, it is important to consider whether this fear is merely theoretical or has a basis in reality—and the evidence does not point in that direction—at least, not in the Western world. As research conducted by the Royal Commission on New Reproductive Technologies has shown,[83] Canadians would like a gender-balanced family, i.e., a "matched set."[84] Furthermore, the Commission found that Canadians have only a "weak preference about the sex of their first-born child,"[85] and even "these preferences were generally seen as unimportant, almost trivial."[86] Similar data come from the U.S.,[87] Germany[88] and Europe in general.[89] Therefore, sex selection on the basis of preference would appear to be ethically defensible in these social contexts.

Cultural Grounds

At the same time, there are data which show that there is a definitive male-oriented preference in some non-Western countries such as China[90] (although that is on the decline),[91] India[92] and Southeast Asia.[93] This raises the issue of the ethics of sex selection that is rooted in cultural values.[94] The reason this is problematic is that it raises the question of the moral legitimacy of cultural values, and the further question of to what degree a society—and particularly a multicultural society such as Canada—should accommodate culture-based values.

Part of the answer was already given in Chapter 1 when dealing with ethical relativism, and in Chapters 4 and 5 when dealing with valuational competence. The same thing that was argued then when considering the ethical legitimacy of privately held values also applies in this connection. (See Chapters 4 and 5, on ethical private values.) As long as values are consistent with fundamental ethical principles, they must be respected, their difference from general social values notwithstanding. However, this condition is not met by sex selection that is based on cultural values. By its very nature, it is grounded in the thesis that one sex is worth less than another. It therefore violates Autonomy and Respect for Persons as well as Equality. It is therefore ethically indefensible.[95]

This conclusion may appear to fly in the face of the Canadian commitment to multiculturalism and the legal requirement of non-interference that is based on sections 2, 15 and 27 of the Charter of Rights and Freedoms.[96] However, section 28 of the Charter explicitly states that

> [n]otwithstanding anything in this Charter, the rights and freedoms referred to in it are guaranteed equally to male and female persons.

Moreover, the prohibition of culture-based sex selection can be defended in terms of section 1 of the Charter. Arguably, a value scheme that denies the equality of persons as persons can never be consistent with the notion of a free and democratic society, because the equality of persons as persons is integral to the concept of democracy itself. Therefore, it is arguable that the prohibition of sex selection based on cultural values can be "demonstrably justified in a free and democratic society."

However, it could be argued that if preference-based sex selection were allowed, culture- and value-based sex selection might be legitimated, so to speak, "by the back door," because people might claim that their use of sex selection was merely the result of personal preference, whereas in actuality it was the result of a cultural or valuational bias.

It is unethical to treat persons who do something ethically legitimate in the same way as persons who act in an ethically indefensible fashion. That would violate the Principle of Equality and Justice. Furthermore, as the Principle of the Least Restrictive Alternative mandates, a right may be interfered with only to the least degree necessary under the circumstances that obtain. Therefore, if there is a way to allow preference-based sex selection without thereby allowing culture-based sex selection under the pretence of preference, it would be ethically mandatory to do so. There is, in fact, a way to do so, and to minimize the danger of such a deceptive practice: It could be achieved by allowing sex selection for non-medical reasons only to create "matched pairs."[97]

POST-MENOPAUSAL MOTHERHOOD

The advances in reproductive technologies have not been confined to IVF and similar techniques. It is now possible—albeit the success rate is very low—to allow post-menopausal women who could not normally become pregnant to become biological mothers. In fact, a whole industry is beginning to appear that is devoted to facilitating post-menopausal pregnancies. The Royal Commission on New Reproductive Technologies has gone on record as questioning the ethical defensibility of using the reproductive technologies to facilitate post-menopausal pregnancy; however, the ethics of post-menopausal motherhood has become the subject of increasing debate, spurred by the fact that there are no legally binding guidelines against it in Canada and that in countries such as Italy, the U.S. and the U.K., post-menopausal pregnancies are on the increase. Since in health care as elsewhere, the technological imperative frequently serves as a driver for applying technological tools once they are available, the use of reproductive technologies in this manner deserves at least some preliminary consideration.

"Naturalness" of the Intervention

One of the most obvious—and at the same time one of the least persuasive—ways of arguing against post-menopausal motherhood is to say that it is "unnatural"—that it is species-normal for women to lose their fertility, just as it is species-normal for men, and the fact that men lose their fertility later than women does not make it unethical or give medicine a mandate to improve on nature.

This line of reasoning is based on the premise that one should not do what is unnatural." However, if "unnatural" is understood as doing something that nature itself does not do, then most of medicine and health care is "unnatural." In a state of unaltered nature, people fall ill, suffer accidents and in general suffer and die in rather unpleasant ways, most of which are alleviated or prevented by modern health care. If, on the other hand, "unnatural" is understood as interfering with what is species-normal, that assumes a view of health that requires separate defence and is not shared by everyone. (See Chapter 9.)

Welfare of Children

Another argument against post-menopausal motherhood begins with the claim that the welfare of children born to post-menopausal mothers is not as good as that of children born to women prior to menopause—indeed, that the children are harmed by the maternal post-menopausal age itself. Since the Principle of non-Malfeasance mandates that one should not knowingly engage in actions that will harm other persons, it follows—so the argument concludes—that post-menopausal motherhood should be prohibited as a matter of social policy.

However, when evaluating this argument one is immediately struck by the fact that there are two ways of understanding this claim of harm: in a biological sense, as involving some health deficit, illness or negative health condition for the child; and in a psycho-social sense, as involving some psychosocial harm experienced by the children of post-menopausal mothers because of the mothers' age. Moreover, anyone who advances this sort of argument has to be able to adduce some evidence for the premise that there is such harm and that it is caused by post-menopausal maternal age.

As to biological harm, there are no data that show that maternal age leads to medical conditions for a child where these can be reliably and uniquely traced to the fact that the mother is post-menopausal. Therefore, the biological version of the argument is hypothetical at best. Likewise, there are no data which show that children raised by post-menopausal women have sustained psychosocial harm as a result of being raised by such mothers. Therefore, the harm-based rejection of post-menopausal motherhood seems to lack any evidentiary basis.

There is a variant of the psychosocial argument, however, which goes like this: Post-menopausal women are likely to die earlier than women who are in their natural child-bearing years. To lose one's mother while young is a traumatic event, and therefore constitutes harm. Consequently, the children born to post-menopausal mothers are knowingly exposed to harm that is not (likely) to befall other children. Therefore, if society were to permit or even facilitate post-menopausal motherhood, it would become complicit in causing harm, thus violating the Principle of non-Malfeasance.

But this argument is not completely persuasive either. There is no right to have a mother, biological or otherwise, for the duration of one's childhood. If there were, every time a child loses his or her mother, something unethical would have happened. In other words, one should not confuse what is tragic with what is unethical. Still, there is the fact that to deliberately bring about a state of affairs that will likely result in such a tragic loss earlier than otherwise would occur is to deliberately maximize the chance of such harm. That may violate the Principle of non-Malfeasance. However, the operant clause in this argument is that to lose one's mother is to sustain harm. Therefore, if reasoning of this argument were adopted consistently, every prospective mother, *irrespective of age*, would have to be medically assessed as to the likelihood of her dying during her offspring's childhood.

Welfare of Mothers

A closely related version of the harm argument focuses not on the child but on the mother. It begins with the premise that the technology involved in producing a post-menopausal pregnancy is not without its dangers to the mother, and that the pregnancy at this stage in her life poses clearly identifiable risks for the woman herself. The hormone regulation and steering that is necessary to facilitate and sustain the pregnancy is not without potentially dangerous side effects, and the stress that sustaining such a pregnancy imposes on aged maternal tissues and organs, etc., can be considerable Therefore, as a sheer matter of non-Malfeasance, such pregnancies should not be permitted.

However, this reasoning is based on several assumptions. *First*, it assumes that all post-menopausal women will be harmed by undergoing the relevant interventions and by being pregnant. The data do not support this claim, and there are many successful post-menopausal pregnancies that have resulted in live births of healthy babies without harm to the mother. *Second*, it would appear to go against the Principle of Autonomy, which allows all persons to have control over their bodies (subject only to the equal and competing rights of others).

In all fairness, however, it is not clear that this last consideration is entirely telling. To be successful, it must assume that autonomy includes the right to use medical technologies for any purpose people see fit—including self-mutilation, self-modification, etc. The question of whether autonomy extends this far, however, cannot be divorced from the question of which model of the physician–patient relationship is appropriate, whether all values are ethically defensible, whether health care is a right or a commodity, the issue of resource allocation and the question of whether the role of medicine is to correct conditions that interfere with species-normal functioning or to improve on species-normal functioning—which, in turn, is inseparable from the issue of the nature of health itself.

Nevertheless, these last considerations notwithstanding, the rejection of this version of the harm argument does have a point. Logically, the harm-based rejection of post-menopausal motherhood is not inherently based on age but on *harm*. Therefore, if the reasoning is applied consistently, under the Principle of Equality and Justice, it would entail that *all* women who wish to become pregnant should be assessed as to the likelihood that they will sustain harm—and very few would defend something like that.

Access to Ova

Another relatively standard argument against facilitating post-menopausal motherhood focuses on the fact that unlike sperm, ova do not freeze well, and that almost invariably, post-menopausal women must use donated ova.[98] Post-menopausal motherhood would therefore take away scarce ova from younger women who do not have viable ova of their own and need donated ova to become pregnant. Post-menopausal women have already had a chance to become pregnant prior to menopause—i.e., they have already had their "fair innings."[99] The fact that they did not avail themselves of the opportunity was their choice. Every choice entails consequences. If one does not like the consequences, one should not make that choice.

Its initial plausibility notwithstanding, however, it is not at all clear that this reasoning is probative. In the first place—as was discussed in Chapter 10—the "fair innings" argument has conditional validity at best. It stands and falls with being able to show that to restrict access to health care modalities based purely on age is ethically defensible—and that is doubtful.

Secondly, it assumes that in fact all post-menopausal candidates for pregnancy have had an equitable opportunity to become pregnant—whereby "equitable opportunity" includes more than merely biological possibility but also the socioeconomic embedding of the woman as candidate for pregnancy. Arguably, this is not the case.[100] Current and evolving socioeconomic realities are pushing more and more women to postpone their child-bearing until they are near or past menopause.

Still, it is very difficult to show that, if one has made a choice that reduces one's downstream options, society must reintroduce that option on the same basis as it existed in the original setting. This is true only if the initial choice was itself forced by unethical social conditions—and that, in turn, requires a separate and distinct analysis of the social embedding of women. While, in the end, such an analysis may substantiate this particular claim, it cannot merely be stated. Moreover, the argument also assumes that there is a right to have children. Only then could one claim that there was a duty to allow access to reproductive technologies as a matter of right.

CONCLUSION

If the preceding analysis is correct, then there is a *prima facie* right to have children (in the full-blooded sense of that phrase) that it is grounded in the biological and social nature of human beings as persons and in the Principle of Autonomy. However, like all rights, it is conditioned and not absolute, and does not belong to everyone under all circumstances. One has to look and see.

Moreover, in the pursuit of this right, one should never lose sight of the fact that the fulfillment of that right involves children, and that children are persons. Therefore, how the children will fare once they are born should be integral to the decision whether to exercise that right.

Finally, it is important to consider that interference with any right, whether by society or by individual persons, always needs ethical justification. Moreover, even when such interference is mandated, it should always be in keeping with the Principle of the Least Restrictive Alternative. That applies not only to the right to have children itself but also to the question of how that right is implemented—whether that be in the traditional manner or through some form of surrogacy. The same thing holds true of preference-based sex selection. If it is not based on ethically objectionable values, then there are also no ethically valid grounds for prohibiting it.

There is an old legal maxim: "What is not forbidden, is allowed!" From an ethical perspective, the maxim is incomplete. It should be completed by adding the clause "and it is important not to forbid the wrong things, because that amounts to an unjustified curtailment of autonomy."

Further Readings

Baird, P. "Individual Interests, Societal Interests, and Reproductive Technologies." *Perspect Biol Med* 40 (1996): 440–451.

Banerjee, A. "Reorienting the Ethics of Transnational Surrogacy as a Feminist Pragmatist." *The Pluralist* 5.3 (2010): 107–127.

Kluge, E.-H. "Sex Selection: Some Ethical and Policy Considerations." *Health Care Analysis* 15.2 (2007): 73–89.

Macklin, R. "The Ethics of Sex Selection and Family Balancing." *Seminars in Reproductive Medicine* 28.4 (2010): 315–321.

Murphy, T.F. "The Ethics of Helping Transgender Men and Women Have Children." *Perspectives in Biology and Medicine* 53.1 (2010): 46–60.

People's Republic of China. *White Paper on Family Planning*, Information Office of the State Council of the People's Republic of China, August 1995, Beijing, available at www.china.org.cn/e-white/familypanning/index.htm

Proclamation of Teheran, Final Act of the International Conference on Human Rights, Teheran, 22 April to 13 May 1968, U.N. Doc. A/CONF. 32/41 at 3 (1968), available at www1.umn.edu/humanrts/instree/l2ptichr.htm

Purdy, L.M. "Genetics and Reproductive Risk: Can Having Children Be Immoral?" in *Reproducing Persons: Issues in Feminist Bioethics*, ed. L.M. Purdy (Ithaca, NY: Cornell University Press, 1996), 39–49.

Royal Commission on New Reproductive Technologies, *Proceed with Care: Final Report of the Royal Commission on New Reproductive Technologies* (2 vols.) (Ottawa: Minister of Government Services Canada, 1993).

Smajdor, A. "The Ethics of IVF over 40." *Maturitas* 69 (2011): 37–40.

van Niekerk, A., and L. van Zyl. "The Ethics of Surrogacy: Women's Reproductive Labour." *Journal of Medical Ethics* 21 (1995): 345–349.

Warnock, M. *Making Babies: Is There a Right to Have Children?* (Oxford: Oxford University Press, 2002).

Zhang, S. "The Morality of Having Children with Disabilities: A Different Perspective on Happiness and Quality of Life." *McGill Journal of Medicine* 8 (2004): 85–88.

Endnotes

1. *Universal Declaration of Human Rights*, accessed 17 Jun 2011 at www.un.org/en/documents/udhr/index.shtml

2. Eugenics is the theory that the genetic characteristics of a species ought to be improved by deliberate interference. It may be either positive, by encouraging the "evolutionary fit" to reproduce abundantly; or negative, by preventing the "evolutionary fit" from reproducing.

3. *Proclamation of Teheran*, Final Act of the International Conference on Human Rights, Teheran, 22 April to 13 May 1968, U.N. Doc. A/CONF. 32/41, at 3 (1968), clause 16, accessed 17 Jun 2011 at www1.umn.edu/humanrts/instree/l2ptichr.htm

4. *The World Population Plan of Action*. Adopted by consensus of the 137 countries represented at the United Nations World Population Conference at Bucharest, August 1974. Clauses 7 and 14 (f); accessed 17 Jun 2011 at www.population-security.org/27-APP1.html#Adoption

5. *Report of the International Conference on Population*, Mexico City, 6–14 August 1984, accessed at www.choike.org/documentos/conf/ICP_mexico84_report.pdf #13

6. People's Republic of China, *Family Planning in China*. Govt. White Paper, accessed 16 Jun 2011 at www.china.org.cn/e-white/familypanning/index.htm

7. The *White Paper* recognizes that exceptions to this rule may be necessary, as for instance in rural contexts where there is an insufficient labour force to produce the foodstuffs necessary to feed the Chinese population and the massive relocation of urban persons into the rural setting would involve more difficulties than it would solve.

8. Compare Great Britain, Dept. of Health and Social Services, *Report of the Committee of Enquiry into Human Fertilisation and Embryology* ("The Warnock Report"), M. Warnock, chair (London: Her Majesty's Stationery Office, 1984). For an extended look at some non-medical issues, see *Should Parents Be Licensed? Debating the Issues,* ed. P. Tittle (Buffalo, NY: Prometheus Books, 2004).

9. See Buck v. Bell, 274 U.S. 200; see also J.L. Waters, "In Whose Best Interest? *New Jersey Division of Youth and Family Services v. V.M. and B.G.* and the Next Wave of Court-Controlled Pregnancies," *Harvard Journal of Law and Gender* 34.1 (2011): 81–111.

10. This usually included dangerous sex offenders. The statutes of Alberta and British Columbia in particular were implicated in this regard, and in the U.S. many states had similar provisions. See also A. McLaren, *Twentieth-Century Sexuality: A History* (Malden, MA: Blackwell, 1999), and Waters, op. cit., *supra.*

11. See A. McLaren, "The Creation of a Haven for 'Human Thoroughbreds': The Sterilization of the Feebleminded and the Mentally Ill in British Columbia," *Canadian Historical Review* 67.2 (1986): 127–150. Similar sterilization laws existed in Alberta until 1972. See also A. McLaren, *Twentieth-Century Sexuality: A History* (Malden, MA: Blackwell, 1999) and *Our Own Master Race: Eugenics in Canada, 1885–1945.* Canadian Social History Series (Toronto: McClelland & Stewart, 1990). See also T.A. Brown, "Forced Abortion and Involuntary Sterilization in China: Are the Victims of Coercive Population Control Measures Eligible for Asylum in the United States?" *San Diego Law Rev* 34 (1995): 745; "Bangladesh: Sterilization Program" *Asian Popul Programme News* 6.3 (1977): 26 337–340, (no authors listed).

12. *Assisted Human Reproduction Act*, S.C. 2004.

13. E. (Mrs.) v. Eve, [1986] 2 S.C.R. 388.

14. Muir v. The Queen in Right of Alberta, D.L.R. 132 (4th series): (1996), 695–762.

15. T.J. Christian, "The Mentally Ill and Human Rights in Alberta: A Study of the Alberta Sexual Sterilization Act," University of Alberta, Faculty of Law, 1973. See also J.M. Grekul, *The Social Construction of the Feebleminded Threat: Implementation of the Sexual Sterilization Act in Alberta 1929–1972.* University of Alberta, PhD Thesis, 2002. British Columbia had a similar sterilization act. See *Sexual Sterilization Act*, Revised Statutes of British Columbia, 1978. For more information, see A. McLaren, *Our Own Master Race*, op. cit.

16. Muir v. The Queen in Right of Alberta, op. cit.

17. The closest Canadian courts came to doing so was in Re K, Supreme Court of B.C. Jan. 30, 1985, Vancouver Registry A 842 616. The Supreme Court took judicial notice of this case in Eve, and cautioned that interference with reproductive capacity, even for therapeutic reasons, "is at best dangerously close to the limits of the permissible" (Eve, at 93).

18. See Ontario Law Reform Commission, *Report on Human Artificial Reproduction and Related Matters* (Toronto, 1985), 153 ff, for a recommendation that surrogacy contracts be legally enforceable.

19. "Out of Africa Revisited," *Science* (13 May 2005): 921.

20. T.L. Wall et al., "Alcohol Metabolism in Asian-American Men with Genetic Polymorphisms of Aldehyde Dehydrogenase," *Annals of Internal Medicine* 127.5 (1997): 376–379.

21. N. Jablonski and G. Chaplin, "The Evolution of Human Skin Coloration," *Journal of Human Evolution* 39.1 (2000): 57–106.

22. L.G. Moore, "Human Genetic Adaptation to High Altitude," *High Alt Med Biol* 2.2 (2001): 257–279.

23. See P. Frost, "European Hair and Eye Color: A Case of Frequency-Dependent Sexual Selection?" *Evolution and Human Behavior* 27 (2006): 85–103. For an analysis of the genetic difference between blue-eyed lemurs and blue-eyed human beings, see B.J. Bradley, A. Pedersen, and

N.I. Mundy, "Blue Eyes in Lemurs and Humans: Same Phenotype, Different Genetic Mechanism," *Am J Phys Anthropol* 139.2 (June 2009): 269–273.

24. E. Juhász, J. Béres, S. Kanizsai and K. Nagy, "The Consequence of a Founder Effect: CCR5-?32, CCR2-64I and SDF1-3'A Polymorphism in Vlach Gypsy Population in Hungary," *Pathol Oncol Res* (2011 Jun 11), Epub ahead of print; M. Samson et al., "Resistance to HIV-1 Infection in Caucasian Individuals Bearing Mutant Alleles of the CCR-5 Chemokine Receptor Gene," *Nature* 382.6593 (August 1996): 722–725.

25. See *Report of the Commission of Inquiry into Human Fertilisation and Embryology*, M. Warnock, chair (London: Her Majesty's Stationery Office, 1984), at 8–9.

26. A. Maslow, "A Theory of Human Motivation," *Psychological Review* 50 (1943): 370–396, and *Motivation and Personality*, 2nd ed. (New York: Harper & Row, 1970).

27. M.A. Wahba and L.G. Bridwell, "Maslow Reconsidered: A Review of Research on the Need Hierarchy Theory," *Organizational Behavior and Human Performance* 15 (1976): 212–240.

28. See Law Reform Commission of Canada, *Sterilization*, at 63. See also E. (Mrs.) v. Eve, [1986] 2 S.C.R. 388, for a version of this argument, focusing on the joy and satisfaction that parenting would bring.

29. For a discussion of some aspects of this, notably the notion of "suitability" to be a parent, see M. Somerville, "Birth Technology, Parenting and 'Deviance,'" *International Journal of Law and Psychiatry* 5 (1982): 123. For a discussion of the issue in relation to techniques of assisted reproduction, see British Columbia, Royal Commission on Family and Children's Law, *Ninth Report of the Royal Commission on Family and Children's Law* (Victoria: 1975), 10, and elsewhere; and Ontario Law Reform Commission, *Report on Human Artificial Reproduction and Related Matters* (Toronto: 1985), 153 ff.

30. B. (B.) v. Child and Family Services, [1989] 1 S.C.R. 291; *Canadian Human Rights Advocate* V: 10 (December 1989), 10.

31. For a similar position adopted by the Supreme Court, see Eve, at 84, *et pass.*

32. See note 29, *supra.*

33. For a classic analysis of some aspects of this reasoning, see R.H. Kenan and R.M. Schmidt, "Stigmatization of Carrier Status: Social Implications of Heterozygote Genetic Screening Programs," *American Journal of Public Health* 68 (1978): 116–120.

34. Eve, at 92.

35. W.S.T. Hays, "Human Pheromones: Have They Been Demonstrated?" *Behavioral Ecology and Sociobiology* 54 (2003): 89–97; C.J. Wysocki and G. Preti, "Pheromonal Influences," *Archives of Sexual Behavior* 27.6 (1998): 627–664.

36. And the *Proclamation of Teheran* and the People's Republic of China's *White Paper*.

37. Cystic fibrosis produces no harm prior to birth because prior to being born the child does not breathe and its oxygen needs are supplied through its umbilical cord by the mother.

38. See L.M. Purdy, "Genetic Diseases: Can Having Children Be Immoral?" in *Genetics Now: Issues in Genetic Research*, ed. J.J. Buckley (Washington, DC: University Press of America, 1978).

39. For a discussion of the ethics of limiting individual rights and freedoms when they conflict with those of others, see Aristotle (384 B.C.E.–322 B.C.E.), *Politics,* Book II, Chapter III, 1261b. For a more contemporary discussion, see the classic article by G. Hardin, "The Tragedy of the Commons," *Science* 162 (1968): 1243–1248.

40. Immanuel Kant, *Metaphysics of Morals* 6: 418.

41. For possible implications regarding the use of abortion as a method of birth control, see *supra.*

42. For a general overview of methods, see A.F. Schrater, "Immunization to Regulate Fertility: Biological and Cultural Frameworks," *Soc Sci Med* 41.5 (1995): 657–671. For a somewhat dated discussion in favour of control, see C.P. Kindregan, "State Power over Human Fertility and Individual Liberty" *Hastings L.J.* 23 (1971/1972): 1401–1426.

43. People's Republic of China, *Family Planning in China*. Govt. White Paper, accessed 16 Jun 2011 at www.china.org.cn/e-white/familypanning/index.htm

44. For another use of the principle in health care, see L.O. Gostin, "Ethical and Legal Challenges Posed by Severe Acute Respiratory Syndrome: Implications for the Control of Severe Infectious Disease Threats," *JAMA* 290.24 (2003): 3229–3237. For a Canadian legal discussion in public health, see S. Trueman, "Community Treatment Orders and Nova Scotia—The Least Restrictive Alternative?" *Health Law Journal* 11 (2003): 1–33.

45. Law Reform Commission of Canada, Working Paper 24, *Sterilization: Implications for Mentally Retarded and Mentally Ill Persons* (Ottawa: Minister of Supply and Services, 1978), 71.

46. See the discussion of non-consensual sterilization, *supra*.

47. *Sterilization*, at 68.

48. *Sterilization*, at 62.

49. Eve, at 84.

50. It should be clear that poverty, marital status, etc., would not be implicated either because these do not rule out society's ability to appropriately assist if necessary or to compensate.

51. E.-H.W. Kluge, "After *Eve*: Whither Proxy Decision-Making?" *Canadian Medical Association Journal* 137 (15 Oct 1987): 715–720.

52. Provincial health care plans differ in their willingness to cover IVF and even the same province may vacillate over time.

53. IVF CANADA/LIFE Program, Fee Schedule, accessed 29 Jun 2011 at www.ivfcanada.com/services/fees/general_fee_schedule.cfm. The additional fee for patients eligible under the provincial health plan is only a fraction of that cost. However, the total cost to the provincial insurer remains the same.

54. S.K. Sunkara et al., "Association between the Number of Eggs and Live Birth in IVF Treatment: An Analysis of 400 135 Treatment Cycles," *Hum Reprod* 26.7 (Jul 2011): 1768–1774; C. Gnoth et al., "Final ART Success Rates: A 10 Uears Survey," *Hum Reprod* (9 Jun 2011), Epub ahead of print; V.C. Wright et al., "Assisted Reproductive Technology Surveillance—United States, 2000," *MMWR Surveill Summ* 52.9 (29 Aug 2003): 1–16.

55. *Assisted Human Reproduction Act*, S.C. 2004, c. 26. 6(1), (2).

56. Baby Manji Yamada v. The Union of India and Anr., [(2008) 13 SCC 518], and Jan Balaz v. Union of India [From L.P.A. No. 2151 of 2009, High Court of Gujarat].

57. Article 6 of the Civil Code of the Ukraine, Articles 627, 628, 629, 639, and 123 of the Family Code of Ukraine, subparagraph 2.2 of paragraph 2 of Order of the Ministry of Justice of Ukraine No. 140/5, dated 18 May 2003.

58. Royal Commission on New Reproductive Technologies, *Proceed With Care: Final Report of the Royal Commission on New Reproductive Technologies*, 2 vols. (Ottawa: Minister of Government Services Canada, 1993), Vol. 2, 670 f, 674.

59. *Proceed*, at 672.

60. *Proceed*, at 677 f.

61. *Proceed*, at 678; American Society of Obstetricians and Gynecologists, Committee on Ethics Opinion, 2008, "Surrogate Motherhood," accessed 23 Jun 2011 at www.acog.org/from_home/publications/ethics/co397.pdf

62. *Proceed*, at 675, 678 f.

63. *Proceed*, at 677.

64. *Proceed*, at 678.

65. India Surrogacy, accessed 23 Jun 2011 at www.weecaresurrogacy.com/surrogate/fees.html; International Surrogacy Partners, accessed 23 Jun 2011 at www.surrogateagency.com/fees.shtml

66. As an aside, this conclusion should prove reassuring for men who marry women because they want to have children. Legally, marriage is a contractual arrangement between two parties. Therefore, if men marry for the sake of having children, they are essentially entering into a contractual fee-for-service arrangement in which they provide material considerations and upkeep in exchange for a child.

67. In what follows, *sex* will be used instead of the increasingly common term *gender*. Gender is a social construct, sex is a biological matter.

68. M. Levitan, *Textbook of Human Genetics* (New York and London: Oxford University Press, 1988); T. Strachan and A.P. Read, *Human Molecular Genetics*, 3rd ed. (New York and London: Garland Science, 2004).

69. See M.B. Mahowald, *Genes, Women, Equality* (Oxford, U.K.: Oxford University Press, 2000); L.M. Purdy, "Genetic Diseases: Can Having Children Be Immoral?," in *Issues in Bioethics*, ed. T.L. Beauchamp and L. Walters (Belmont CA: Wadsworth Publishing Company, 1978), 243–247; and L.M. Purdy, *Reproducing Persons: Issues in Feminist Bioethics* (Ithaca, NY: Cornell University Press, 1996).

70. Mahowald, op. cit.; M. Shaw, "Preconception and Prenatal Tests," in *Genetics and the Law II*, ed. A. Milunsky and A. Annas (New York: Plenum Press, 1980); C. Perry, "Wrongful Life and Comparison of Harms," *Westminster Institute Review* 1.4 (1982): 7–9.

71. *Donum Vitae*: "Instruction on Respect for Human Life in Its Origin and on the Dignity of Procreation—Replies to Certain Questions of the Day," given at Vatican City, Rome, from the Sacred Congregation for the Doctrine of the Faith, approved and ordered for publication by the Supreme Pontiff, John Paul II, 22 Feb 1987; Pope Paul VI, Encyclical Letter, "Humanae Vitae," *Acta Apostolicae Sedis* LX: 9 (1968).

72. D.C. Wertz and J.C. Fletcher, "Sex Selection through Prenatal Diagnosis," in *Feminist Perspectives in Medical Ethics*, ed. N. Holmes and L. Purdy (Bloomington: Indiana University Press, 1992), 240–253; Mahowald, op. cit.

73. L. Kass, "Implications of Prenatal Diagnosis for the Human Right to Life," in *Biomedical Ethics*, ed. T.A. Mappes and J.S. Zembatty (New York and London: McGraw-Hill, 1978).

74. Compare Anglican Church of Canada, *On Dying Well* (Toronto: Anglican Church Information Office, 1975); Campbell, op cit.

75. See D. Schiff, "Trouble Ahead: Decision Making Corners in Neonatology," *The Bioethics Bulletin* 2.4 (1990): 1, for an application of the notion of differential quality of life to the neonatal setting. See also K. Bennett and D. Feeny, "Clinical and Economic Evaluation of Therapeutic Technologies: The Case of Neonatal Intensive Care Programs," in *Health Care Technology: Effectiveness, Efficiency and Public Policy*, ed. D. Feeny, G. Guyatt and P. Tugwell (Montreal: The Institute for Research on Public Policy, 1988), 199–223.

76. This is the device suggested by John Rawls, in his *Theory of Justice*, where the individual knows neither her place in society, her class position or social status, nor her natural assets or natural abilities (such as strength, looks, and intelligence), and has to make a choice on that basis.

77. For an extended discussion of this, see D. Benatar, *Better Never to Have Been: The Harm of Coming into Existence* (Oxford, U.K.: Oxford University Press, 2006). For a critical review of Benatar, see E. Harman, *Nous* 43.4 (2009): 776–785, and E.-H. Kluge, *Philosophy in Review* 28.5 (Oct 2008): 317–319.

78. G.R. Dunstan, "On selecting the sex of the child to be born," in *The Status of the Human Embryo*, ed. G.R. Dunstan and M.J. Seller (London: King Edward's Hospital Fund, 1988); J. Glover, *Ethics of New Reproductive Technologies: The Glover Report to the European Commission* (DeKalb: Northern Illinois University Press, 1989); E.-H W. Kluge and C. Lucock, *New Reproductive Technologies: A Preliminary Perspective of the Canadian Medical Association* (Ottawa: CMA, 1991); Mahowald, 2000; B.K. Rothman, *The Book of Life: A Personal and Ethical Guide to Race, Normality, and the Implications of the Human Genome Project* (Boston: Beacon Press, 2001); Purdy, 1996; Society of Obstetricians and Gynaecologists of Canada, *In Vitro Fertilization and Embryo Transfer: Report to the Royal Commission on New Reproductive Technologies* (Ottawa: Society of Obstetricians

and Gynecologists of Canada, 1991); D.C. Wertz and J.C. Fletcher, "Fatal Knowledge? Prenatal Diagnosis and Sex Selection," *Hastings Center Report* 19.3 (1989): 21–27.

79. *Shorter Oxford English Dictionary.*

80. *Shorter Oxford English Dictionary.*

81. R.A. Crouch, "Letting the Deaf Be Deaf: Reconsidering the Use of Cochlear Implants in Prelingually Deaf Children," *Hastings Center Report* 27.4 (1997): 14–21; R. Sparrow, "Defending Deaf Culture: The Case of Cochlear Implants," *The Journal of Political Philosophy* 13.2 (2005): 135–152.

82. For a different approach leading to a similar conclusion as the one argued here, see T.F. Murphy, "Reproductive Controls and Sexual Destiny," *Bioethics* 4.2 (Apr 1990): 121–142. See also R.L. Reid, *Ethical Considerations of the New Technologies: A Report of the Combined Ethics Committee of the Canadian Fertility and Andrology Society and the Society of Obstetricians and Gynaecologists of Canada* (Toronto: Ribosome, 1990).

83. *Proceed*, Vol. 2, Chapter 28, "Sex Selection for Non-Medical Reasons," 890 f.

84. Ibid.

85. Ibid., 890.

86. Loc. cit.

87. T. Jain et al., "Preimplantation Sex Selection Demand and Preferences in an Infertility Population," *Fertility and Sterility* 83.3 (2005): 649–658.

88. E. Dahl et al., "Preconception Sex Selection for Nonmedical Reasons: A Representative Survey from Germany," *Human Reproduction* 18.10 (2003): 2231–2234.

89. J. Cohen, "Gender Selection: Is There a European View?" *Journal of Assisted Reproduction and Genetics* 19.9 (2002): 417–419.

90. Yu Xie, "Measuring Regional Variation in Sex Preference in China: A Cautionary Note," *Social Science Research* 18.3 (1989): 291–305; M.J. Graham, U. Larsen and X. Xu, "Son Preference in Anhui Province, China," *International Family Planning Perspectives* 24.2 (1998): 72–77.

91. C. Zhou et al., "Son Preference and Sex-Selective Abortion in China: Informing Policy Options," *Int J Public Health* (17 Jun 2011), Epub ahead of print.

92. R. Kansal et al., "A Hospital-Based Study on Knowledge, Attitude and Practice of Pregnant Women on Gender Preference, Prenatal Sex Determination and Female Feticide," *Indian J Public Health* 54.5 (Oct–Dec 2010): 209–212.

93. F.G. Abrejo, B.T. Shaikh, and N. Rizvi, "'And they kill me, only because I am a girl' . . . A Review of Sex-Selective Abortions in South Asia," *Eur J Contracept Reprod Health Care* 14.1 (Feb 2009): 10–16.

94. See also N.E. Williamson, "Boys or Girls? Parents' Preferences and Sex Control," *Population Bulletin* 33:1 (Jan 1978): 3–35, for some dated but still relevant data; as well as R. Steinbacher, "Futuristic Implications of Sex Preselection," in *The Custom-Made Child? Women-Centered Perspectives*, ed. H.B. Holmes, B.B. Hoskins and M. Gross (Clifton, NJ: Human Press, 1981), 188, *et pass.*; and V. Patel, "Sex-Determination and Sex Preselection Tests in India: Recent Techniques in Femicide," *Reproductive and Genetic Engineering: Journal of International Feminist Analysis* 2.2 (1989): 111–119.

95. For an argument against non-medical sex selection that centres in slippery-slope considerations, see J. Egozcue, "Preimplantation Social Sexing: A Problem of Proportionality and Decision Making," *Journal of Assisted Reproduction and Genetics* 19.9 (2002): 440–442.

96. R.S.C. 1985, Appendix II, No. 44.

97. See also American Society of Reproductive Medicine, Ethics Committee, "Sex Selection and Preimplantation Genetic Diagnosis," *Fertil Steri* 72 (1999): 595–598. American Society of Reproductive Medicine, Ethics Committee, "Preconception Gender Selection for Nonmedical Reasons," *Fertil Steril* 75 (2001): 861–864.

98. For a critical analysis of this and related arguments against post-menopausal motherhood, see A. Smajdor, "The Ethics of IVF over 40," *Maturitas* 69 (2011): 37–40.

99. A. Williams, "Rationing Health Care by Age," *British Medical Journal* 314 (15 Mar 1997): 820.

100. J.A. Parks, "A Closer Look at Reproductive Technology and Postmenopausal Motherhood," *CMAJ* 154.8 (1996): 1189–1191.

SAMPLE CASES

1. Crispina Calvert (whose uterus had been removed for medical reasons but who still had functioning ovaries) and her husband Mark wanted children. They contracted with Anna Johnson to act as gestational surrogate mother for their child, which would be conceived though IVF, the embryo being implanted in Ms. Johnson's uterus. The negotiated fee was $10,000. In the seventh month of the pregnancy, Ms. Johnson told the Calverts that she was not going to give up the child. The Calverts countered by saying that the child was biologically theirs and that Ms. Johnson was not biologically related to the child she carried. They also reminded her that she had signed a contract. The California Supreme Court found that Ms. Johnson had no parental rights because she was not the "natural mother" and that she would have to surrender the baby (Johnson v. Calvert, 5 Cal.4th 84 P.2d 776).

2. The funerary customs of C and A's religion demand that the eldest son of the dead person act as chief mourner and take flaming pieces of kusha grass to light the pyre upon which C and A respectively would be laid to be cremated after they were dead, for their souls to ascend to heaven. The customs also demand that the son circumambulate the pyre counter-clockwise while his sacred thread, which usually hangs from the left shoulder, hangs from the right. C and A had no sons, only daughters. According to A and C's understanding of their religion, this meant that they would not achieve heavenly beatitude, because no son would perform the appropriate rite. C and his wife therefore agreed to go to a fertility clinic and have sex selection done, so that this calamity might not befall them.

3. In 2010, Canada decided that its foreign aid to countries such as Somalia (which are experiencing unprecedented mortality and morbidity rates because of starvation caused by crop failures due to insufficient rainfall) would not include birth control information, devices or medications. Some criticized this and said that it would guarantee the continued rise of mortality and morbidity rates, since people could then not stop pregnancies from occurring and every new mouth to feed would make the situation worse. One of the replies to this has been that under such conditions, responsible people would refrain from intercourse and not have children.

Chapter 12
Biotechnology

Advances in health care are not confined to such things as surgery, pharmacology and diagnostics. They include technologies such as genetic screening, testing and gene therapy, and are poised to expand into cloning and ectogenesis. These developments have implications for more than health care. They have the potential to reshape the very understanding of what it is be human. This chapter gives a brief overview of the technologies, outlines some of their more important implications and puts them into the context of health care in general.

Questions to Keep in Mind While Reading this Chapter:

1. What are some arguments for ectogenesis? Against? Would it be ethical for Canada to import ectogenetic technology even though the *Assisted Human Reproduction Act* effectively prohibits its development?

2. What are some arguments in favour of cloning? Against? Is the Canadian prohibition of reproductive cloning ethically defensible?

3. What ethical issues—if any—are raised by genetic screening and genetic testing respectively? How do they relate to the ethics of health care in general?

4. What is genetic engineering? What are some of the arguments for genetic engineering? Against? Is there an ethical difference between somatic cell and germ line genetic engineering? How do they, respectively, relate to the ethics of health care?

5. What ethical issues are raised by the development and use of biotechnologies in human reproduction in general?

INTRODUCTION

Common perception and official pronouncements notwithstanding, what health care is delivered is not simply a function of patient needs and available resources. It is also driven by public attitudes and values, as well as by the agendas of health care professionals, health care administrators and politicians. This is a volatile mix and is subject to many influences. One of the most profound of these is the technological imperative: If something is technologically new and sophisticated, and promises to provide a "rational" solution to a particular problem, then it must be better than what has been used so far, and it must be tried.[1]

Newer may be better, and technology may solve hitherto intractable problems, but this does not mean that its use does not have ethical implications—particularly in health care. The reason is simple: Technology that is used in health care is technology that is used on people. It therefore raises two fundamental questions: Is the technology ethically appropriate in itself? and Does its use potentiate a paradigm shift in the concept of a human being and of a patient? For instance, rightly or wrongly, the medical technologies that are designed to facilitate abortions[2] or euthanasia[3] raise ethical issues because of their very nature, and arguably tend to foster a view of human beings as disposable entities and of patients as individuals who, when all else fails, may be killed. Do genetic engineering, cloning and artificial uteruses fall into the same pattern? And more particularly, are they ethically acceptable in and of themselves?

The discussion that follows looks at some of these issues. It begins with ectogenesis and cloning, and then considers genetic screening and testing. It concludes with a brief look at genetic engineering both as a means of therapy and as a method of enhancement. A recurrent background to the discussion is the question of whether these technologies have the potential for initiating a paradigm shift in the concept of the patient as person— and whether that is a good thing or a bad one.

ECTOGENESIS

The word *ectogenesis* means "generating outside." It is a scientific term for what is essentially an artificial uterus. The last few decades have seen a steady rise in interest— and increasing success—in trying to develop this technology.[4] It began as very limited research with opossum and goat fetuses in the late 1970s and early 1980s,[5] and has since come to include such other animals as mice and lambs. It is an active area of research not only in Japan and the U.S.[6] but also in Europe,[7] and it is speculated that it is only a matter of time before the technology is perfected and becomes available for human use. So far, of course, ectogenesis from fertilization to birth is still in the realm of science fiction—but it is science fiction that is quickly becoming reality. And because of its potential human use, it is important to gain some insight into its ethical implications.

Arguments Pro

There are several reasons for trying to develop the technology for human use. The most important is probably to provide a means for saving extremely premature infants. Children who are born prematurely usually die of development-related conditions. These may include insufficiently developed lungs, immature immune systems, gastrointestinal systems that are not developed enough to absorb nutrients, and the inability to maintain body heat. Other potential problems are heart defects (e.g., patent ductus arteriosus) and retinopathy of prematurity (an eye disorder that may lead to blindness)—the list is extensive.

Currently, premature babies are placed into incubators. The problem with incubators is that they do not supply all of the premature infants' needs and that they carry their own risks. For instance, the high oxygen atmosphere in incubators—which is necessary for proper oxygenation because of the immaturity of the lungs—can lead to retrolental fibroplasia; the electromagnetic fields of the incubator machinery itself may interfere with proper cardiac and lung rhythms;[8] the noise levels may negatively affect cardiac function;[9] and the incubator environment itself may give rise to iatrogenic infections. If the technology were developed to mimic a human uterus, most of these problems would be resolved or entirely avoided. In other words, it would be a beneficial adjunct to current neonatal intensive care.

The development of an artificial uterus would also solve the ethical problem that some see with abortions.[10] Instead of killing the fetus—as is currently the case in most abortions—the fetus could be removed from the woman's uterus by a hysterotomy and placed into the artificial uterus. There it could be allowed to gestate until term and then be given up for adoption. Therefore, it would expand the autonomy of women with unwanted pregnancies whose belief in the sanctity of human life prevented them from terminating their pregnancies.[11] It would also increase the number of babies that would be available for adoption.[12]

Development of the technology would also have the advantage of dealing with the current Canadian prohibition of commercial surrogacy.[13] At present, prospective parents who cannot have children by "natural" means have to find an altruistic surrogate mother. In most cases, this is impossible. Ectogenesis would solve the problem at one stroke. Anyone who wanted their own biological offspring could then—at least in principle— have a child. Paying for such a service might be problematic if ectogenesis was not funded by the public health care system. However, once the success rate of this technology had reached a sufficiently high level, there would in principle be no reason why it could not be funded, much as other successful technologies currently are, as an insured service under the rubric of infertility.

Finally, ectogenesis has the potential of solving at least part of the organ shortage that bedevils contemporary organ transplantation.[14] That is to say, organ transplantation is one of the most cost-effective ways of dealing with end-stage renal disease, and it is really the only way of dealing with end-stage liver failure and of helping patients in end-stage heart failure who remain symptomatic despite optimal medical therapy. However, the need for organs by far and away exceeds the supply. That is why potential transplant recipients are put on waiting lists, where they may sometimes languish for years and die before a suitable organ becomes available. Very young children are particularly implicated in this regard, since pediatric organs are in exceedingly short supply. Ectogenesis would solve at least part of this problem in that the fetuses from unwanted pregnancies could be allowed to develop in artificial uteruses. The full-term fetuses would then be harvested for suitable pediatric organs.

Arguments Contra

However, as those who reject ectogenesis for human use point out, the technology would not come without an ethical price. In the first instance, the technology would introduce an artificial element into human reproduction and essentially technologize it. It would also empty a personal female function, where each stage of fetal development is fraught with personal meaning and significance, of all human significance and turn having a baby into a matter of mechanics.[15]

Moreover, by doing that, it would shift the paradigm of what it is to be human. Human beings would no longer be seen as embodied rational beings of incommensurable worth but as mere biological organisms that could be treated like pieces of flesh grown under controlled conditions in an artificial environment. They would be more complicated than, but essentially similar to, vat-grown meat.[16] Ironically—and contrary to the values of care and compassion that supposedly drive the development of the technology—the humane desire to minimize harm for premature infants would be replaced by utilitarian considerations of organic damage and design specifications. Similarly, the tragedy of fetal loss and the notion of care that is demanded by premature infants—which is grounded in seeing them as people—would be replaced by frustration over manufacturing flaws.

Moreover, as was made clear in Chapter 6 on experimentation, research that has been conducted on animal models cannot simply be transferred to human beings. It has to undergo controlled human testing. Ectogenesis, therefore, would have to undergo human trials if it were to be used in the human setting. That, in turn, raises a whole series of ethical issues that centre in consent. If ectogenesis were to save premature infants, it would have to use premature infants during its experimental phases. Premature infants, however, in the later phases of gestation—say, after twenty to twenty-four weeks—would be persons. Since they would lack capacity, their involvement in the research would require substitute consent. It is unclear, however, how substitute consent for Phase I trials in ectogenesis would be ethically possible, given that such trials would be non-therapeutic in nature and, moreover, that they would produce greater than minimal harm—because they would likely lead to the fetuses' death.

As an aside, it may be worth pointing out that the relevant research could not legally be conducted in Canada. The *Assisted Human Reproduction Act* stipulates at section 5 (d) that it is a criminal offence to

> maintain an embryo outside the body of a female person after the fourteenth day of its development following fertilization or creation, excluding any time during which its development has been suspended

This would raise the interesting (and difficult) question of whether Canada could ethically allow the importation of artificial uteruses if it prohibits their development.

Discussion[17]

Legal considerations, of course, are just that, and carry no inherent ethical weight. Likewise, the fact that the technology would introduce an artificial element into human reproduction does not itself constitute an ethically grounded objection. The fact that something is artificial does not in itself mark it as unethical unless it is presumed to be so by definition. It is its development and use that may be unethical—which means that one must look and see in each particular case.[18]

To untangle the ethics of what is here at issue, let us begin with the claim that one could not ethically engage in Phase I trials because this would involve the non-therapeutic use of human incompetent beings (and their possible destruction): This could be countered simply by suggesting that Phase I trials be dispensed with. One could proceed straight from research with animal models to Phase III trials or even to therapeutic use. The relevant substitute consent protocols could here be structured along the same lines as when substitute decision-makers have to decide whether a non-validated therapy should be used when other options offer little or no chance of success. Fidelity, Beneficence and non-Malfeasance would be engaged, and it would be strictly a matter of balancing.

Nor would the development and use of an artificial uterus for therapeutic purposes undermine the paradigm of what it is to be a human person, or replace the concept of a being with intrinsic worth with that of an object that may be used to achieve a certain end. Instead, it would be precisely because the paradigm remains the same—because human beings are considered entities of inestimable worth and not mere objects—that such development would be undertaken and that substitute decision-makers could entertain the use of an artificial uterus for prematurely born infants as a last-ditch effort to save their lives.

Likewise—and irrespective of the position one may adopt on the status of the human fetus—it is arguably appropriate to avoid killing living things when it is unnecessary to do so. Therefore, an abortion-related use of an artificial uterus would fall under the rubric of harm reduction.[19] Of course, the technology may alter how abortions are performed. Here, the developmental stage of the fetus would become important. If ectogenesis were a reality, then a pregnant woman who did not wish to carry her fetus to term could agree to a hysterotomy and have the fetus implanted in an artificial uterus once the fetus had reached the twenty- to twenty-four-week stage. If it was done against her will, that would arguably constitute an interference with her autonomy and the integrity of her person. However, if the gradualistic perspective enunciated in *Morgentaler* is correct (see Chapter 8), that would not necessarily be unethical.

By contrast, the use of an artificial uterus for non-therapeutic purposes would be ethically more problematic. If the aim was to produce pediatric organs for transplantation, this would treat the developing fetus as a commodity to be harvested.[20] Since it is highly unlikely that the relevant organs would be usable before the third trimester, this would mean that the fetus would have passed the stage of personhood that was identified in

Chapter 8. Harvesting its organs would therefore be ethically tantamount to murder, the absence of legal provisions that would allow this—i.e., section 223(1) of the *Criminal Code of Canada*, which would deny such a fetus legal status—notwithstanding. In other words, it would be difficult to reconcile this with a deontological perspective. (For more on fetal development and its ethical relevance, see Chapter 8.) The only way to avoid such ethical complications would be to pith the developing fetus, thus preventing its neurological development. That might also avoid any issues arising from using fetuses without consent for experimental purposes. However, it is at least *prima facie* plausible to argue that this would facilitate a paradigm shift towards an instrumentalistic view of human beings beyond anything that occurs when abortions are justified by claiming that fetuses may be killed so that the aims and aspirations of women who do not want to be pregnant can be realized.

The use of an artificial uterus for reproductive purposes would, of course, not encounter these ethical problems. It would also solve some of the issues that surround surrogate motherhood. Moreover if, as some feminists maintain, motherhood is a burden, then this technology would be liberating for women[21] and would be perfectly in keeping with the Principles of Autonomy and Equality.[22]

At the same time, it would leave unresolved the experimental-use issue already referred to above, and it is at least arguable that if it were widely employed, ectogenesis could facilitate the objectification of fetuses and children. It might also lead to a fundamental dichotomization of personhood and biological embodiment, in which the human body is seen merely as a tool or object without any moral significance. It may be that such a denouement is ethically defensible—the point will be addressed more fully later— but at least it deserves close consideration.

HUMAN CLONING

Cloning is the production of genetically identical animals, and was first successfully performed in 1996 in Dolly, a Finn-Dorset sheep. It may be performed in several ways. In somatic cell nuclear transfer (SCNT) the nuclear DNA of a donor somatic cell is transferred into an enucleated ovum *in vitro*. The resultant zygote may then be transferred into the uterus of the surrogate mother or, if an artificial uterus has been developed—which is not currently the case—into an artificial uterus. Clones produced in this way are not strictly identical with their donor animals, because nuclear DNA of the donors' somatic cells may contain mutations that are not present in the whole donor animals. Moreover, the mitochondrial DNA of the enucleated ova—which will lay the basis for the mitochondrial DNA of the cloned organisms—will not be the same as that of the donor animals.

Cloning may also be performed by embryo splitting—sometimes called embryo twinning—whereby a zygote is split at around the six- to eight-cell stage. The resultant multiple zygotes are allowed to grow *in vitro* and are then transferred to a uterus. Cloning by embryo splitting gives rise to genetically truly identical individuals, because both their nuclear and their mitochondrial DNA are identical.

There are two different reasons for contemplating human cloning: therapeutic and reproductive. The purpose of therapeutic cloning would be to provide tissues that would not be rejected by the recipient because clone and recipient would be genetically identical;[23] the purpose of reproductive cloning, as the term implies, would be to produce a genetically identical offspring.

Cloning of either type is specifically prohibited by the *Assisted Human Reproduction Act*:

> **5.** (1) No person shall knowingly
>
> (a) create a human clone by using any technique, or transplant a human clone into a human being or into any non-human life form or artificial device

But again, this is merely the law, which may be changed if Parliament so decides, and it gives no indication as to the ethics of the matter—and there is argumentation on both sides.

Arguments Pro

Argumentation in favour of reproductive cloning usually begins with the claim that procreative freedom is a fundamental right of every person in a (democratic) society.[24] It then points out that some people, either because of an injury, a medical condition or age, cannot produce viable and functional gametes. Without cloning that uses somatic cell nuclear transfer (SCNT) technology—in which the nuclear DNA of the persons to be cloned replaces the nuclear DNA of stem cells—they could never have biological offspring.[25] Therefore, if there is a right to have children (as the preceding chapter argued), and if the technology is available, then not to allow cloning would be to discriminate on the basis of disability. Moreover, there are cases in which people produce viable gametes, but in such small numbers that fertilization rarely occurs. Cloning through embryo splitting would increase the number of embryos and maximize the chance of having biological offspring. This would be of particular interest in assisted human reproduction, where quite often the number of recovered healthy ova is very small and the likelihood of *in vitro* fertilization is correspondingly low.

More fanciful is the argument that SCNT cloning using DNA from eminent persons who have contributed a great deal to society would preserve the genetic basis of that greatness in the offspring. With appropriate nurturing, these offspring would have a good chance of expressing their parents' personalities and traits and of following in their footsteps.[26] If SCNT cloning were combined with embryo splitting, it would maximize the chances of preserving that genetic heritage. In a similar vein, resistance to diseases such as HIV would be a boon to humanity. Cloning individuals who have such resistance[27] would maximize the chances of the trait spreading through the population even if the relevant persons were cloned only a few times. Normal reproductive practices and genetic drift would ensure the increased spread of the gene.[28]

Finally, arguments in favour of therapeutic cloning generally point to the obvious advantage it would have for organ transplantation. Tissues derived from clones would not be rejected.[29] Not only would this be financially more prudent than engaging in lifelong immunosuppressant therapy, it would also lead to a much better quality of life for the recipients. In that sense, it would be mandated by the Principles of Beneficence and non-Malfeasance.[30]

Arguments Contra

Arguments against reproductive cloning can take several forms. One begins with the claim that everyone has the right to a unique genetic identity, and that to deliberately bring about genetically identical persons, whether through SCNT cloning or embryo splitting, is an affront to their dignity as persons.[31] Another maintains that allowing reproductive SCNT cloning is to cater to an extreme form of narcissism[32]—which is neither a good reason to have a child nor a good reason to expose potential human beings to the dangers inherent in the cloning procedure itself. Finally, because of their identical genetic heritage, reproductive cloning would lock the children into personality developments with their identical forebears. This would be inconsistent with the right of every person to choose his or her own life plan. In a word, they would not have an "open future."[33] This would not only produce psychological harm but also violate their autonomy.[34]

As to therapeutic cloning, it would require the use of stem cells. Although some advances have been made in deriving stem cells from somatic tissue, the usual source would either be embryos that have been specifically developed for that purpose or so-called supernumerary embryos: embryos that would have been left over from assisted reproduction and would otherwise be destroyed. Even if those embryos would be destroyed anyway, that would not justify using them as means to advance the welfare of others.[35]

Finally, it has been argued that to allow cloning of any sort would be to potentiate a paradigm shift in what it is to be human.[36] Human beings would essentially cease to be seen as persons and become nothing more nor less than biological machines to be replicated at will. This would strike at the very basis of our ethical interrelations.

Discussion

Any analysis of the ethics of reproductive cloning must begin by acknowledging that cloning occurs naturally. Monozygotic twins (who are clones of each other) occur naturally in approximately 1 per 1,000 births[37] and, unlike fraternal twins (whose incidence ranges from 4 per 1,000 in Japan to 15 per 1,000 in India[38]), the incidence is invariant around the world.[39] No one would suggest even for a moment that having monozygotic siblings was unethical—or even that using folk remedies or other "natural" means to increase the likelihood of having identical twins was unethical. Therefore, the fundamental question that any argument against reproductive cloning has to face is why producing identical twins artificially using modern biotechnologies should be unethical.

An obvious reply is that all sorts of things occur naturally: death, illness, natural disasters and global warming are good examples. This does not, however, mean that one should either potentiate their occurrence or bring them about deliberately. To do so is to produce harm—and that violates the Principle of non-Malfeasance.

However, the validity of this reply really hinges on the somewhat dubious assumption that having the same genetic makeup as one's sibling constitutes harm. This seems to be assumed by the United Nations *Declaration on Human Cloning*,[40] which states that human cloning is "incompatible with human dignity and the protection of human life" and the European Parliament's 1998 resolution that "every individual has the right to his own genetic identity and that human cloning must be prohibited."[41] However, if that assumption were granted, it would follow that all multiple monozygotic pregnancies would have to be reduced to single pregnancies. Not to do so would be to become a passive agent of harm.[42] While this reply does not show that the argument is invalid, it does suggest that its premise has to be examined more carefully before any conclusion can be based on it.

The "open future" argument, in turn, assumes that genetic heritage determines personality. Demonstrably, that is not the case. While personality traits are genetically potentiated, they also depend on the neurological development of the individual—which is functionally dependent on environmental factors such as sensory stimulation, social embedding and personal experiences. All monozygotic siblings differ in this respect already *in utero*, where their difference in position exposes them to different stimuli, and these differences are multiplied as they go through life.[43]

The objection to reproductive cloning by embryo splitting could be sustained only if one could show on independent grounds that deliberately having offspring with identical genetic makeup was "incompatible with human dignity." As was pointed out, that may be difficult to do. Dignity is a concept that primarily applies to individuals as persons, not as bodies. And even if one granted that genetic identity entailed identical personhood—and it was shown a moment ago that this is not the case—it is unclear how having similar or even the same personalities would amount to an indignity. If it did, then trying to model oneself as closely as possible on someone one admired—for instance, Mother Teresa or Madame Curie—would be ethically questionable. While this reply to the argument does not constitute a logical refutation, it at least shows that the underlying premise may not be all that compelling.

As to the claim that it would be unethically narcissistic to want an offspring who is biologically like oneself, this assumes that it is never acceptable to want children that are biologically as much like oneself as possible. However, such an assumption may not be generalizable. For instance, suppose that because of the success of modern medicine in providing supportive care for those with serious genetic conditions, what in previous centuries had been self-correcting lethal genes such as Pompe disease, cystic fibrosis, galactosemia and phenylketonuria (because the infants who carried them would die in childhood) had spread throughout the population and become quite common. Suppose further that someone who did not carry the relevant gene wanted to have offspring that were biologically like her. It is unclear that this would be unethical.

It would also be wrong to say that therapeutic cloning would lead to a paradigm shift in the concept of a human person. To be sure, therapeutic cloning requires that one distinguish between the concept of a human person as an embodied being and a mere body, for it is only if one accepts this distinction that one can adopt an instrumentalistic stance towards zygotes and fetuses and treat them as mere biological entities. However, the germ of that distinction is already inherent in the claim that human persons are not identical with their bodies. It also underlies the gradualistic approach to fetal development, which legitimates abortion prior to a certain developmental stage. (See Chapter 8.)

Moreover, if it is a paradigm shift, it is not a new one but goes back to the Middle Ages. Already St. Augustine and St. Thomas Aquinas distinguished between a "formed" human body—one that has acquired a soul because it is neurologically sufficiently developed to sustain the "properly human activity" of self-awareness and rational thought— and a mere animal body that has not yet reached that stage.[44] That is why they said that abortion prior to that stage of fetal development is not murder—and why a similar position is adopted by almost all major religions. (See Chapter 8.)

The real conceptual issue that therapeutic cloning moves to centre stage is that of whether the human body, at any stage of development, deserves ethical consideration or valuational concern. In other words, the real issue is whether human beings *as biological organisms* are ethically distinct from other animals or merely—like all similar biological organisms—subjects of serious valuational concern. If human beings as biological organisms are located somewhere on a spectrum that includes all biological organisms, then the respect that is due human bodies is not a matter of kind but a matter of degree. One can then easily argue that while tremendous respect is due human bodies, that degree is commensurate with their stage of development relative to that spectrum. By that token, therapeutic cloning is not ruled out if it is done for serious reasons and in keeping with the guidelines that apply to all other biological organisms of a similar stage of development. To put it in a nutshell: as long as guidelines such as those promulgated by the Canadian Council on Animal Care were followed.[45]

On the other hand, if human beings as biological organisms are ethically distinctive as such, irrespective of stage of development, then the difference from other biological organisms is one of a kind, and entirely different considerations apply. By that very token, however, abortion and organ harvesting from brain-dead human bodies would also become seriously problematic.

GENETIC TESTING AND GENETIC INFORMATION

Another important biotechnology that has momentous implications for human health and reproduction—and one which, by contrast, is currently employed—is genetic testing and genetic screening. It identifies the molecular basis of somatic characteristics and diseases, and in many cases is integral to adjusting reproductive practices and treatment options for persons with genetically grounded diseases or conditions.

The idea that underlies this technology is of course not new. From the earliest times, people have known that the characteristics of living organisms depend at least partly on those of their parents. They put this knowledge to use by breeding selectively for desirable traits in cereals, vegetables, fruits and livestock. They knew *how* to do it, but they did not know *why* it worked. The mechanism that was responsible began to be unravelled only in the 19th century when Mendel, through controlled cross-pollination, traced the generational inheritance of the characteristics of peas. His work marked the beginning of the scientific study of genetics, which was soon applied in the medical field to assist in diagnosing and dealing with heritable human diseases.

In the beginning, medical genetics was confined to the application of statistical tools to family histories. Its practical application was essentially limited to preventing births when it was likely that the offspring would suffer from serious debilitating diseases or conditions or, when that was not considered an option, to prepare appropriate ways of dealing with the situation ahead of time. However, in 1959, Krick and Watson discovered the double-helix nature of deoxyribonucleic acid (DNA), and with this the road was opened to the genetic identification and detection of debilitating or fatal human conditions. Not surprisingly, human genetic screening soon became a legitimate medical tool to complement traditional, family-based statistical approaches. It allowed the definite detection and identification of genetically grounded medical conditions in parents and in fetuses prior to birth, so that either appropriate treatment could be provided as soon as the child was born—PKU is a good example—or the birth of an affected infant could be prevented. The list of human conditions and diseases that can be identified has steadily grown and currently numbers in the hundreds. It includes Huntington's disease, hemophilia, cystic fibrosis, sickle cell anemia and the like.

Arguments Pro and Contra

While medically very useful, the technology immediately raises several important ethical concerns. One centres in the privacy implications that surround the information resulting from genetic testing; another involves the question of whether the knowledge that one carries deleterious genes entails an obligation to adjust one's reproductive behaviour accordingly; a third is the question of whether, if one has reasonable grounds to suppose that one carries genes that would result in serious and debilitating diseases in one's offspring, one has a duty to screen one's offspring *in utero* to determine whether that is the case and, upon a positive finding, to terminate the pregnancy. Logically distinct but closely associated is the question of whether the ability to identify the genetic basis of serious heritable diseases entails a general social obligation to fund research into developing means of correcting genetic flaws. There is also the question whether, if it is possible to engage in genetic manipulation as such, it is ethical to use these techniques to alter and improve human capacities such as strength, intelligence, body shape and size, etc.: in a word, whether it is ethically permissible to engage in genetic engineering for not only therapeutic but also enhancement purposes.

Some of these questions have already been considered in the preceding chapters (see Chapters 8 and 11, which dealt with abortion and with the right to have children respectively) and require no further discussion. As was pointed out then, the right to reproductive autonomy is conditioned by the obligation not to initiate a causal chain that predictably will lead to harm for any person who might be born. Consequently, if one has reasonable grounds to believe that one carries a deleterious gene, one has an obligation to be tested for that gene and, if one is a carrier, to adjust one's reproductive behaviour accordingly.

For instance, Huntington's disease is a neurodegenerative disease that is caused by an autosomal dominant mutation on either of an individual's two copies of a gene called Huntingtin. This means that any child of an affected parent has a 50 percent risk of inheriting the disease.[46] Physical symptoms of Huntington's disease can begin at any age from infancy to old age, but usually start to manifest themselves between the ages of thirty-five and forty-four. It has been argued that if one has reasonable grounds to believe that one is a carrier, one has an obligation to use prenatal genetic screening and to abort an affected fetus, so as to avoid future pain and suffering. It has also been argued that one has an obligation to share the information with consanguineous relatives, so that they can adjust their lives accordingly.

However, this position is not universally shared, and various reasons are given for rejecting it. *First*, regarding oneself, it is argued that there is no duty to know one's genetic condition, even if one has reasons to suppose that one has a genetic disease such as Huntington's—because there is nothing that one can do to avert the onset of the disease. In other words, as is stated in the UNESCO *Universal Declaration on Bioethics and Human Rights*[47] (and as the World Medical Association concurs), there is a right not to know.[48] *Second*, genetic information is "uniquely private" because it is about the specific individual; therefore, it should lie completely under the control of the individual from whose tissue it is obtained, and sharing it is a strictly voluntary matter.[49] *Third*, making it obligatory for people to disclose genetic information about themselves may discourage them from seeking genetic testing.[50] *Fourth*, the information that would be obtained through genetic testing may well be misleading, because the way in which a particular genetic trait is expressed is not an absolute matter but, depending on the gene, may vary from individual to individual even with the same trait. Therefore, sharing such information might well cause unnecessary worries. *Fifth*, in most cases genetic screening for carrier status would be a monumental waste of resources. Thus, in a Canadian study of the incidence and prevalence of Tay-Sachs in which 21,071 individuals were screened, only 24 couples were identified as both being carriers, three pregnancies were monitored and only one fetus was aborted—at a total cost of over $100,000. While the cost for other screening programs may not be quite as high, it may be argued that in view of the scarcity of medical resources, funding such programs would be extravagant.[51]

Moreover, most genetic characteristics are cross-linked in such a way that the elimination of one entails the elimination of others. Therefore, to eliminate cross-linked deleterious genes would mean the loss of desirable characteristics as well—in which case, by "improving" the genotype, one would in fact make it worse. Also, what may be a deleterious gene under one set of circumstances may be advantageous in another. The gene for sickle cell anemia is a case in point: When the person who inherits it is not heterozygous for it, it makes that person more resistant to malaria.

Still others have focused on the nature of the physician–patient relationship and have emphasized the duty of confidentiality that physicians have towards their patients. The argument here is that physicians do not have a fiduciary duty towards third parties. Consequently, in the absence of such a duty, the duty of confidentiality towards their patients is paramount.[52]

Finally, it has been argued that not sharing the information with (consanguineous) third parties does not violate non-Malfeasance, because this will not result in additional harm. The harm is caused by the expression of the genetic predisposition, and that will occur whether the individual knows about it or not.[53]

Discussion

However, it is unclear how the claim of a "right not to know" one's own carrier status even if one has reason to suspect it, is compatible with the *Declaration of Teheran* and the injunction that one should be responsible in one's reproductive practice. (See Chapter 11.) Logically, it would seem that responsible persons who have reasonable grounds to suspect that they carry a deleterious gene would want to know whether this was the case so that they could adjust their reproductive behaviour accordingly. As to the claim that making it obligatory to disclose the information may discourage people from getting tested, there are no data that support such a claim. Furthermore, it is a standard requirement of contemporary genetic screening that it be accompanied by genetic counselling. Therefore, the danger of misunderstanding the implications of a particular test are relatively small.

It is also not true that all hereditary diseases are genetically cross-linked or multifactorial. Cystic fibrosis is a case in point, as is hemophilia. Therefore, this argument against carriers' status testing has limited applicability at best. Moreover, the cost involved in testing for Tay-Sachs is not representative of the incidence and prevalence of genetically based diseases such as cystic fibrosis. Therefore, again, the acceptability of the argument depends on a very careful selection of premises.

As to not sharing genetic information, that would deprive affected persons of the opportunity to adjust their conduct and to arrange their lives.[54] For instance—as in the case of Huntington's disease—the information would allow a couple to make appropriate plans concerning their own future and, if they have not yet had children, to adjust their reproductive behaviour by either not having any children or by insisting on prenatal screening of any children that the woman might conceive or that the man might father, and then taking appropriate steps—whatever these might be.

In this connection, it is also interesting to note that while the UNESCO and WMA declarations do insist on the right not to know, they also state that there are limits on the right to privacy. They stipulate that if there is a high likelihood of serious harm to third parties, then the right to privacy is overruled. They even go so far as to say that if affected persons refuse to disclose such information to relevant third parties, their physicians have a duty to disclose it—a position that is consistent with the CMA Code of Ethics. The Code states that, normally, an ethical physician should disclose patients' health information to third parties "only with their consent," but it goes on to state that disclosure is mandatory "when the maintenance of confidentiality would result in a significant risk of substantial harm to others."[55] The underlying reason here is the Principle of non-Malfeasance. Under the circumstances, non-disclosure of the relevant information to third parties would be unethical because it would put them at preventable risk.[56] With due alteration of detail, analogous reasoning applies in the case of genetic information. Furthermore, as the Supreme Court of Canada stated in *McInerney v. MacDonald*,[57]

> prima facie, the patient has a right to require that professional secrets acquired by the practitioner shall not be divulged. This right is absolute *unless there is some paramount reason that overrides it.* For example, there may be cases in which reasons connected with the safety of individuals or of the public, physical or moral, would be sufficiently cogent to supersede or qualify the obligations prima facie imposed by the confidential relation. [Emphasis added]

Therefore, both ethically and legally, if there is a high likelihood of serious harm, the physician has an ethical duty to make sure that the relevant parties receive the information in question.[58]

This, of course, raises the question of what constitutes a "high likelihood of serious harm." There appears to be no consensus on the subject. One line of reasoning takes the position that in some cases—Huntington's disease is here cited as an example—non-Malfeasance itself entails that the information should not be shared, because suicide rates among people who carry the Huntingtin gene are higher than among the average population.[59] Therefore, if the information were shared, the affected parties might well commit suicide to avoid the tragic fate of terminal Huntington's sufferers. However, this statistic cannot in itself be considered indicative of harm. One also has to ask whether suicide is always a harm, and whether it would be rational to commit suicide under such circumstances. As was pointed out in the discussion of euthanasia and assisted suicide, there may be situations in which suicide would be quite rational. (See the case of Sue Rodriguez, Chapter 7, who was diagnosed as rational despite "suicidal ideations.") Therefore, if someone is told that he or she has the Huntingtin gene and subsequently commits suicide, this does not necessarily mean the disclosure caused the harm. It all depends on how the disclosure is made and on the perspective of the individual in question.

To sum up, non-disclosure is arguably unethical if the information has relevance for reproductive practice. If it does not, then the important issue is probably whether disclosure of the information would increase individual autonomy—for instance, by opening up choices that would not be obvious if the person was unaware of his or her condition and its implications. In all cases, however, it would be appropriate to explore, prior to disclosure, ways of minimizing the impact, so that it would not interfere with rational decision-making.

Genetic Information and Biological Parentage

Ethical issues surrounding genetic information are not confined to questions that centre in traits and conditions. They may also involve questions of parenthood. For instance, it is estimated that approximately 3 percent of children cannot have the father their mothers say they have.[60] What, then, should a health care professional do who becomes aware that, genetically, a patient's father, as identified by the patient's mother, cannot in fact be the biological father?

At first glance, this is a matter of social significance only and has nothing to do with the delivery of health care; therefore, it does not fall within the purview of the physician as professional. However, to argue thus is to overlook the fact that parental misattribution may have serious medical implications. Genetic parentage can play an important role in the identification and treatment of diseases or conditions from which children may suffer or that they are likely to develop. In fact, it is for precisely this reason that children who have been conceived by IVF from donor sperm have claimed that they have a right to know the identity of their genetic parents.[61] Arguably, therefore, the fiduciary nature of the physician–patient relationship entails that in a case like this, the physician must take reasonable steps to ensure that the patient is aware that his or her social father and biological father are not the same person. Autonomy and Respect for persons, of course, entails that, all other things being equal—for instance, the maternal parent not being deceased—the maternal parent should be given the option of disclosing that information herself. It is only when that is not possible—or when the maternal parent refuses to disclose the information—that Beneficence and non-Malfeasance oblige the physician to disclose the information.

But again, the matter is not that clear. One could argue that there is a difference between knowing the identity of one's biological parents and having access to genetic or other relevant health information about them. The latter is what is important from a health care perspective; the former is not. That is why it is arguable that, from a health perspective, the most this reasoning could establish is that there is a right to genetic (and health) information about one's biological parents. Their identity is another matter.

However, there is a counter-argument to this as well. One could reply that if one was unaware of the identity of one's biological parent, one might unwittingly have children with someone who in fact was a sibling. This would not only constitute incest, the children might also carry two copies of a deleterious gene that was inherited from the unknown biological progenitor—with potentially disastrous consequences for the children.

If accepted, however, this last point would have potentially unsettling consequences. If the above statistics about the misattribution of biological parentage are correct, then these dangers exist irrespective of whether someone was conceived through IVF. In fact, one could argue that since the number of people conceived through IVF is several orders of magnitude smaller than the number of those conceived naturally, the likelihood of this danger materializing is much greater for people who are conceived in the normal manner.

Therefore, if mandatory disclosure of biological parentage held only for children who were conceived by IVF, that would discriminate against everyone who was not conceived in that way. This would violate the Principle of Equality and Justice. At the same time if, in agreement with the *Convention on the Rights of the Child*, one were to say that "every child has the right to . . . know his or her parent"[62] and if this was consistently applied across the board, it would potentially have serious social repercussions.[63]

The Implications of Genetic Knowledge: A Paradigm Shift

The preceding considerations notwithstanding, it seems undeniable that genetic testing and screening technology provides a useful and potentially very important tool for health care and for reproductive decision-making. Of course, it is far from clear what those decisions should be. In that respect, it is like all biotechnologies: It provides options and, by so doing, increases the complexity of the ethical landscape. Moreover—so it has been argued—it does more than that: It potentiates a subtle paradigm shift in the concept of a person.

That is to say, the traditional concept of persons is that of members of the biological species *homo sapiens*. On that understanding, their identities are functionally related to what might be called their spatio-temporal footprint. This footprint is unique to each individual and is not shared with anyone else. Privacy and integrity considerations, therefore, are traditionally defined by the material being of individuals, which in turn defines the sphere of privacy that surrounds them.

However, with the advent of genetic technology, people have also come to be seen as genetic entities. As such, their identity is no longer defined by their spatio-temporal footprint but also by their genetic makeup. This means that while as human beings their uniqueness is functionally defined in terms of their spatio-temporal footprint, as genetic beings their uniqueness is functionally defined by the degree to which they are genetically distinct from each other. Therefore, from this perspective, the genetic identity of an individual is not self-contained, and the sphere of genetic privacy is not the same as the sphere of material privacy that he or she enjoys as a material being. Instead, it overlaps with that of others to the degree that they share the same genetic structures. In that sense, people as genetic beings cannot be wholly separated from their next-of-kin. As one commentator put it, they have a "joint genetic account."[64]

To really understand what this means, and to see its implications for privacy, it may be useful to do a bit of metaphysics and go back to Aristotle's notion of a form.[65] Aristotle defined a form as a principle of structure, and he argued that all substances that have the same principle of structure—for instance, all rubber balls and all warthogs— share the same form, and *in that sense* are the same. However, Aristotle distinguished between forms as such and substances or instantiations of forms. Forms as such are universal or generic. To go back to the example of rubber balls and warthogs, the form of a rubber ball or of a warthog is something general, not something specific like an individual ball or an individual warthog. It is the instantiations of these forms—the individual substances—that are unique and distinct.

If one applies this to the distinction between personal identity and genetic identity, one can see that, just as Aristotelian substances "overlap" at the level of forms, so persons as genetic beings overlap at the level of genes. In that sense, they share an identity at the level of principles of structure (i.e., genes) to the degree that they share the same principles of structure (genes). Further, just as Aristotelian substances are unique as instantiations of forms, so individual persons are unique at the level of actually expressed genes (instantiated forms). Therefore, while each person *as an embodied material being* is surrounded by a sphere of privacy as that unique being (i.e., as that instantiated set of principles of structure, or genes), each person as a *genetic* entity (i.e., considered at the level of genes, or principles of structure) is not so surrounded, because the genes or principles are shared. That is why the privacy concerns of individuals as unique embodied persons are distinct from the privacy concerns of individuals as genetic entities. The two function at different levels, and different standards apply. This has been expressed in the literature as the notion that genetic information constitutes a "joint account" because of joint presence/ownership.[66]

GENETIC ENGINEERING

Another example of a biotechnology that has caused a fair bit of controversy even though, for the most part, it is only in the developmental stages is genetic engineering. Genetic engineering is the alteration of the genome of an individual by either the deletion of a particular gene sequence, the addition of a new gene sequence or the alteration of its expression at the molecular level. The central question here is, whether this technology—which was originally developed for animal and plant use—could ethically be used to modify the human genome.

Some Historical Considerations

To put the issue of genetic engineering into historical context, it may be useful to recall that humanity has always actively changed its genetic heritage, even before the advent of modern genetics. It may not have done so consciously, but standards of beauty combined with success in survival channelled mate selection into certain lines, with results such as distinct body types—steatopygia among the Khoisan of Africa or the rounded body shape of the Inuit,[67] being merely two examples.

Long ago, utopian social planners such as Plato had toyed with the idea of deliberate breeding programs to make for healthier human beings.[68] At the turn of the 20th century, the idea moved from the realm of philosophical theory into the public arena. Prominent public figures such as Oliver Wendell Holmes began to espouse the concept[69] and gave impetus to the so-called "eugenics movement," which maintained that deleterious genes should be removed from the human gene pool. The movement gained such popular support that the U.S. enacted eugenic sterilization laws.[70] When Germany later became interested in the issue as a matter of social policy, it turned to the U.S. for information and advice.[71] Canada had adopted similar measures in the 1920s and 1930s (and its legislation was not repealed until the 1970s).[72]

The eugenics movement advocated both positive and negative eugenics. *Positive eugenics* consists in encouraging those with "good" or "desirable" genes to have children. The population policy of Nazi Germany in the 1930s, which honoured "Aryan" women who had more than four living children with the "Order of the Mother" (*Mutterorden*), and the1920s policy of France, which honoured women with many children with the *médaille d'honneur de la famille française* (and which is still awarded to this day), are here good examples.[73] *Negative eugenics* is the attempt to actively delete what have been identified as undesirable genes, either by sterilizing those who carry them or by otherwise discouraging them from having children.[74] The eugenic sterilization laws of Canada and the U.S. were illustrative examples of negative eugenics.

Eugenics was embraced not only by social reformers, but also by the scientific community. However, most scientists rejected the notion of coercive eugenics legislation. They envisioned a voluntary program based on the responsible exercise of human freedom. J. Muller, one of the foremost geneticists of his time and one of the most outspoken scientific proponents of eugenics, emphasized this clearly when he rejected any attempt to impose forcible control by the state.[75] However, he was pessimistic that such voluntary control would be effective:[76]

> However, it seems asking almost too much to expect those individuals who are really less well equipped than the average in mentality or disposition to acknowledge to themselves that they are genetically inferior to their neighbours in these respects and then publicly to admit this low appraisal of themselves by raising no family at all or a smaller one than normal, especially since at the same time they would often be thwarting a natural urge to achieve the deep fulfilment, accorded to their superiors, that go with having little ones to care for and bring up. Moreover, those with physical impairments would likewise tend to rationalize the situation, by thinking that they possessed some superior psychological qualities that more than compensated for their physical defects.

In other words, Muller foresaw the ironic possibility that people with the very traits to be enhanced would be motivated by a sense of social responsibility and practise restraint in their reproductive habits, so as not to stretch resources beyond their limit, whereas those who lacked these traits would not control their reproductive behaviour.

Genetic Engineering with Modern Tools

The eugenics movement of the early 20th century is no longer in vogue, and the ideal of "improving" humanity as a species has been replaced with the ideal of correcting genetic flaws that lead to disease and disability on an individual basis. Moreover, the venue for implementing this ideal has moved from the setting of social programs to that of the clinic, where it is supported by new technologies that allow clinicians to identify individual genes and—at least in principle—to directly manipulate human DNA.

There are two ways of doing this: by *somatic cell therapy* and by *germ line therapy*. In somatic cell therapy, the defective gene is identified, and a functional version of the gene is constructed and then inserted into the affected person. This usually involves modifying a virus and infecting the patient's cells, where the virus integrates the modified gene into the patient's DNA. The cells, which now have a healthy copy of the relevant gene, can then function normally, and the illness is cured without need for treatment or medication. If gene therapy is carried out late enough—after the development of the ovaries in the case of women, and after the development of testes in the case of men—the genetic modification will not be passed on to any offspring. In *germ line genetic therapy*, the genetic modification is made either to the cells that produce the gametes—which includes zygotes and embryos—or to the gametes themselves. These genetic modifications are therefore heritable and are passed on to any offspring.

The *Assisted Human Reproduction Act* allows somatic cell therapy, but it prohibits germ line therapy on pain of criminal sanction. Specifically, it stipulates that

> **5.** (1) No person shall knowingly
>
> (f) alter the genome of a cell of a human being or *in vitro* embryo such that the alteration is capable of being transmitted to descendants

This position is based on—although it goes further than—the recommendation of the Royal Commission on New Reproductive Technologies which, in its 1993 Report to Parliament, suggested that "no research involving alteration of the DNA of human zygotes [should] be permitted or funded in Canada."[77] The Tri-Council Guidelines, which provide the ethical grounding for most research protocols in Canada, are essentially silent on the whole issue of genetic engineering. Most countries agree with Canada in allowing somatic cell therapy and in prohibiting germ line therapy.

This new genetic technology raises two important questions. *First*, are there any ethical problems with the application of genetic engineering technology to human beings? *Second*, is there an ethical difference between somatic cell therapy and germ line therapy? To this, one could add a *third* question: If genetic engineering is ethically defensible at all, should it be confined to dealing with diseases, or may it be extended to enhance traits such as intelligence, sensory acuity, physical ability and the like?

Arguments Pro   One can easily see why genetic engineering is considered ethical by its proponents. If successful—and so far it is mainly in the developmental stage for human beings—it would be a much more cost-effective way of dealing with genetically based human diseases than current approaches. To use cystic fibrosis as an example, the Canadian prevalence of the diseases lies around 2.8 per 10,000 births.[78] The (2006) cost for cystic fibrosis per patient per year ranges from $10,000 to $21,842,[79] depending on the severity, and the median survival age is 36.7 years for men and 27.8 years for women.[80] This means that, as a low estimate, the cost of treating cystic fibrosis symptomatically is approximately $300,000 over the lifetime of a patient.[81] If cystic fibrosis could be cured through genetic engineering, it would free up a sizable amount of resources for other health care.[82]

But expense is not the major reason for considering the use of genetic engineering to treat such diseases: It is the fact that current treatments are inherently symptomatic. To revert to the example of cystic fibrosis, people who suffer from cystic fibrosis have short-ened lifespans despite medication, and are forced to lead a restricted lifestyle with a com-paratively reduced quality of life. To cure the disease once and for all, therefore, would be entirely in keeping with the Principles of Beneficence and non-Malfeasance. Cystic fibrosis is only one of several single-gene disorders or single-locus diseases. Others include Huntington's disease, hemochromatosis, fragile X syndrome, and Duchenne and Becker muscular dystrophy. All of them lead to a reduced quality of life. It is arguable that in all these cases not to explore possible treatment options that would cure the diseases is to perpetuate a harm through inaction—and that is unethical.

Arguments Contra Of course, this reasoning does not stand unopposed. Counter-arguments include the claim that there are too many uncertainties about long-term effects, because we know so little about the cross-linkages between the various genes.[83] Then there is the paradigm-shift argument: To approach the human genetic code as something to be fixed, to be repaired and to be manipulated, bespeaks a view of humanity that sees human beings like pieces of machinery: to be designed, redesigned and moulded.

It also gives rise to eugenic concerns.[84] Specifically, it is feared that if genetic engineering were to become standard therapy, then the genetically unimproved or non-regularized individual would have lower value in the eyes of others and would lose all dignity as a being of inherent worth. Some have even argued that genetic engineering could become a tool for social oppression.[85]

Then there is the slippery-slope argument. It maintains that if the inviolability of the genetic code were to be abandoned in some cases, then the door would be opened to further changes. What began as a matter of therapy would slowly devolve into genetic modification for any and all reasons—including enhancement.[86] In a similar vein, it has also been suggested that once genetic engineering was regarded as an ethically acceptable technology for medical conditions, it would be a short step to using it for economic purposes. For instance, instead of correcting unsafe working conditions that involve dan-gerous chemicals, radiation and the like, workers would be required to submit to genetic engineering so that they would no longer be susceptible to illnesses brought about by unhealthy conditions.[87]

Discussion However, these objections either miss the point or draw unwarranted conclusions on the basis of insufficient evidence. For instance, there are no data to sup-port the claim of positive cross-linkages in the case of single-locus diseases such as cystic fibrosis or hemochromatosis. As to the slippery slope from genetic engineering to genetic modification and enhancement, it is entirely possible that the success of therapeutic genetic engineering might lead to non-therapeutic uses such as enhancement of normal capacities. However, this does not show that either the therapeutic or the non-therapeutic uses are unethical. The claim that this extension of use is unethical has to be argued on independent grounds. The suggestion that somatic cell therapy might be expanded to deal with unsafe working conditions does, of course, paint a logically possible picture. However, there is a difference between being logically possible and being likely. The likelihood of this occurring is directly proportional to the likelihood that the global move towards safer working conditions as a matter of human rights will be reversed.[88]

The argument from the fear of eugenics also has little factual basis. More importantly, however, and from a logical perspective, it is potentially self-defeating. The point of eugenics is to prevent people with serious genetic loads from having children that would run the danger of spreading the gene throughout the gene pool and thereby lowering the evolutionary fitness of the species. However, that danger would be minimized if, every time the genetically grounded condition surfaced, it could be corrected through somatic cell therapy—much in the way that any other disease is dealt with at the present time. Of course, it would be ideal if the condition could be eradicated once and for all— which would be a good argument in favour of germ line gene therapy—but at least with somatic cell therapy, there would be no reason to adopt drastic eugenic measures.

On the other hand, the suggestion that the use of somatic cell therapy might lead to a paradigm shift in the concept of a person does have some merit. It is consonant with the previous suggestion that the development and use of genetic screening and testing technology might lead to a paradigm shift. However, just as that shift would not be a shift in content but in focus, this shift would also be one of focus. The newly focused paradigm would not reduce human beings to mere pieces of biological machinery, to be designed, redesigned and moulded. Instead, it would focus attention on the fact that as embodied rational entities, their characteristics as rational beings are functionally related to their embodiment, and would make it clear that the genetic endowment of the body can interfere with the exercise of the capacities that they have as rational entities. Therefore, the use of somatic cell therapy to correct genetically grounded biological flaws that interfere with the exercise of these capacities would be perfectly consistent with the overall paradigm of human beings as embodied persons, and would not change it. It would merely focus it on the genetic grounding of the embodiment.

Germ Line Gene Therapy

The discussion so far has focused on somatic cell therapy. Some people have argued that while somatic cell therapy may be ethically acceptable, germ line therapy is certainly not, the reason being that its effects transcend the individual who is treated and extend to future generations. This consideration was foundational to Parliament's passage of section 5(1)(f) of the *Assisted Human Reproduction Act*, which was quoted above. A somewhat similar perspective is reflected in the claim of the Royal Commission on

New Reproductive Technologies that "[t]he risk of passing on genetic disease is inherent in the human condition. It makes no sense to try to alter this in any way."[89]

In a similar vein, some have argued that humanity lacks the wisdom to identify the traits that should be altered permanently—which, of course, would be the case if germ line gene therapy were to be practised.[90] There is the very real possibility that by permanently altering the genomic makeup of the species, one would inadvertently threaten its very survival—the reason being that this alteration would not only permanently remove certain genes from the overall genome but also destroy important genetic cross-linkages. That would lower the species' overall ability to respond to evolutionary threats.[91]

Moreover, germ line alteration would be performed without the consent of those who are most affected: namely, future generations.[92] In the words of C.S. Lewis,[93]

> [i]f any one age really attains, by eugenic means and scientific education, the power to make its descendants what it pleases, all men who live after it are patients of that power. They are weaker, not stronger . . . Man's conquest of Nature, if the dreams of the scientific planners are realized, means the rule of a few hundreds of men over billions upon billions of men.

It has also been argued that germ line gene therapy violates the right to an unmodified genetic heritage, and thereby constitutes an affront to human dignity.[94] Its use also increases the danger of eugenics, as has already been pointed out above.[95] Finally, it has been suggested that germ line genetic therapy would be the first step down a slippery slope that would end with the integration of non-human genes into the human genome.[96]

Some of these considerations are already familiar from the discussion of somatic cell therapy and therefore require little additional comment. For instance, the cross-linkage argument is no more trenchant when dealing with germ line therapy than with somatic cell therapy. The therapy is intended for single-locus diseases only, and no linkages have ever been identified or even suggested in this connection. As to the spectre of eugenics, it is no more reasonable here than in the previous context. The point of single-locus germ line gene therapy would be to eliminate diseases—to do away with genes that interfere with the health of human beings, irrespective of race, sex or any other characteristics. The only way this would differ from non-genetic ways of dealing with these conditions— and even from somatic cell therapy—is that it would deal with the relevant diseases permanently, rather than treating them on a symptomatic and recurrent basis.

The claim that everyone has the right to an unmodified genetic heritage, in turn, is logically interesting because it entails some very peculiar consequences. If one grants its basic premise, this entails that people who suffer from cystic fibrosis have the right to suffer from the disease, that children who are born with Tay-Sachs have a right to die a rather painful death at a very early age and that people who carry the gene for hemochromatosis have the right to a dysfunctional pancreas and to cirrhosis, polyarthropathy, adrenal insufficiency, heart failure and diabetes. It is unclear in what sense suffering from these conditions is a right. Of course, this does not show that the argument is invalid. It merely shows that the premise is rather suspect.

At the same time, however, even if (for whatever reason) one does grant the premise, the conclusion still does not follow. The reason lies in the logic of rights and the ethics of substitute decision-making. Any right can be waived. (See Chapter 1.) Therefore, if, purely for the sake of argument, one assumes that zygotes, fetuses and future generations have rights; and further, if one assumes that they have the right to an unmodified genetic heritage, then they need substitute decision-makers to exercise that right for them. (See Chapter 5.) Since unborn persons do not have values of their own, the substitute decision-makers would have to use the values of the objective reasonable person when making their decisions. It follows that unless the objective reasonable person's values include suffering from these conditions because of their unmodified genetic heritage, the substitute decision-makers could not ethically insist on retaining the flawed genetic structures that lead to these diseases if a treatment was available to prevent it. That holds both for unborn persons here and now (i.e., to fetuses and embryos) as well as for future generations (who would be born with the genetic flaws if these were not corrected in the embryos and fetuses).

Moreover, the appeal to the Council of Europe's statement that everyone has the right to an unmodified genetic heritage is really quite disingenuous. That very statement is qualified, in the very same document, by the statement that "the explicit recognition of this right must not impede development of the therapeutic applications of genetic engineering (gene therapy), which holds great promise for the treatment and eradication of certain diseases which are genetically transmitted."[97]

As to the issue of human dignity, the *Universal Declaration on the Human Genome and Human Rights* states that everyone has the right to respect for their dignity *irrespective* of their genetic characteristics.[98] This stance is meaningful only if the signatories of the *Declaration* saw a distinction between individuals and their genetic makeup. That, in turn, makes it logically impossible to say that modifying someone's genetic makeup is an affront to his or her dignity as a person.

As to the argument that allowing genetic engineering would hold all future humanity subject to the values of people who are alive today, the underlying logic of this reasoning applies to everything that is done in health care. Every time that medicine saves people and keeps them alive to have children, the future of the species is affected. Whatever genetically grounded conditions they have will be passed on to the next generation. Moreover, having children *with a particular partner* does the same thing. Over the years, such choices have resulted in the evolutionary development of *homo sapiens*. This was neither good nor bad—unless, of course, one were to argue that early humans should have refrained from having children with anyone whose genome had changed in any way from the original model. It is unclear how one would go about establishing such a contention.

Finally, the significance of the claim about a slippery slope to incorporating non-human genes into the human genome is unclear. Quite irrespective of any evidence for the slippery slope itself, there is the fact that the human genome already shares significant parts with other animals and even with some plants—and has always done so.[99] Without further specifying what counts as human as opposed to non-human, and without indicating which non-human genes are implicated and why, the argument lacks cogency.

Overall, then, it seems that the arguments against germ line gene therapy trade more on fear than on fact, and are not logically very persuasive. They do, of course, have a point. As with all biotechnology, if germ line gene therapy is used at all, it should be used with great care and only after less drastic options have been explored. However, that does not mean that it should not be explored as a possible way of dealing with genetic conditions for which either no treatment is available or the treatment available is merely symptomatic and does not result in a quality of life similar to that of people without these particular genetic burdens.

In fact, some have argued that there exists something like a therapeutic imperative to explore gene therapy. That is to say, in any situation that requires therapy, the physician has an obligation to identify the options that are reasonably available, evaluate which are more likely to provide a therapeutically beneficial result and pose the least danger of harm, and offer these options to the duly empowered decision-maker. This lies in the fiduciary nature of the physician–patient relationship. Moreover, as was pointed out above, the duly empowered decision-maker has a duty to choose the option that is in keeping with the values of the objective reasonable person, provides the greatest benefit and entails the least harm, and is consistent with otherwise ethically applicable values—and then to integrate the choice into an appropriate treatment plan. This becomes even more compelling for both the health care professional and the decision-maker when a particular option—in this case, germ line gene therapy—is less resource intensive than the competing alternatives.

Finally—and this is perhaps the strongest argument in favour of germ line gene therapy—there is an ethical difference between allowing a preventable injury to occur and then treating it, and preventing the injury in the first place. Allowing a preventable injury to occur is to become a passive agent of harm. Applied to germ line gene therapy, this means that not performing germ line therapy when doing so is an option is to say that harm must occur first before it will be treated. The fact that the preventable injury will be treated once it occurs does not detract from the fact that a preventable injury will have occurred. To draw an analogy, to refuse to use germ line gene therapy when it becomes available because the relevant condition can be treated once it has occurred is like saying that it is all right not to push someone out of the way of a falling brick (and thereby prevent an injury) because the resulting skull fracture can be treated after it has occurred. That violates the Principle of non-Malfeasance.[100] The refusal to develop and apply germ line therapy falls into the same category. Of course, this does not mean that such therapy should not be developed and applied with caution. However, caution is the watchword for any type of medical intervention and does not make germ line gene therapy unique.

Genetic Therapy versus Genetic Enhancement

Genetic enhancement, as distinct from genetic therapy, is the non-therapeutic use of genetic engineering technology. Its purpose is to modify the human genome either to optimize attributes or capabilities beyond the level normally associated with it in the particular genome or, alternatively, to introduce attributes or capabilities that humans do not currently possess.

Before going any further in this discussion, it is important to acknowledge that unlike (some) somatic cell therapy and like germ line gene therapy, genetic enhancement is currently entirely in the realm of science fiction. It has not been attempted in human beings and, unlike germ line genetic therapy for single-locus diseases, it is not even on the drawing board. The reasons for this are manifold and interrelated. No funding has been released for the relevant research because the attributes and capabilities in question—intelligence, life extension, physical endurance, social confidence and the like—involve a multiplicity of genes, not all of which have been identified and whose interrelationship, even where they have been identified, is far from clear. Moreover, the ethics of gene enhancement is even less clear than the ethics of therapeutic gene therapy, which, in turn, contributes to the lack of research funding. Therefore, the debate over gene enhancement is a debate over what might be possible if the technical problems were solved. In short, it is a debate about hypotheticals. The discussion that follows is an attempt to sketch the major arguments pro and con, to clarify some of their assumptions and implications, and to identify possible ways of dealing with the issue itself.

Arguments Pro Arguments in favour of gene enhancement generally centre in the Principles of Beneficence and Equality and Justice. With the possible exception of monozygotic siblings, all human beings differ in their genetic endowment. However, some differ more radically from the norm than others, and this may impact significantly on their ability to compete on an equal footing with other members of society. Thus, someone who lacks intelligence, physical endurance or beauty cannot compete on an equal footing with a genius, someone who is genetically endowed with greater muscle capabilities or someone who has greater beauty,[101] etc. Therefore, if one believes in Equality and Justice, and if the means are available to correct such inequalities, then there is a duty to use genetic engineering if it could make for a level playing field. It would not only correct a *de facto* injustice, it would also result in good for the individual person.[102] By the same token, it would also raise the overall capabilities of society as a whole and thereby contribute to the evolutionary fitness of society.[103] Not only that, it would also make for a happier social fabric.[104]

Some also argue that evolution has been less than kind to human beings, and that enhancement would merely supplement what a niggardly Nature has failed to provide.[105] Others have argued that the distinction between gene therapy and gene enhancement is unclear and therefore cannot carry the burden of a negative argument placed on it.[106] Still others have suggested that gene enhancement would satisfy the Rawlsian requirement of choice behind a veil of ignorance,[107] or that a ban would be "unstable,"[108] or that enhancement is inevitable in any case.[109]

Arguments Contra Arguments against genetic enhancement tend to be equally varied. They range from religiously based arguments that condemn interference with Creation[110] to arguments that focus on the eugenic potential of such a practice.[111] Other objections maintain that it would lead to a stratification of society into those who are enhanced and those who are not, and thus would contribute to genetically based and hence permanently entrenched social inequality.[112] Still others have argued that it would lead to an exclusionary approach to disability because of a spillover effect, and that it would be unjust on its own terms, because not everyone would have access to the technology itself.[113]

Both sides of the debate make important points. On the pro side, the issue of Beneficence and non-Malfeasance is really unassailable. To draw an analogy: the point of allowing private schooling and tutoring is to enhance intellectual capacities that otherwise would be insufficient or not as great as they could be; the rationale of sport training and conditioning is to enhance physical abilities; and the enhancement of physical characteristics such as beauty (and even size) has spawned veritable industries devoted to this task—none of which is considered unethical. Even Equality and Justice are satisfied by enhancement, in that the technology merely supplies what is otherwise provided through social programs that are intended to level the socioeconomic playing field through accommodation for disabilities or provision of other assistance. Finally, the very point of medicine and medical care, as it is currently understood, is to correct the evolutionary flaws that have left humanity subject to disease, and that have limited its development. From this perspective, then, the principle of genetic technology for enhancement purposes shares the same justification as all these other practices.

But the negative side also makes valid points. As a matter of principle, levelling the playing field is certainly ethically defensible, but herein lies the problem: Before one even considers levelling the playing field, one should be certain that the playing field that one is trying to level is identified correctly. Are intelligence, beauty, physical capacities and the like really the correct determinants of the field that is to be levelled? According to whose point of view? Is there here a cultural—or even a personal—bias? In other words, how does one ensure—"guarantee" is too strong a word, because nothing in life can be guaranteed—that enhancement does not become a tool of cultural hegemony, in the sense that standards of what is considered good, healthy or beautiful are globally imposed by the success of economically interested and politically powerful players? Moreover, how does one ensure that enhancement is not restricted to those who can afford it, and that the playing field is thereby in fact not levelled but made even more uneven? And finally, how does one ensure that the paradigm shift in the concept of what it is to be human—a paradigm shift that may just be acceptable if it occurs along the lines that are hinted at by screening and therapeutic modification technology—does not become slanted solely towards the physical, at the expense of what makes human beings persons?

CONCLUSION

The advancement of knowledge and technology may be a desirable thing, and their application may well improve the state of humanity. However, their development is desirable only if it is not bought at the price of unethical behaviour, and their application is to be welcomed only if it does not imperil the ethical status of society itself. A fundamental precept, therefore, that should guide the advancement of scientific knowledge and that should steer the development of technology is the understanding that scientific and technological developments do not occur in isolation. They take place in a social context. It is this context that makes them possible and that is influenced by them in turn.

Therefore, in any scientific or technological development—and this is particularly the case with the biotechnologies, since they go to the very essence of what it is to be human—it is important that a balance be struck between what society can do and what it should do: between what it should encourage, allow or forbid. Unless such a balance is struck, the nature of humanity, and possibly its identity and survival, will become subject to the vagaries of an uncontrolled process that assumes a life of its own. Such a balance, however, is not a matter of serendipity. It is the product of a deliberate stance that gets to the facts, and then strives to understand and harmonize the conflicting concerns. It requires the identification of relevant issues, the reconciliation of distinct perspectives and of varying points of view—and the determination of their importance and weight.

Ectogenesis and cloning, genetic screening and gene therapy are all Janus-faced biotechnologies. That is to say, they have the potential to be both beneficial and detrimental. Which of these it is, is not a function of the technology itself but of how it is used—and, indeed, of whether it is used at all. The discussion in this chapter cannot and does not claim to have provided definitive answers. Indeed, how could it? Its sole purpose has been to present an overview of the technologies, sketch the discussion that surrounds them, outline some of the more important ethical considerations that shape the debate, and to put them into the overall context of health care in general.

Further Readings

Allhoff, F. "Germ-Line Genetic Enhancement and Rawlsian Primary Goods." *Kennedy Inst Ethics J* 15.1 (Mar 2005): 39–56.

Baylis, F., and J.S. Robert. "The Inevitability of Genetic Enhancement Technologies." *Bioethics* 18.1 (2004): 1–26.

Chan, S., and J. Harris. "The Ethics of Gene Therapy." *Current Opinions in Molecular Therapy* 8.5 (2006): 377–383.

Dickens, B.M., N. Pei and K.M. Taylor. "Legal and Ethical Issues in Genetic Testing and Counseling for Susceptibility to Breast, Ovarian and Colon Cancer." *CMAJ* 154.6 (1996): 813–818.

McLaren, A. "The Creation of a Haven for 'Human Thoroughbreds': The Sterilization of the Feebleminded and the Mentally Ill in British Columbia." *Canadian Historical Review* 67.2 (1986): 127–150.

Nussbaum, M.C. *Clones and Clones: Facts and Fantasies about Human Cloning* (New York: Norton, 1998).

Parker, M., and A. Lucassen. "Genetic Information: A Joint Account?" *British Medical Journal* 329 (2004): 165–167.

Purdy, L. "What Can Progress in Reproductive Technology Mean for Women?" *Journal of Medicine and Philosophy* 21.5 (1996): 499–514.

Savulescu, J. "Should We Clone Human Beings? Cloning as a Source of Tissue Transplantation." *Journal of Medical Ethics* 25.2 (1999): 87–95.

Singer, P., and D. Wells. "Ectogenesis" in *Ectogenesis: Artificial Womb Technology and the Future of Human Reproduction*, ed. S. Gelfand and J.S. Shook (Amsterdam: Rodopi, 2006), 9–26.

Zhang, S. "The Morality of Having Children with Disabilities: A Different Perspective on Happiness and Quality of Life." *McGill Journal of Medicine* 8 (2004): 85–88.

Endnotes

1. M.J. Hanson, "The Idea of Progress and the Goals of Medicine," in *The Goals of Medicine: The Forgotten Issues in Health Care Reform*, ed. M.J. Hanson and D. Callahan (Washington, DC: Georgetown University Press, 1999), 137–151; B. Hoffman, "Is There a Technological Imperative in Health Care?" *International Journal of Technology Assessment in Health Care* 18.3 (2002): 675–689; S. Wolf and B.B. Berle, *The Technological Imperative in Medicine* (New York: Plenum Press, 1981), 125.

2. Vacuum aspiration machines would fall into this category; see *A Book for Midwives*, (2010), Chapter 23, "Manual Vacuum Aspiration MVA," accessed 4 Jul 2011 at www.hesperian.info/assets/Midwives/Midwives_Ch23.pdf

3. Drs. J. Kevorkian and P. Nitschke each devised machines that would allow patients to kill themselves.

4. S. Gelfand and J.R. Shook (eds.), *Ectogenesis: Artificial Womb Technology and the Future of Human Reproduction* (Amsterdam: Rodopi, 2006); S. Colman, *The Ethics of Artificial Uteruses: Implications for Reproduction and Abortion* (Burlington, VT: Ashgate Publishing Company, 2004).

5. D.A.T. New and M. Mizell, "Opossum Fetuses Grown in Culture," *Science* 175.4021 (1972): 533–536. See also Y. Kuwabara et al., "Artificial Placenta: Long-Term Extrauterine Incubation of Isolated Goat Fetuses," *Artificial Organs* 13.6 (1989): 527–553.

6. B. George, "Development of an Artificial Placenta," Grant 5R03HD062713-02 from the Eunice Kennedy Shriver National Institute of Child Health & Human Development, University of Michigan, Ann Arbor, MI, starting date 2010-04-01.

7. R.H. Bartlett, "Extracorporeal Life Support: History and New Directions," *Seminars in Perinatology* 29.1 (2005): 2–7.

8. S. Ciesielski and J. Kopka, "Kidawa B. Incubator Noise and Vibration—Possible Iatrogenic Influence on Neonate," *Int J Pediatr Otorhinolaryngol* 1.4 (Feb 1980): 309–316.

9. Ibid.

10. For extended exploration of this use, see P. Singer and D. Wells, *Making Babies* (New York: C. Scribner's Sons, 1987); for a reply to some of their points, see D.N. James, "Ectogenesis: A Reply to Singer and Wells," *Bioethics* 1.1 (Jan 1987): 80–99.

11. For further discussion of this and related issues, see A. Smajdor, "In Defense of Ectogenesis," *Cambridge Quarterly of Healthcare Ethics* 21 (Jan 2012): 90–103.

12. See S. Coleman, *The Ethics of Artificial Uteruses: Implications for Reproduction and Abortion* (Hants, U.K.: Ashgate Publishing, 2004), 57 ff.

13. See *Assisted Human Reproduction Act*, s. 5.

14. See P. Singer and D. Wells, "Ectogenesis," in *Ectogenesis: Artificial Womb Technology and the Future of Human Reproduction*, ed. S. Gelfand and J.R. Shook (Amsterdam: Rodopi, 2006), 9–26.

15. J.S. Murphy, "Is Pregnancy Necessary? Feminist Concerns about Ectogenesis," in Gelfand and Shook, op. cit., 27–46.

16. For a discussion of advances in vat-grown meat, see M.A. Benjaminson, J.A. Gilchriest and M. Lorenzet, "In Vitro Edible Muscle Protein Production System (mpps): Stage 1, Fish," *Acta Astronautica* 51.12 (2002): 879–889; Z.F. Bhat and H. Bhat, "Tissue Engineered Meat—Future Meat," *Journal of Stored Products and Postharvest Research* 2.1 (2011): 1–10.

17. See Gelfand and Shook (eds.), op. cit.; see also S. Coleman, *The Ethics of Artificial Uteruses: Implications for Reproduction and Abortion* (Hants, U.K.: Ashgate Publishing, 2004).

18. See Singer and Wells, "Ectogenesis," in Gelfand and Shook, op. cit.,9–26, at 19 f.

19. See Singer and Wells, op. cit.

20. See Singer and Wells, at 18 f.

21. See S. Firestone, *The Dialectic of Sex* (New York: William Morrow and Company, 1970), 27, *et pass.*; see also A. Smajdor, "The Moral Imperative of Ectogenesis," *Cambridge Quarterly of Healthcare Ethics* 16.3 (2007): 336–345.

22. For a contrary view, see J.S. Murphy, "Is Pregnancy Necessary? Feminist Concerns about Ectogenesis," in Gelfand and Shook, op. cit., 27–46.

23. F. Bowring, "Therapeutic and Reproductive Cloning: A Critique," *Soc Sci Med* 58.2 (2005): 401–409; M.B. Mahowald, "Self-Preservation: An Argument for Therapeutic Cloning, and a Strategy for Fostering Respect for Moral Integrity," *Am J Bioeth* 4.2 (2004): 56–66; J. Savulescu, "Should We Clone Human Beings? Cloning as a Source of Tissue for Transplantation," *J Med Ethics* 25.2 (1999): 87–95; R. Sparrow, "Therapeutic Cloning and Reproductive Liberty," *J Med Philos* 34.2 (2009): 102–118.

24. R. Dworkin, *Life's Dominion* (New York: Alfred A. Knopf, 1993), at 167, *et pass.*

25. See J. Harris, "'Goodbye Dolly?' The Ethics of Human Cloning," *J Med Ethics* 23 (1997): 353–360, at 358.

26. For personality studies on monozygotic twins and personality, see W. Weitten et al., *Psychology Applied to Modern Life*, 9th ed. (Belmont, CA: Wadsworth, 2009), at 56, *et pass.*

27. R. Liu et al., "Homozygous Defect in HIV-1 Coreceptor Accounts for Resistance of Some Multiply-Exposed Individuals to HIV-1 Infection," *Cell* 86 (9 Aug 1996): 367–377; M. Dean et al., "Genetic Restriction of HIV-1 Infection and Progression to AIDS by a Deletion Allele of the CKR5 Structural Gene," *Science* 273.5283 (1996): 1856–1862.

28. D. Futuyma, *Evolution* (Sunderland, MA: Sinauer Associates, 1998): 226–288.

29. Z. Han, C.A. Vandevoort and K.E. Latham, "Therapeutic Cloning: Status and Prospects," *Curr Opin Mol Ther* 9.4 (Aug 2007): 392–397.

30. F. Svenaeus, "A Heideggerian Defense of Therapeutic Cloning," *Theor Med Bioeth* 28.1 (2007): 31–62.

31. Resolution on Human Cloning, European Parliament, 1998 O.J. (C 34) 164 (15 Jan 1998), accessed 7 Jul 2011 at www1.umn.edu/humanrts/instree/cloning2.html

32. M. Häyry, "Philosophical Arguments For and Against Human Reproductive Cloning," *Bioethics* 17 (2003): 447–459.

33. J. Feinberg, "The Child's Right to an Open Future," in *Whose Child? Children's Rights, Parental Authority, and State Power*, ed. W. Aiken and H. LaFollette (Totawa, NJ: Rowman & Littlefield, 1980), 124–153.

34. For a rebuttal of this, see M. Mameli, "Reproductive Cloning, Genetic Engineering and the Autonomy of the Child: The Moral Agent and the Open Future," *J Med Ethics* 33.2 (2007): 87–93. See also J.C. Havstad, "Human Reproductive Cloning: A Conflict of Liberties," *Bioethics* 24.2 (2010): 71–77.

35. See Bowring, op. cit. See also Savulescu, op. cit., and M.J. Radin, "Cloning and Commodification," *Hastings Law J* 53.5 (2002): 1123–1132. For an argument that therapeutic cloning would be unethical unless it was done with parental consent, see Sparrow, op. cit.

36. P. Ramsey, *Fabricated Man: The Ethics of Genetic Control* (New Haven: Yale University Press, 1970).

37. K. Illmensee et al., "Human Embryo Twinning with Applications in Reproductive Medicine," *Fertil Steril* 93.2 (2009): 423–427.

38. J.J. Oleszczuk et al., "Projections of Population-Based Twinning Rates through the Year 2100," *The Journal of Reproductive Medicine* 44.1 (1999): 913–921.

39. R. Bortolus et al., "The Epidemiology of Multiple Births," *Human Reproduction Update* (European Society of Human Reproduction and Embryology) 5.2 (1999): 179–187.

40. United Nations Declaration on Human Cloning, UN General Assembly, accessed 7 Jul 2011 at http://daccess-dds-ny.un.org/doc/UNDOC/GEN/N04/493/06/PDF/N0449306.pdf?OpenElement

41. Resolution on Human Cloning, European Parliament, 1998 O.J. (C 34) 164 (15 Jan 1998), accessed 7 Jul 2011 at www1.umn.edu/humanrts/instree/cloning2.html

42. It would also raise the question of which twin to kill.

43. A.M. Torgersen and H. Janson, "Why Do Identical Twins Differ in Personality: Shared Environment Reconsidered," *Twin Res* 5.1 (2002): 44–52; N.L. Segal, S.L. Hershberger and S. Arad, "Meeting One's Twin: Perceived Social Closeness and Familiarity," *Evolutionary Psychology* 1 (2003): 70–95; C.S. Bergeman et al., "Genotype–Environment Interaction in Personality Development: Identical Twins Reared Apart," *Psychology and Aging* 3.4 (1988): 399–406.

44. St. Thomas Aquinas, *Summa Contra Gentiles* II:89:3. See also *Quaestiones disputatae de potentia* IIIa:11–12. Aquinas maintained that the fetus develops its organ systems "by a formative power acting by virtue of the generative soul of the father." (*Summa contra gentiles* II:89:9 and *Commentarium in quattuor lobros sententiarum Magistri Petri Lobardi* IIId3q.5a2s.

45. For guidelines developed by the Canadian Council on Animal Care, see www.ccac.ca.

46. When both parents have an affected copy—which is rare—the risk increases to 75 percent. When either parent has two affected copies of the gene, the risk is 100 percent and all of the children will be affected.

47. UNESCO, *Universal Declaration on Bioethics and Human Rights*, 19 Oct 2005, Article 10 (2).

48. Council of Europe, *Convention for the protection of human rights and dignity of the human being with regard to the application of biology and medicine: Convention on human rights and biomedicine* (Oviedo: Council of Europe, 1997). See also UNESCO, International Bioethics Committee (IBC): *International declaration on human genetic data* (Paris: UNESCO, IBC, 2003); World Health Organization (WHO): *Genetic Databases: Assessing the Benefits and the Impact on Human and Patient Rights* (Geneva: World Health Organization, 2003). See also World Medical Association (WMA), *World Medical Association Declaration on the Rights of the Patient* (Lisbon: World Medical Association, 1981), available at www.wma.net/e/policy/l4.htm. For a review of the duty to disclose genetic information in research, see B.M. Knoppers et al., "The Emergence of an Ethical Duty to Disclose Genetic Research Results: International Perspectives," *European Journal of Human Genetics* 14 (2006): 1170–1178. For a critical stance, see F.A. Miller et al., "Duty to Disclose What? Querying the Putative Obligation to Return Research Results to Participants," *J Med Ethics* 34 (2008): 210–213.

49. G.J. Annas et al., "Drafting the Genetic Privacy Act: Science, Policy and Practical Considerations," *J Law Med Ethics* 23 (1995): 360–366.

50. House of Commons, U.K., *Human Genetics: The Science and the Consequence* (London, U.K.: Her Majesty's Stationery Office, 1995).

51. J.H. Swint et al., "The Economic Returns to a Community and Hospital Screening Program for a Genetic Screening," *Preventive Medicine* 8 (1979): 465–470. See also J.T.R. Clark, "Screening for Carriers of Tay-Sachs Disease: Two Approaches," *Canadian Medical Association Journal*, 119 (1978): 450.

52. N. Park and B. Dickens, "Legal and Ethical Issues in Genetic Prediction and Genetic Counselling for Breast, Ovarian and Colon Cancer Susceptibility," in *Critical Choices: Ethical, Legal and Social Behavioural Implications of Heritable Breast, Ovarian and Colon Cancer* (Toronto: International Research and Policy Symposium, 1995); S. Suter, "Whose Genes Are These Anyway?: Familial Conflicts over Access to Genetic Information," *Michigan Law Rev* 91 (1993): 1881–1854.

53. G. Laurie, "Obligations Arising from Genetic Information: Negligence and the Protection of Family Interests," *CFLQ* 11 (1999): 109–124.

54. For a legal expression of this point, see Safer v. Estate of Pack, 677 A2d 1188 (NJ Super Ct App Div 1996), at 1192, where the Court talked about a "duty to warn of avertible risk from genetic causes," and said that this was "by definition a matter of familial concern" and that the notion was "sufficiently narrow to serve the interests of justice." See also World Medical Association (WMA), *Declaration on the Human Genome Project* (Marbella: World Medical Association, 1992), and the HUGO declaration, which states that genetic research protocols should be structured in such a way that if it becomes clear that a subject carries a deleterious gene, "special considerations should be made for access by immediate relatives." See also World Health Organization (WHO), *Proposed International Guidelines on Ethical Issues in Medical Genetics and Genetic Services* (Geneva: World Health Organization, 1997); Suter, op. cit.; Park and Dickens, op. cit.

55. CMA Code, clause 35.

56. For a discussion of Canadian law, see E.I. Picard and G.B. Robertson, *Legal Liability of Doctors and Hospitals in Canada,* 4th ed. (Carswell: Toronto, 2007), at 31–40. The leading case here is Tarasoff v. Regents of the University of California, 551 P. 2d. 334 (Cal. 1976).

57. McInerney v. MacDonald, [1992] 2 S.C.R., emphasis added.

58. For a similar conclusion, see B.M. Knoppers et al., "Professional Disclosure of Familial Genetic Information," *Am J Hum Gene* 62 (1998): 474–483.

59. M. Schoenfeld et al., "Increased Rate of Suicide among Patients with Huntington's Disease, " *J Neurol Neurosurg Psychiatry* 47.12 (1984): 1283–1287.

60. The incidence of misattribution of biological paternity ranges from 0.8 to 30 percent (median 3.7 percent). However, the range shifted from 17 to 33 percent (median of 26.9 percent) when paternity was tested because of suspicion of misattribution; see M.A. Bellis et al., "Measuring Paternal Discrepancy and Its Public Health Consequences," *J Epidemiol Community Health* 59.9 (2005): 749–754.

61. See Pratten v. British Columbia (Attorney General), 2011 BCSC 656.

62. United Nations, *Convention on the Rights of the Child,* adopted and opened for signature, ratification and accession by General Assembly resolution 44/25 of 20 Nov 1989, accessed 11 Jul 2011 at www2.ohchr.org/english/law/crc.htm

63. See S. Besson, "Enforcing the Child's Right to Know Her Origins: Contrasting Approaches under the Convention on the Rights of the Child and the European Convention on Human Rights," *Int Jnl of Law, Policy and the Family* 21.2 (2007): 137–159.

64. M. Parker and A. Lucassen, "Genetic Information: A Joint Account?" *BMJ* 329 (2004): 165–167, at 166.

65. Aristotle, *Categories* 5, *et pass.*

66. Parker and Lucassen, op cit., at 166.

67. S. Andersen et al., "Body Proportions in Healthy Adult Inuit in East Greenland in 1963," *Int J Circumpolar Health* 63 (2004): 73–76.

68. Plato, *The Republic*, 457c10-d3.

69. J. Beckwith, "Social and Political Uses of Genetics in the United States: Past and Present," *Annals of the New York Academy of Sciences* 265 (1976): 46–58.

70. Op. cit., at 48 ff.

71. Beckwith, at 49 f.

72. A. McLaren, "The Creation of a Haven for 'Human Thoroughbreds': The Sterilization of the Feeble-minded and the Mentally Ill in British Columbia," *Canadian Historical Review* 67.2 (1986): 127–150. Similar sterilization laws existed in Alberta until 1972. See also A. McLaren, *Twentieth-Century Sexuality: A History* (Malden, MA: Blackwell, 1999), and *Our Own Master Race: Eugenics in Canada, 1885–1945.* Canadian Social History Series (Toronto: McClelland & Stewart, 1990).

73. For a description, see www.villebon-sur-yvette.fr/pdfs/med-familles.pdf

74. For a discussion of more recent proposals along similar lines, see T.M. Powledge, "Genetic Screening and Personal Freedom," in *Intervention and Reflection*, ed. R. Munson (Belmont, CA: Wadsworth, 1979), 371–375.

75. H.J. Muller, "Genetic Progress by Voluntary Conducted Germinal Choice," quoted in P. Ramsey, *Fabricated Man: The Ethics of Genetic Control* (New Haven and London: Yale University Press, 1970), 162 n.

76. H.J. Muller, "Human Evolution by Voluntary Choice of Germ Plasm," in *Intervention and Reflection*, ed. R. Munson (Belmont, CA: Wadsworth, 1999), 352.

77. Op. cit., at 942.

78. Which, interestingly enough, is down from 3.7 in 1987 because of increasing use of genetic screening. See A. Dupuis et al., "Cystic Fibrosis Birth Rates in Canada: A Decreasing Trend since the Onset of Genetic Testing," *Journal of Pediatrics* 147:3 (2005): 312–315.

79. V. Horvais et al., "Cost of Home and Hospital Care for Patients with Cystic Fibrosis Followed Up in Two Reference Medical Centers in France," *International Journal of Technology Assessment in Health Care* 22 (2006): 525–531.

80. M. Corey and V. Farewell, "Determinants of Mortality from Cystic Fibrosis in Canada, 1970–1989," *Am J Epidemiol* 143.10 (1996): 1007–1017.

81. For a similar estimate from the U.S., see C. Krauth et al., "Cystic Fibrosis: Cost of Illness and Considerations for the Economic Evaluation of Potential Therapies," *Pharmacoeconomics* 21.14 (2003): 1001–1024.

82. P.L. Sinn, R. Anthony and P.B. McCray, Jr., "Genetic Therapies for Cystic Fibrosis Lung Disease," *Hum Mol Genet* (21 Mar 2011), published online; L.G. Johnson et al., "Efficiency of Gene Transfer for Restoration of Normal Airway Epithelial Function in Cystic Fibrosis," *Nature (Genetics)* 2 (1992): 21–25.

83. European Medical Research Council, *Draft Guidelines for the Application of Gene Therapy to Human Beings* (Strasbourg: undated); NIH Recombinant DNA Advisory Committee, Human Gene Therapy Subcommittee, *Points to Consider in the Design and Submission of Protocol for the Transfer of Recombinant DNA into Human Subjects* (Bethesda, VA: Nat. Inst. Health, 21 Jun 1989); World Council of Churches, Working Group Sub-Unit on Church and Society, "Manipulating Life," *Church and Society* (Sep/Oct 1982); President's Commission for the Study of Ethical Problems in Medicine and Biomedical and Behavioral Research, *Splicing Life: A Report on the Social and Ethical Issues of Genetic Engineering with Human Beings* (Washington, DC: U.S. Government Printing Office, 1982), 63; Medical Research Council of Canada, *Guidelines for Research on Somatic Cell Gene Therapy in Humans* (Ottawa: Medical Research Council, 1990).

84. N. Agar, "Designing Babies: Morally Permissible Ways to Modify the Human Genome," *Bioethics* 9.1 (Jan 1995): 1–15; S. Chan and J. Harris, "The Ethics of Gene Therapy," *Current Opinion in Molecular Therapeutics* 8.5 (2006): 377–383; *Tri-Council Policy Statement: Ethical Conduct for Research Involving Humans*, 8:E.

85. M. Häyry and T. Lehto, "Genetic Engineering and the Risk of Harm," paper presented at the Twentieth World Congress of Philosophy, Boston, MA, U.S.A., 10–15 Aug 1998, accessed 13 Jul 2011 at www.bu.edu/wcp/index.html

86. P. Ramsay, *Fabricated Man: The Ethics of Genetic Control* (New Haven and London: Yale University Press, 1970); see also *Report of the Commission of Enquiry of the German Bundestag, Prospects and Risks of Genetic Engineering*, Parts I and II (Bonn: Deutscher Bundestag, 10. Wahlperiode, 1987), 188b–189b.

87. Cf. President's Commission for the Study of Ethical Problems in Medicine and Biomedical and Behavioral Research, *Splicing Life: The Social and Ethical Issues of Genetic Engineering with Human Beings* (Washington, DC: U.S. Government Printing Office, 1982), 72.

88. For international pronouncements on the right to safe working conditions, see European Union Charter of Fundamental Rights, Article 31(1): "Every worker has the right to working conditions which respect his or her health, safety and dignity." Accessed 14 Jul 2011 at www.eucharter.org/home.php?page_id=38; see also *Universal Declaration of Human Rights*, Article 23, which, *inter alia*, stipulates the right to "favourable conditions of work."

89. *Proceed*, at 942. See also Recommendations 269 and 270.

90. Ramsey, at 124.

91. L. Kass, "New Beginnings in Life," in *The New Genetics and the Future of Man*, ed. M.P. Hamilton (Grand Rapids, MI: Wm. B. Eerdmans Publ., 1972), 13–63, at 61.

92. J.C. Fletcher, "Moral Problems and Ethical Issues in Prospective Human Gene Therapy," *Virginia Law Review* 69 (1983): 538–540; M. Lappe, "Ethical Issues in Manipulating the Human Germ Line," *The Journal of Medicine and Philosophy* 16 (1991): 621–639.

93. C.S. Lewis, *The Abolition of Man* (New York: Collier-Macmillan, 1965), 70.

94. Council of Europe, Parliamentary Assembly, Recommendation 934 (1982)[1] on genetic engineering, sec. 4 (a) ff, available at http://assembly.coe.int/Main.asp?link=/Documents/AdoptedText/ta82/EREC934.htm

95. *Proceed*, at 940–941.

96. H.J.J. Leenen, "Genetic Manipulation with Human Beings," *Medicine and the Law* 7 (1988); 73–79, at 75; President's Commission (1982), 57–60.

97. Council of Europe, op. cit., at 4 (c).

98. UNESCO, *Universal Declaration on the Human Genome and Human Rights*, Article 2, available at http://portal.unesco.org/en/ev.php-URL_ID=13177&URL_DO=DO_TOPIC&URL_SECTION=201.html

99. International Human Genome Sequencing Consortium, "Human Genome," *Nature* 409 (15 Feb 2001): 860–921.

100. Arguably, in Quebec this may even amount to a duty under the *Charte des droits et libertés de la personne (Charter of Rights and Freedoms of the Person) L.R.Q. c. C-12*, which stipulates a duty to help if one can do so without undue danger to oneself.

101. J.H. Langlois et al., "Maxims or Myths of Beauty? A Meta-Analytic and Theoretical Review," *Psychological Bulletin* 126.3 (2000): 390–423; S.J. Solnick and M.E. Schweitzer, "The Influence of Physical Attractiveness and Gender on Ultimatum Game Decisions," *Organizational Behavior and Human Decision Processes* 79.3 (1999): 199–215.

102. See A. Sandberg, "Genetic Modifications," accessed 14 Jul 2011 at www.aleph.se/Trans/Individual/Body/genes.html. See also European Parliament, Policy Department Economic and Scientific Policy, *Technology Assessment on Converging Technologies* (IP/A/STOA/SC/2005-183) at iii, evidence of Baroness Susan Greenfield, accessed 14 Jul 2011 at www.europarl.europa.eu/stoa/publications/studies/stoa183_en.pdf; for an argument along these lines but focusing on prenatal selection, see J. Savulescu, "Procreative Beneficence: Why We Should Select the Best Children," *Bioethics* 15 (2001): 413–426.

103. For a discussion of various arguments, see F. Baylis and J.S. Robert, "The Inevitability of Genetic Enhancement Technologies," *Bioethics* 18.1 (2004): 1–26.

104. N. Agar, "Designing Babies: Morally Permissible Ways to Modify the Human Genome," *Bioethics* 9.1 (Jan 1995): 1–15.

105. N. Brostrom and R. Roache, "Human Enhancement: Ethical Issues in Human Enhancement," in *New Waves in Applied Ethics*, ed. J. Ryberg, T.S. Petersen and C. Wolf (Houndmills, U.K.: Macmillan, 2007), accessed 14 Jul 2011 at www.nickbostrom.com/ethics/human-enhancement.pdf

106. Agar, op. cit.; N. Holtug, "Equality and the Treatment-Enhancement Distinction," *Bioethics* 25.3 (Mar 2011): 137–144.

107. F. Allhoff, "Germ-Line Genetic Enhancement and Rawlsian Primary Goods," *Kennedy Institute of Ethics Journal* 15.1 (Mar 2005): 39–56.

108. W. Gardner, "Can Human Genetic Enhancement Be Prohibited?" *J Med Philos* 20.1 (1995): 65–84.

109. Baylis and Robert, op. cit.

110. R. Cole-Turner, "Genes, Religion, and Society: The Developing Views of the Churches," *Science and Engineering Ethics* 3.3 (1997): 273–288; National Council of Churches, *Human Life and the New Genetics* (New York: National Council of Churches of Christ in the U.S.A., 1980); T. Peters *Playing God?: Genetic Determinism and Human Freedom* (London: Routledge, 2003); Ramsey, op. cit. But see S.M. Glick, "Some Jewish Thoughts on Genetic Enhancement," *J Med Ethics* 37 (2011): 415–419, for a mitigated Jewish perspective.

111. S. Chan and J. Harris, "The Ethics of Gene Therapy," *Curr Opin Mol Ther* 8.5 (2006): 377–383.

112. M.H. Shapiro, "The Impact of Genetic Enhancement on Equality," *Wake Forest Law Review* 34 (1999): 561–637.

113. A. Buchanan, D. Brock, N. Daniels and D. Wikler, *From Chance to Choice* (Cambridge, U.K.: Cambridge University Press, 2000); Chan and Harris, op cit.

114. A. McLaren, "Cloning: Pathways to a Pluripotent Future," *Science* 288.5472 (2000): 1775–1780.

SAMPLE CASES

1. In October and December 2002, the Necker Hospital in Paris announced that the two youngest boys enrolled into a gene therapy study for the treatment of X-linked severe combined immunoinsufficiency disease (X-SCID), which is caused by a mutation in the IL2RG gene, had developed leukemia. Boys with X-linked SCID are prone to recurrent and persistent opportunistic infections by bacteria, viruses and fungi that do not ordinarily cause illness in people who do not carry this disorder. Without treatment, children who suffer from it usually do not live beyond infancy. A retroviral vector had been used to insert the modified retrovirus near the gene LMO2, which encodes a transcription factor whose over-expression has been implicated in childhood T-cell acute lymphoblastic leukemia. Unfortunately, the over-expression was stimulated in this case. One child has died. A third infant later also developed leukemia. This has prompted the U.S. Food and Drug Administration to suspend three gene-therapy trials on SCID in the U.S. The U.S. Panel has announced that gene therapy for X-linked SCID may proceed only if patients have failed to respond to other treatments. This restriction does not apply to non-X-linked SCID cases.

2. In 1978 David Rorvik, in his book *In His Image: The Cloning of a Man*, claimed that after several years of research and experimentation, a wealthy businessman had been successfully cloned by means of somatic cell nuclear transfer into an enucleated human ovum, which had then been implanted into the uterus of a commercial surrogate mother. Rorvik did not cite sources because he claimed that he was allowed to tell the story only on condition of source anonymity. The publisher of the book was sued by an Oxford University geneticist who claimed that the author had plagiarized his PhD thesis. (The suit was ultimately settled out of court.) In 1996, Dolly the

Sheep was successfully cloned at the Roslin Institute in Scotland by somatic cell nuclear transfer and the details were confirmed in *Science*.[114] Irrespective of whether Rorvik's account is true, would it have been unethical for the industrialist to have cloned himself?

3. The *Criminal Code* of Canada, at section 223(1) states that

> [a] child becomes a human being within the meaning of this Act when it has completely proceeded, in a living state, from the body of its mother, whether or not
>
> (a) it has breathed;
>
> (b) it has an independent circulation; or
>
> (c) the navel string is severed.

What would be the implications of this if an artificial uterus were to be developed and used in Canada?

Note: *n* indicates endnote number